EMBRYOLOGY

4TH EDITION

EMBRYOLOGY

4TH EDITION

Ronald W. Dudek, PhD

Full Professor of Anatomy and Cell Biology
Department of Anatomy and Cell Biology
Brody School of Medicine
East Carolina University
Greenville, North Carolina

Questions Contributor:
H. Wayne Lambert, Ph.D.

James D. Fix, PhD

Professor Emeritus of Anatomy
Marshall University School of Medicine
Huntington, West Virginia

Wolters Kluwer | Lippincott Williams & Wilkins
Health
Philadelphia · Baltimore · New York · London
Buenos Aires · Hong Kong · Sydney · Tokyo

Acquisitions Editor: Crystal Taylor
Managing Editor: Kathleen Scogna
Marketing Manager: Emilie Moyer
Production Editor: Gina Aiello
Designer: Holly McLaughlin
Compositor: Nesbitt Graphics
Printer: Data Reproductions Corp

Fourth Edition

Copyright © 2008 <1994, 1998, 2005> Lippincott Williams & Wilkins, a Wolters Kluwer business.

351 West Camden Street
Baltimore, MD 21201

530 Walnut Street
Philadelphia, PA 19106

9 8 7 6 5 4 3 2 1

Library of Congress Cataloging-in-Publication Data

Dudek, Ronald W., 1950-
  Embryology / Ronald W. Dudek, James D. Fix. -- 4th ed.
    p. ; cm. -- (Board review series)
  Includes bibliographical references and index.
  ISBN-13: 978-0-7817-7116-0 (alk. paper)
  ISBN-10: 0-7817-7116-1 (alk. paper)
  1. Embryology, Human--Examinations, questions, etc. I. Fix, James D.
II. Title. III. Series.
  [DNLM: 1. Embryology--Outlines. QS 618.2 D845e 2008]
  QM601.F68 2008
  612.6'40076--dc22
                                                            2007006971

To Connor, Sean, and Katherine

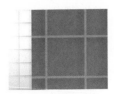

Preface

The fourth edition of *BRS Embryology* has afforded us the opportunity to further fine-tune a work that was already a highly rated course review book as well as an excellent review for the USMLE Step 1. This fine-tuning is a result of the many students who have contacted us by email to point out errors and give suggestions for improvement. We appreciate this student feedback very much.

In the fourth edition, the major change has been to revise the end-of-chapter tests and the Comprehensive Examination at the end of the book. We have revised the questions to reflect the USMLE Step 1 format.

We hope that students will continue to find *BRS Embryology* a clear and thorough review of embryology. After taking the USMLE Step 1, we invite our readers to e-mail Dr. Dudek at *dudekr@ecu.edu* to convey any comments or to indicate any area that was particularly represented on the USMLE Step 1, so that future editions of this book may improve.

Ronald W. Dudek
James D. Fix

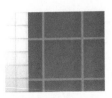

Contents

Prefertilization Events

I.   Sexual Reproduction

Sexual reproduction occurs when female and male gametes (oocyte and spermatozoon, respectively) unite at fertilization. Gametes are direct descendants of **primordial germ cells**, which are first observed in **the wall of the yolk sac** at week 4 of embryonic development and subsequently migrate into the future gonad region. Gametes are produced by **gametogenesis** (called **oogenesis** in the female and **spermatogenesis** in the male). Gametogenesis employs a specialized process of cell division, **meiosis**, which uniquely distributes chromosomes among gametes.

II.   Chromosomes (Figure 1-1)

A single chromosome consists of two characteristic regions called **arms (p arm = short arm; q arm = long arm)**, which are separated by a **centromere**. During meiosis I, **single chromosomes** undergo DNA replication, which essentially duplicates the arms. This forms **duplicated chromosomes**, which consist of two sister **chromatids** attached at the centromere.

A. Ploidy and "N" number   Ploidy refers to **the number of chromosomes** in a cell. The "N" number refers to the **amount of DNA** in a cell.

    1. **Normal somatic cells and primordial germ cells** contain **46 single chromosomes** and **2N amount of DNA**. The chromosomes occur in **23 homologous pairs**; one member (homologue) of each pair is of maternal origin and the other is of paternal origin. The term "diploid" is classically used to refer to a cell containing 46 single chromosomes. Chromosome pairs 1 to 22 are **autosomal (non-sex) pairs**. Chromosome pair 23 consists of the **sex chromosomes** (XX for a female or XY for a male).

    2. **Gametes** contain **23 single chromosomes** (22 autosomes and 1 sex chromosome) and **1N amount of DNA**. The term "haploid" is classically used to refer to a cell containing 23 single chromosomes. Female gametes contain only the X sex chromosome. Male gametes contain either the X or Y sex chromosome; therefore, the male gamete determines the genetic sex of the individual.

B. The X chromosome   A normal female somatic cell contains **two X chromosomes (XX)**. The female cell has evolved a mechanism for permanent **inactivation** of one of the X chromosomes, which occurs during week 1 of embryonic development. The choice of which X chromosome (maternal or paternal) is inactivated seems to be random. The inactivated X chromosome, which can be seen by light microscopy near the nuclear membrane, is called the **Barr body**.

C. The Y chromosome   A normal male somatic cell contains **one X chromosome** and **one Y chromosome (XY)**.

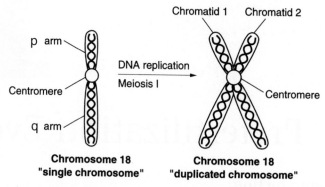

Figure 1-1. A schematic diagram of chromosome 18 shown in its "single chromosome" state and "duplicated chromosome" state that is formed by DNA replication during meiosis I. It is important to understand that both the "single chromosome" state and "duplicated chromosome" state will be counted as one chromosome 18. As long as the additional DNA in the "duplicated chromosome" is bound at the centromere, the structure is counted as one chromosome 18, even though it has twice the amount of DNA.

III. Meiosis (Figure 1-2)

Meiosis is a specialized process of cell division that occurs only in the production of gametes. It consists of two divisions, meiosis I and meiosis II, which result in the formation of four gametes, each of which contains half the number of chromosomes (23 single chromosomes) and half the amount of DNA (1N) found in normal somatic cells (46 single chromosomes, 2N).

A. **Meiosis I**   Events that occur during meiosis I include:
  • **Synapsis**: pairing of 46 homologous duplicated chromosomes.
  • **Crossing over**: large segments of DNA are exchanged.
  • **Alignment**: 46 homologous duplicated chromosomes align at the metaphase plate.
  • **Disjunction**: 46 homologous duplicated chromosomes separate from each other; **centromeres do not split.**
  • **Cell division**: two secondary gametocytes (23 duplicated chromosomes, 2N) are formed.

B. **Meiosis II**   Events that occur during meiosis II include:
  • **Synapsis**: absent.
  • **Crossing over**: absent.
  • **Alignment**: 23 duplicated chromosomes align at the metaphase plate.
  • **Disjunction**: 23 duplicated chromosomes separate to form 23 single chromosomes; **centromeres split.**
  • **Cell division**: four gametes (23 single chromosomes, 1N) are formed.

IV. Oogenesis: Female Gametogenesis

A. **Primordial germ cells (46, 2N)** from the wall of the yolk sac arrive in the ovary at **week 4** and differentiate into **oogonia (46, 2N)**, which populate the ovary through mitotic division.

B. Oogonia enter meiosis I and undergo DNA replication to form **primary oocytes (46, 4N)**. All primary oocytes are formed by **month 5 of fetal life**. No oogonia are present at birth.

C. Primary oocytes remain **dormant in prophase (diplotene) of meiosis I** from month 5 of fetal life until puberty. After puberty, from 5 to 15 primary oocytes begin maturation with each ovarian cycle, usually with only one reaching full maturity in each cycle.

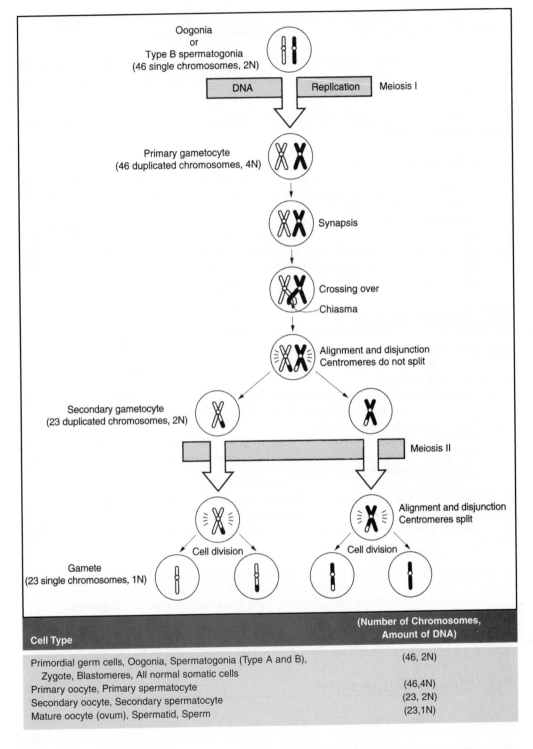

Cell Type	(Number of Chromosomes, Amount of DNA)
Primordial germ cells, Oogonia, Spermatogonia (Type A and B), Zygote, Blastomeres, All normal somatic cells	(46, 2N)
Primary oocyte, Primary spermatocyte	(46, 4N)
Secondary oocyte, Secondary spermatocyte	(23, 2N)
Mature oocyte (ovum), Spermatid, Sperm	(23, 1N)

Figure 1-2. Schematic representation of meiosis I and meiosis II, emphasizing the changes in chromosome number and amount of DNA that occur during gametogenesis. Only one pair of homologous chromosomes is shown (*white* = maternal origin and *black* = paternal origin). The point at which DNA crosses over is called the chiasma. Segments of DNA are exchanged, thereby introducing genetic variability to the gametes. In addition, various cell types along with their appropriate designation of number of chromosomes and amount of DNA are shown.

D. During the ovarian cycle, a primary oocyte completes meiosis I to form two daughter cells: the **secondary oocyte (23, 2N)** and the **first polar body,** which degenerates.

E. The secondary oocyte promptly begins meiosis II but is **arrested in metaphase of meiosis II** about 3 hours before ovulation. The secondary oocyte remains arrested in metaphase of meiosis II until fertilization occurs.

F. At fertilization, the secondary oocyte completes meiosis II to form a **mature oocyte (23, 1N)** and a **second polar body.**

G. Approximate number of oocytes
1. **Primary oocytes.** At month 5 of fetal life, 7 million primary oocytes are present. At birth, 2 million are present (5 million have degenerated). At puberty, 40,000 are present (1.96 million more have degenerated).
2. **Secondary oocytes.** Twelve are ovulated per year, up to 480 over the entire reproductive life of the woman (40 years × 12 secondary oocytes per year = 480). This number (480) is obviously overly simplified since it is **reduced** in women who take birth control pills (which prevent ovulation), in women who become pregnant (ovulation stops during pregnancy), and in women who may have anovulatory cycles.

V. Spermatogenesis

Male gametogenesis is classically divided into three phases.

A. Spermatocytogenesis
1. **Primordial germ cells (46, 2N)** form the wall of the yolk sac, arrive in the testes at **week 4,** and remain **dormant until puberty.** At puberty, primordial germ cells differentiate into **Type A spermatogonia (46, 2N).**
2. Type A spermatogonia undergo mitosis to provide a continuous supply of stem cells throughout the reproductive life of the male. Some Type A spermatogonia differentiate into **Type B spermatogonia (46, 2N).**

B. Meiosis Type B spermatogonia enter meiosis I and undergo DNA replication to form **primary spermatocytes (46, 4N).** Primary spermatocytes complete meiosis I to form **secondary spermatocytes (23, 2N).** Secondary spermatocytes complete meiosis II to form four **spermatids (23, 1N).**

C. Spermiogenesis Spermatids undergo a **postmeiotic series of morphologic changes** to form **sperm (23, 1N).** These changes include formation of the acrosome; condensation of the nucleus; and formation of head, neck, and tail. The total time of sperm formation (from spermatogonia to spermatozoa) is about 64 days. Newly ejaculated sperm are incapable of fertilization until they undergo **capacitation,** which occurs in the female reproductive tract and involves the unmasking of sperm glycosyltransferases and the removal of proteins coating the surface of the sperm.

VI. Clinical Considerations

A. Offspring of older women Prolonged dormancy of primary oocytes may be the reason for the high incidence of chromosomal abnormalities in offspring of older women. Since all primary oocytes are formed by month 5 of fetal life, a female infant is born with her entire supply of gametes. Primary oocytes remain dormant until ovulation; those ovulated late in the woman's reproductive life may have been dormant for as long as 40 years. The incidence of **trisomy 21 (Down syndrome)** increases with advanced age of the mother. The primary cause of Down syndrome is maternal meiotic nondisjunction. Clinical findings include: severe mental retardation, epicanthal folds, Brushfield spots, simian creases, and association with a decrease in α fetoprotein.

B. Offspring of older men   An increased incidence of **achondroplasia** (a congenital skeletal anomaly characterized by retarded bone growth) and **Marfan syndrome** is associated with advanced paternal age.

C. Male fertility   This depends on the number and motility of sperm. Fertile males produce from 20 million to more than 100 million sperm/mL of semen. Sterile males produce less than 10 million sperm/mL of semen. Normally up to 10% of sperm in an ejaculate may be grossly deformed (two heads or two tails), but these sperm probably do not fertilize an oocyte owing to their lack of motility.

D. Hormonal contraception
1. **Oral contraceptives**
   a. **Combination pills** contain a combination of estrogen and progesterone. They are taken for 21 days and then discontinued for 7 days. The primary mechanism of action is the inhibition of gonadotropin-releasing hormone (GnRH), follicle-stimulating hormone (FSH), and luteinizing hormone (LH) secretion, thereby preventing ovulation.
   b. **Progesterone-only pills** contain only progesterone. They are taken continuously without a break. The primary mechanism of action is not known, but thickening of cervical mucus (hostile to sperm migration) and thinning of the endometrium (unprepared for conceptus implantation) are known to occur.
2. **Medroxyprogesterone acetate (Depo-Provera)** is a progesterone-only product that offers a long-acting alternative to oral contraceptives. It can be injected **intramuscularly** and prevents ovulation **for 2–3 months.**
3. **Levonorgestrel (Norplant)** is a progesterone-only product that offers an even longer-acting alternative to Depo-Provera. The capsules containing levonorgestrel can be implanted **subdermally** and prevent ovulation for **1–5 years**.
4. **Seasonale** is a combined ethinyl estradiol (0.03 mg) and levonorgestrel (0.15 mg) product that is an **extended cycle** oral contraceptive. Seasonale is a 91-day treatment cycle whereby the woman should expect to have four menstrual periods per year.
5. **Ortho Evra** is a combined ethinyl estradiol (0.75 mg) and norelgestromin (6.0 mg) product that is a transdermal contraceptive patch.
6. **Emergency contraceptive pills (ECPs) or postcoital contraception.** ECPs are sometimes called "**morning-after pills**," but the pills can be started right away or up to 5 days after the woman has had unprotected sex. The therapy is more effective the earlier it is initiated within a **120-hour window.** There are two types of ECPs:
   a. **Combined ECPs** contain both estrogen and progesterone in the same dosage as ordinary birth control pills. In many countries (but not the United States), combined ECPs are specially packaged and labeled for emergency use. However, not all brands of birth control pills can be used for emergency contraception (for more information, see *www.not-2-late.com*). The dosage of **Ogestrel** and **Ovral** is two pills within 120 hours after unprotected sex followed by two more pills 12 hours later. Combined ECPs are associated with a high incidence of nausea and vomiting.
   b. **Progesterone-only ECPs** contain only **progesterone.** The brand name in the United States is **Plan B** (0.75 mg levonorgestrel). The dosage of Plan B is one pill within 72 hours of unprotected sex; the second pill should be taken 12 hours after the first pill. Plan B shows a reduced incidence of nausea and vomiting.
   c. **Diethylstilbestrol (DES)** was used as an ECP in the past but has been discontinued since it is associated with reproductive tract anomalies and vaginal cancers in exposed offspring. **Clear cell adenocarcinoma of the vagina** occurs in daughters of women who were exposed to DES therapy during pregnancy. A precursor to clear cell adenocarcinoma is **vaginal adenosis** (a benign condition) where stratified squamous epithelium is replaced by mucosal columnar epithelial-lined crypts.
7. **Luteinizing hormone–releasing hormone (LH-RH) analogues.** Chronic treatment with a LH-RH analogue (e.g., **buserelin**) paradoxically results in a down-regulation of FSH and LH secretion, thereby preventing ovulation.

E. Anovulation is the absence of ovulation in some women caused by inadequate secretion of FSH and LH. **Clomiphene citrate** is a drug that competes with estrogen for binding sites in the adenohypophysis, thereby suppressing the normal negative feedback loop of estrogen on the adenohypophysis. This stimulates FSH and LH secretion and induces ovulation.

F. The estimated chance of pregnancy (fertility) in the days surrounding ovulation is shown in Table 1-1.

TABLE 1-1	*Chance of Pregnancy in Days Near Ovulation*
Time	**Chance of Pregnancy**
5 days before ovulation	10%
4 days before ovulation	16%
3 days before ovulation	14%
2 days before ovulation	27%
1 day before ovulation	31%
Day of ovulation	33%
Day after ovulation	0%

STUDY QUESTIONS FOR CHAPTER 1

*Directions: Each of the numbered items or incomplete statements in this section is followed by answers or by completions of the statement. Select the **one** lettered answer or completion that is **best** in each case.*

1. Which of the following is a major characteristic of meiosis I?
(A) Splitting of the centromere
(B) Pairing of homologous chromosomes
(C) Reducing the amount of DNA to 1N
(D) Achieving the diploid number of chromosomes
(E) Producing primordial germ cells

2. A normal somatic cell contains a total of 46 chromosomes. What is the normal complement of chromosomes found in a sperm?
(A) 22 autosomes plus a sex chromosome
(B) 23 autosomes plus a sex chromosome
(C) 22 autosomes
(D) 23 autosomes
(E) 23 paired autosomes

3. Which of the following describes the number of chromosomes and amount of DNA in a gamete?
(A) 46 chromosomes, 1N
(B) 46 chromosomes, 2N
(C) 23 chromosomes, 1N
(D) 23 chromosomes, 2N
(E) 23 chromosomes, 4N

4. Which of the following chromosome compositions in a sperm normally results in the production of a genetic female if fertilization occurs?
(A) 23 homologous pairs of chromosomes
(B) 22 homologous pairs of chromosomes
(C) 23 autosomes plus an X chromosome
(D) 22 autosomes plus a Y chromosome
(E) 22 autosomes plus an X chromosome

5. In the process of meiosis, DNA replication of each chromosome occurs thereby forming a structure consisting of two sister chromatids attached to a single centromere. What is this structure?
(A) A duplicated chromosome
(B) Two chromosomes
(C) A synapsed chromosome
(D) A crossover chromosome
(E) A homologous pair

6. All primary oocytes are formed by
(A) week 4 of embryonic life
(B) month 5 of fetal life
(C) birth
(D) month 5 of infancy
(E) puberty

7. When does formation of primary spermatocytes begin?
(A) During week 4 of embryonic life
(B) During month 5 of fetal life
(C) At birth
(D) During month 5 of infancy
(E) At puberty

8. In the production of female gametes, which of the following cells can remain dormant for 12 to 40 years?
(A) Primordial germ cell
(B) Primary oocyte
(C) Secondary oocyte
(D) First polar body
(E) Second polar body

9. In the production of male gametes, which of the following cells remains dormant for 12 years?
(A) Primordial germ cell
(B) Primary spermatocyte
(C) Secondary spermatocyte
(D) Spermatid
(E) Sperm

10. Approximately how many sperm are ejaculated by a normal fertile male during sexual intercourse?
(A) 10 million
(B) 20 million
(C) 35 million
(D) 100 million
(E) 350 million

11. A young woman enters puberty with approximately 40,000 primary oocytes in her ovary. About how many of these primary oocytes will be ovulated over the entire reproductive life of the woman?

(A) 40,000
(B) 35,000
(C) 480
(D) 48
(E) 12

12. Fetal sex can be diagnosed by noting the presence or absence of the Barr body in cells obtained from the amniotic fluid. What is the etiology of the Barr body?

(A) Inactivation of both X chromosomes
(B) Inactivation of homologous chromosomes
(C) Inactivation of one Y chromosome
(D) Inactivation of one X chromosome
(E) Inactivation of one chromatid

13. How much DNA does a primary spermatocyte contain?

(A) 1N
(B) 2N
(C) 4N
(D) 6N
(E) 8N

14. During meiosis, pairing of homologous chromosomes occurs, which permits large segments of DNA to be exchanged. What is this process called?

(A) Synapsis
(B) Nondisjunction
(C) Alignment
(D) Crossing over
(E) Disjunction

15. During ovulation, the secondary oocyte resides at what specific stage of meiosis?

(A) Prophase of meiosis I
(B) Prophase of meiosis II
(C) Metaphase of meiosis I
(D) Metaphase of meiosis II
(E) Meiosis is completed at the time of ovulation

16. Concerning maturation of the female gamete (oogenesis), when do the oogonia enter meiosis I and undergo DNA replication to form primary oocytes?

(A) During fetal life
(B) At birth
(C) At puberty
(D) With each ovarian cycle
(E) Following fertilization

17. Where do primordial germ cells initially develop?

(A) In the gonads at week 4 of embryonic development
(B) In the yolk sac at week 4 of embryonic development
(C) In the gonads at month 5 of embryonic development
(D) In the yolk sac at month 5 of embryonic development
(E) In the gonads at puberty

ANSWERS AND EXPLANATIONS

1. B. Pairing of homologous chromosomes (synapsis) is a unique event that occurs only during meiosis I in the production of gametes. Synapsis is necessary so that crossing over can occur.

2. A. A normal gamete (sperm in this case) contains 23 single chromosomes. These 23 chromosomes consist of 22 autosomes plus 1 sex chromosome.

3. C. Gametes contain 23 chromosomes and 1N amount of DNA, so that when two gametes fuse at fertilization a zygote containing 46 chromosomes and 2N amount of DNA are formed.

4. E. A sperm contains 22 autosomes and 1 sex chromosome. The sex chromosome in sperm may be either the X or Y chromosome. The sex chromosome in a secondary oocyte is only the X chromosome. If an X-bearing sperm fertilizes a secondary oocyte, a genetic female (XX) is produced. Therefore, sperm is the arbiter of sex determination.

5. A. The structure formed is a duplicated chromosome. DNA replication occurs so that the amount of DNA is doubled (2 × 2N = 4N). However, the chromatids remain attached to the centromere forming a duplicated chromosome.

6. B. During early fetal life, oogonia undergo mitotic divisions to populate the developing ovary. All the oogonia subsequently give rise to primary oocytes by month 5 of fetal life; at birth no oogonia are present in the ovary. At birth, a female has her entire supply of primary oocytes to carry her through reproductive life.

7. E. At birth, a male has primordial germ cells in the testes that remain dormant until puberty, at which time they differentiate into Type A spermatogonia. At puberty, some Type A spermatogonia differentiate into Type B spermatogonia and give rise to primary spermatocytes by undergoing DNA replication.

8. B. Primary oocytes are formed by month 5 of fetal life and remain dormant until puberty, when hormonal changes in the young woman stimulate the ovarian and menstrual cycles. From 5 to 15 oocytes then begin maturation with each ovarian cycle throughout the woman's reproductive life.

9. A. Primordial germ cells migrate from the wall of the yolk sac during week 4 of embryonic life and enter the gonad of a genetic male, where they remain dormant until puberty (about age 12) when hormonal changes in the young man stimulate the production of sperm.

10. E. A normal fertile male ejaculates about 3.5 mL of semen containing about 100 million sperm/mL (3.5 mL × 100 million = 350 million).

11. C. Over her reproductive life, a woman ovulates approximately 480 oocytes. A woman ovulates 12 primary oocytes per year provided that she is not using oral contraceptives, does not become pregnant, or does not have any anovulatory cycles. Assuming a 40-year reproductive period, 40 × 12 = 480.

12. D. The Barr body is formed from inactivation of one X chromosome in a female. All somatic cells of a normal female contain two X chromosomes. The female has evolved a mechanism for permanent inactivation of one of the X chromosomes presumably because a double dose of X chromosome products would be lethal.

13. C. Type B spermatogonia give rise to primary spermatocytes by undergoing DNA replication, thereby doubling the amount of DNA (2 × 2N = 4N) within the cell.

14. D. Synapsis (pairing of homologous chromosomes) is a unique event that occurs only during meiosis I in the production of gametes. Synapsis is necessary so that crossing over, in which large segments of DNA are exchanged, can occur.

15. D. The secondary oocyte is arrested in metaphase of meiosis II about 3 hours before ovulation, and it will remain in this meiotic stage until fertilization occurs.

16. A. All primary oocytes are formed by month 5 of fetal life, so no oogonia are present at birth.

17. B. Primordial germ cells, the predecessors to gametes, are first seen in the wall of the yolk sac at week 4 of embryonic development, and they will migrate into the gonads at week 6.

Week 1 of Human Development (Days 1–7)[a]

I.   Fertilization

Fertilization occurs in the **ampulla of the uterine tube** and includes three phases.

A. Phase 1   Sperm penetration of corona radiata is aided by the action of sperm and uterine tube mucosal enzymes.

B. Phase 2   Sperm binding and penetration of zona pellucida occur during phase 2.
  1. **Sperm binding** occurs through interaction of sperm glycosyltransferases and ZP3 receptors located on the zona pellucida. Sperm binding triggers the **acrosome reaction**, which entails the fusion of the outer acrosomal membrane and sperm cell membrane resulting in the release of acrosomal enzymes.
  2. **Penetration of zona pellucida** is aided by acrosomal enzymes, specifically **acrosin**. Sperm contact with the cell membrane of a secondary oocyte triggers the **cortical reaction**, which entails the release of cortical granules (lysosomes) from the oocyte cytoplasm. This reaction renders both the zona pellucida and the oocyte membrane impermeable to other sperm.

C. Phase 3   Fusion of sperm and oocyte cell membranes occurs with subsequent breakdown of both membranes at the fusion area.
  1. The entire sperm (except the cell membrane) enters the cytoplasm of the secondary oocyte arrested in metaphase of meiosis II. The sperm mitochondria and tail degenerate. The sperm nucleus is now called the **male pronucleus.** Since all sperm mitochondria degenerate, all mitochondria within the zygote are of maternal origin (i.e., **all mitochondrial DNA is of maternal origin).**
  2. The secondary oocyte completes meiosis II, forming a mature ovum and a second polar body. The nucleus of mature ovum is now called the **female pronucleus.**
  3. Male and female pronuclei fuse, thereby forming a **zygote** (a new cell whose genotype is an intermingling of maternal and paternal chromosomes).

---

[a]The age of a developing conceptus can be measured either from the estimated day of fertilization (fertilization age) or from the day of the last normal menstrual period (LNMP age). In this book, age is presented as the fertilization age.

II.   Cleavage and Blastocyst Formation (Figure 2-1)

A. **Cleavage** is a series of **mitotic** divisions of the zygote.
   1. Zygote cytoplasm is successively partitioned (cleaved) to form a blastula consisting of increasingly smaller **blastomeres** (2-cell, 4-cell, 8-cell, and so on). Blastomeres are considered **totipotent** (capable of forming a complete embryo) up to the 4- to 8-cell stage (important when considering monozygotic twinning).
   2. Blastomeres form a **morula** by undergoing **compaction**; that is, tight junctions are formed between the cells in the **outer cell mass**, thereby sealing off the **inner cell mass**. **Uvomorulin**, a glycoprotein found on the surface of blastomeres, is involved in compaction.

B. **Blastocyst formation** involves fluid secreted within the morula that forms the **blastocyst cavity**. The conceptus is now called a **blastocyst**.
   1. The inner cell mass is now called the **embryoblast** (becomes the embryo).
   2. The outer cell mass is now called the **trophoblast** (becomes fetal portion of the placenta).

C. **Zona pellucida degeneration** occurs by day 4 after conception. The zona pellucida must degenerate for implantation to occur.

III.   Implantation (see Figure 2-1)

The blastocyst usually implants within the **posterior superior wall of the uterus** by day 7 after fertilization. Implantation occurs in the **functional layer of the endometrium** during the **progestational (secretory) phase** of the menstrual cycle. The trophoblast proliferates and differentiates into the **cytotrophoblast** and **syncytiotrophoblast**. Failure of implantation may involve immune rejection (graft-versus-host reaction) of the antigenic conceptus by the mother.

IV.   Clinical Considerations

A. **Ectopic tubal pregnancy (ETP)** occurs when the blastocyst implants within the uterine tube owing to **delayed transport**. The **ampulla of the uterine tube** is the most common site of an ectopic pregnancy. The **rectouterine pouch (pouch of Douglas)** is a common site for an ectopic abdominal pregnancy. ETP is most commonly seen in women with **endometriosis** or **pelvic inflammatory disease**. ETP leads to uterine tube rupture and hemorrhage if surgical intervention (i.e., salpingectomy) is not performed. An ETP presents with **abnormal uterine bleeding, unilateral pelvic pain, increased levels of HCG** (but lower than originally expected with uterine implantation pregnancy), and a **massive 1st first trimester bleed**. An ETP must be differentially diagnosed from **appendicitis**, an **aborting intrauterine pregnancy**, or a **bleeding corpus luteum** of a normal intrauterine pregnancy.

B. **In vitro fertilization (IVF)** requires the sequential application of a number of steps as indicated:
   1. **Clomiphene citrate** is administered to stimulate multiple ovulation.
   2. Oocytes are collected by needle aspiration from the ovary assisted by ultrasound visualization.
   3. Sperm are collected by masturbation, separated from seminal fluid, and capacitized by exposure to ionic solutions. In cases of oligospermy (infertility due to low number of sperm), multiple samples may be obtained over an extended period of time.
   4. Sperm and oocytes are cultured together. The success of in vitro fertilization is judged by the presence of two pronuclei with the oocyte.
   5. Cleavage is allowed to proceed in vitro to the **8-cell stage** embryo.

6. Typically, at least three embryos are transferred to the uterus, since there is a low success rate of implantation.

7. The remaining embryos are frozen for future use if the first embryo transfer does not result in a pregnancy.

C. Teratocarcinoma (TC)   Spontaneous TCs are **gonadal tumors** that contain both differentiated cell types and undifferentiated pluripotent stem cells called **embryonic carcinoma (EC) cells.** TCs can be experimentally produced by implanting a blastocyst in an extrauterine site. The ability of blastocysts to form TCs suggests a relationship between the inner cell mass and EC cells. This relationship has been confirmed by isolation of cell lines from blastocysts called **embryonic stem (ES) cells,** which have biochemical characteristics remarkably similar to EC cells.

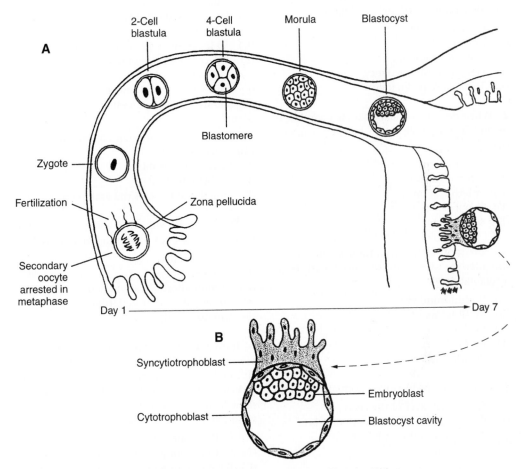

Figure 2-1.   (A) The stages of human development during week 1. (B) A day 7 blastocyst.

STUDY QUESTIONS FOR CHAPTER 2

*Directions: Each of the numbered items or incomplete statements in this section is followed by answers or by completions of the statement. Select the **one** lettered answer or completion that is **best** in each case.*

1. A 20-year-old woman presents at the emergency department with severe abdominal pain on the right side with signs of internal bleeding. She indicated that she has been sexually active without contraception and missed her last menstrual period. Based on this information, which of the following disorders must be included as an option in the diagnosis?

(A) Ovarian cancer
(B) Appendicitis
(C) Normal pregnancy
(D) Ectopic tubal pregnancy
(E) Toxemia of pregnancy

2. When does a secondary oocyte complete its second meiotic division to become a mature ovum?

(A) At ovulation
(B) Before ovulation
(C) At fertilization
(D) At puberty
(E) Before birth

3. How soon after fertilization occurs within the uterine tube does the blastocyst begin implantation?

(A) Within minutes
(B) By 12 hours
(C) By day 1
(D) By day 2
(E) By day 7

4. Where does the blastocyst normally implant?

(A) Functional layer of the cervix
(B) Functional layer of the endometrium
(C) Basal layer of the endometrium
(D) Myometrium
(E) Perimetrium

5. Which of the following events is involved in cleavage of the zygote during week 1 of development?

(A) A series of meiotic divisions forming blastomeres
(B) Production of highly differentiated blastomeres
(C) An increased cytoplasmic content of blastomeres
(D) An increase in size of blastomeres
(E) A decrease in size of blastomeres

6. Which of the following structures must degenerate for blastocyst implantation to occur?

(A) Endometrium in progestational phase
(B) Zona pellucida
(C) Syncytiotrophoblast
(D) Cytotrophoblast
(E) Functional layer of the endometrium

7. Which of the following is the origin of the mitochondrial DNA of all human adult cells?

(A) Paternal only
(B) Maternal only
(C) Combination of paternal and maternal
(D) Either paternal or maternal
(E) Unknown origin

8. Individual blastomeres were isolated from a blastula at the 4-cell stage. Each blastomere was cultured in vitro to the blastocyst stage and individually implanted into four pseudopregnant foster mothers. Which of the following would you expect to observe 9 months later?

(A) Birth of one baby
(B) Birth of four genetically different babies
(C) Birth of four genetically identical babies
(D) Birth of four grotesquely deformed babies
(E) No births

9. Embryonic carcinoma (EC) cells were isolated from a yellow-coated mouse with a teratocarcinoma. The EC cells were then microinjected into the inner cell mass of a blastocyst isolated from a black-coated mouse. The blastocyst was subsequently implanted into the uterus of a white-coated foster mouse. Which of the following would be observed after full-term pregnancy?

(A) A yellow-coated offspring
(B) A black-coated offspring
(C) A white-coated offspring
(D) A yellow- and black-coated offspring
(E) A yellow- and white-coated offspring

10. In oogenesis, which of the following events occurs immediately following the completion of meiosis II?

(A) Degeneration of the zona pellucida
(B) Sperm penetration of corona radiata
(C) Formation of a female pronucleus
(D) Appearance of the blastocyst
(E) Completion of cleavage

ANSWERS AND EXPLANATIONS

1. D. Ectopic tubal pregnancy must always be an option in the diagnosis when a woman in her reproductive years presents with such symptoms. Ninety percent of ectopic implantations occur in the uterine tube. Ectopic tubal pregnancies result in rupture of the uterine tube and internal hemorrhage, which presents a major threat to the woman's life. The uterine tube and embryo must be surgically removed. The symptoms may sometimes be confused with appendicitis.

2. C. At ovulation, a secondary oocyte begins meiosis II, but this division is arrested at metaphase. The secondary oocyte remains arrested in metaphase until a sperm penetrates it at fertilization. Therefore, the term "mature ovum" is somewhat of a misnomer, because it is a secondary oocyte that is fertilized and, once fertilized, the new diploid cell is known as a zygote. If fertilization does not occur, the secondary oocyte degenerates.

3. E. The blastocyst begins implantation by day 7 after fertilization.

4. B. The blastocyst implants in the functional layer of the uterine endometrium. The uterus is composed of the perimetrium, myometrium, and endometrium. Two layers are identified within the endometrium: (1) the functional layer, which is sloughed off at menstruation, and (2) the basal layer, which is retained at menstruation and serves as the source of regeneration of the functional layer. During the progestational phase of the menstrual cycle, the functional layer undergoes dramatic changes; uterine glands enlarge and vascularity increases in preparation for blastocyst implantation.

5. E. Cleavage is a series of mitotic divisions whereby the large amount of zygote cytoplasm is successively partitioned among the newly formed blastomeres. Although the number of blastomeres increases during cleavage, the size of individual blastomeres decreases until they resemble adult cells in size.

6. B. The zona pellucida must degenerate for implantation to occur. Early cleavage states of the blastula are surrounded by a zona pellucida, which prevents implantation in the uterine tube.

7. B. The mitochondrial DNA of all human adult cells is of maternal origin only. In human fertilization, the entire sperm enters the secondary oocyte cytoplasm. However, sperm mitochondria degenerate along with the sperm's tail. Therefore, only mitochondria that are present within the secondary oocyte (maternal) remain in the fertilized zygote.

8. C. This scenario would result in four genetically identical children. Blastomeres at the 4-cell to 8-cell stage are totipotent, that is, capable of forming an entire embryo. Since blastomeres arise by mitosis of the same cell (zygote), they are genetically identical. This phenomenon is important in explaining monozygotic (identical) twins. About 30% of monozygotic twins arise by early separation of blastomeres. The remaining 70% originate at the end of week 1 of development by a splitting of the inner cell mass.

9. D. This scenario would result in a yellow- and black-coated offspring. Because EC cells and inner cell mass cells have very similar biochemical characteristics, they readily mix with each other and development proceeds unencumbered. Because the mixture contains cells with yellow-coat genotype and black-coat genotype, offspring with coats of two colors (yellow and black) will be produced. The offspring are known as mosaic mice.

10. C. The secondary oocyte is arrested in metaphase of meiosis II, and it will remain in this meiotic stage until fertilization occurs. Following fertilization, the secondary oocyte completes meiosis II, forming a mature ovum and a polar body. The nucleus of the mature ovum is called the female pronucleus, which fuses with the male pronucleus to form a zygote.

Week 2 of Human Development (Days 8–14)

I. Further Development of the Embryoblast (Figure 3-1)

During week 2, the embryoblast differentiates into two distinct cellular layers: the dorsal **epiblast** layer (columnar cells) and the ventral **hypoblast** layer (cuboidal cells). The epiblast and hypoblast together form a flat, ovoid-shaped disk known as the **bilaminar embryonic disk.** Within the epiblast, clefts begin to develop and eventually coalesce to form the **amniotic cavity.** Hypoblast cells begin to migrate and line the inner surface of the cytotrophoblast forming the **exocoelomic membrane,** which delimits a space called the **exocoelomic cavity** (or **primitive yolk sac**). This space is later called the **definitive yolk sac** when a portion of the exocoelomic cavity is pinched off as an **exocoelomic cyst.**

At the future site of the mouth, hypoblast cells become columnar-shaped and fuse with epiblast cells to form a circular, midline thickening called the **prochordal plate.**

II. Further Development of the Trophoblast (see Figure 3-1)

A. Syncytiotrophoblast The syncytiotrophoblast is the outer multinucleated zone of the trophoblast where no mitosis occurs (i.e., it arises from the cytotrophoblast). During this time period, the syncytiotrophoblast continues its invasion of the endometrium, thereby eroding endometrial blood vessels and endometrial glands. Lacunae form within the syncytiotrophoblast and become filled with maternal blood and glandular secretions. In addition, endometrial stromal cells (**decidual cells**) at the site of implantation become filled with glycogen and lipids and also supply nutrients to the embryoblast. The isolated lacunae fuse to form a **lacunar network** through which maternal blood flows, thus establishing early **uteroplacental circulation.** Although a primitive circulation is established between the uterus and future placenta, the embryoblast receives its nutrition via **diffusion** only at this time.

B. Cytotrophoblast The cytotrophoblast is mitotically active as new cytotrophoblastic cells migrate into the syncytiotrophoblast, thereby fueling its growth. In addition, cytotrophoblastic cells produce local mounds called **primary chorionic villi** that bulge into the surrounding syncytiotrophoblast.

III. Development of Extraembryonic Mesoderm (see Figure 3-1)

The extraembryonic mesoderm develops from the epiblast and consists of loosely arranged cells that fill the space between the exocoelomic membrane and the cytotrophoblast. Large spaces develop in the extraembryonic mesoderm and coalesce to form the **extraembryonic coelom.** The extraembryonic coelom divides the extraembryonic mesoderm into the **extraembryonic somatic mesoderm** and **extraembryonic visceral mesoderm.** The extraembryonic somatic mesoderm lines the trophoblast, forms the connecting stalk, and covers the amnion. The extraembryonic visceral mesoderm covers the yolk sac. As soon as the extraembryonic somatic mesoderm and extraembryonic visceral mesoderm form, one can delineate the **chorion,** which consists of the extraembryonic somatic mesoderm, cytotrophoblast, and syncytiotrophoblast. As the chorion is delineated, the extraembryonic coelom is now called the **chorionic cavity.** The conceptus is suspended by the **connecting stalk** within the chorionic cavity.

IV.   Clinical Considerations (Figure 3-2)

A. Human chorionic gonadotropin (hCG) is a glycoprotein **produced by the syncytiotrophoblast** that stimulates the production of progesterone by the corpus luteum (i.e., maintains corpus luteum function). This is clinically significant because progesterone produced by the corpus luteum is essential for the maintenance of pregnancy until week 8. The placenta then takes over progesterone production. hCG can be assayed in **maternal blood at day 8** or **maternal urine at day 10** and is the basis of pregnancy testing. hCG is detectable throughout a pregnancy. **Low hCG values** may predict a spontaneous abortion or may indicate an ectopic pregnancy. **Elevated hCG values** may indicate a multiple pregnancy, hydatidiform mole, or gestational trophoblastic neoplasia.

B. Hydatidiform mole (complete or partial) represents an abnormal placenta characterized by marked enlargement of chorionic villi. A complete mole is distinguished from a partial mole by the amount of chorionic villus involvement. The hallmarks of a complete mole include gross generalized edema of chorionic villi forming grapelike, transparent vesicles, hyperplastic proliferation of surrounding trophoblastic cells, and absence of an embryo/fetus. Clinical signs diagnostic of a mole include preeclampsia during the first trimester, elevated hCG levels (>100,000 mIU/mL), and an enlarged uterus with bleeding. Follow-up visits after a mole are essential because 3–5% develop into gestational trophoblastic neoplasia.

C. Gestational trophoblastic neoplasia (GTN; or choriocarcinoma) is a malignant tumor of the trophoblast that may occur after a normal or ectopic pregnancy, an abortion, or a hydatidiform mole. With a high degree of suspicion, elevated hCG levels are diagnostic. Nonmetastatic GTN (i.e., confined to the uterus) is the most common form of the neoplasia, and treatment is highly successful. However, the prognosis of metastatic GTN is poor if it spreads to the liver or brain.

D. RU-486 (mifepristone [Mifeprix]) initiates menstruation when taken within 8–10 weeks of the start of the last menstrual period. If implantation of a conceptus has occurred, the conceptus is sloughed along with the endometrium. RU-486 is a **progesterone receptor antagonist (blocker)** used in conjunction with **misoprostol (Cytotec; a PGE_1 analogue)** and is 96% effective at terminating pregnancy.

E. Oncofetal antigens (Table 3-1) are cell surface antigens that normally appear only on embryonic cells, but for unknown reasons reexpress themselves in human malignant cells. Monoclonal antibodies directed against specific oncofetal antigens provide an avenue for cancer therapy.

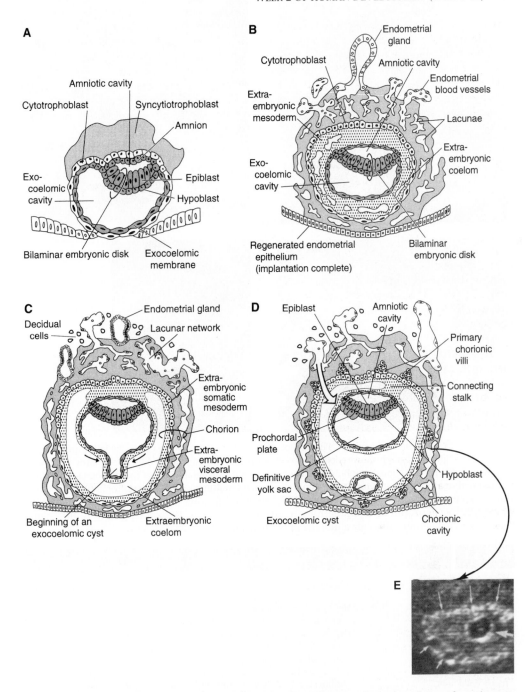

Figure 3-1. **(A)** Day 8 blastocyst is shown partially implanted into the endometrium. Extraembryonic mesoderm (EEM) has not formed yet. **(B)** Day 12 blastocyst is shown completely implanted within the endometrium, and epithelium has regenerated. This type of implantation is known as interstitial implantation. EEM begins to form. **(C)** Day 13 blastocyst. A lacunar network forms, establishing an early uteroplacental circulation. An exocoelomic cyst begins to pinch off (*small arrows*). **(D)** Day 14 blastocyst. The embryoblast can be described as two balloons (amniotic cavity and yolk sac) pressed together at the bilaminar embryonic disk. The *curved open arrow* indicates that the embryoblast receives maternal nutrients via diffusion. **(E)** A sonogram at about week 3 shows a hyperechoic rim representing the chorion (*thick arrow*) surrounding the chorionic cavity (or gestational sac). Within the chorionic cavity, two tiny cystic areas (i.e., the amnion and yolk sac) separated by a thin echogenic line (i.e., embryonic disk) can be observed. Note the hyperechoic base of the endometrium (*long arrows*) and two endometrial cysts (*short arrows*).

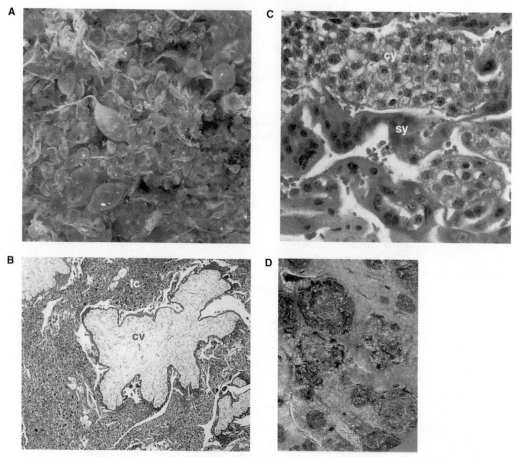

Figure 3-2. (A, B) Hydatidiform mole. Photograph shows gross edema of the chorionic villi forming grape-like vesicles. Light micrograph shows edema of the chorionic villi (*cv*) surrounded by hyperplastic trophoblastic cells (*tc*). (C, D) Gestational trophoblastic neoplasia. Light micrograph shows the distinctive alternating arrangement of mononuclear cytotrophoblastic cells (*cy*) and multinucleated syncytiotrophoblastic cells (*sy*). Photograph shows hemorrhagic nodules metastatic to the liver. This is due to the rapid proliferation of trophoblastic cells combined with marked propensity to invade blood vessels. The central portion of the lesion is hemorrhagic and necrotic with only a thin rim of trophoblastic cells at the periphery.

TABLE 3–1	*Oncofetal Antigens and Tumor Markers*
Antigen	**Associated Tumor**
α-Fetoprotein (AFP)	Hepatocellular carcinoma, germ cell neoplasms, yolk sac or endodermal sinus tumors of the testicle or ovary
AAT	Hepatocellular carcinoma, yolk sac or endodermal sinus tumors of the testicle or ovary
Carcinoembryonic antigen (CEA)	Colorectal cancer, pancreatic cancer, breast cancer, and small cell cancer of the lung; bad prognostic sign if elevated preoperatively
β_2-Microglobulin	Multiple myeloma (excellent prognostic factor), light chains in urine (Bence Jones protein)
CA 125	Surface-derived ovarian cancer
CA 15-3	Breast cancer
CA 19-9	Pancreatic cancer (excellent marker)
Neuron-specific enolase (NSE)	Small cell carcinoma of the lung, seminoma, neuroblastoma
Prostate-specific antigen (PSA)	Prostate cancer
hCG	Trophoblastic tumors; hydatidiform mole (benign); choriocarcinoma (malignant)
Bombesin	Small cell carcinoma of the lung, neuroblastoma
LDH	Hodgkin's disease

CA = cancer antigen.

STUDY QUESTIONS FOR CHAPTER 3

Directions: Each of the numbered items or incomplete statements in this section is followed by answers or by completions of the statement. Select the **one** lettered answer or completion that is **best** in each case.

1. Which of the following components plays the most active role in invading the endometrium during blastocyst implantation?

(A) Epiblast
(B) Syncytiotrophoblast
(C) Hypoblast
(D) Extraembryonic somatic mesoderm
(E) Extraembryonic visceral mesoderm

2. Between which two layers is the extraembryonic mesoderm located?

(A) Epiblast and hypoblast
(B) Syncytiotrophoblast and cytotrophoblast
(C) Syncytiotrophoblast and endometrium
(D) Exocoelomic membrane and syncytiotrophoblast
(E) Exocoelomic membrane and cytotrophoblast

3. During week 2 of development, the embryoblast receives its nutrients via

(A) diffusion
(B) osmosis
(C) reverse osmosis
(D) fetal capillaries
(E) yolk sac nourishment

4. The prochordal plate marks the site of the future

(A) umbilical cord
(B) heart
(C) mouth
(D) anus
(E) nose

5. Which of the following are components of the definitive chorion?

(A) Extraembryonic somatic mesoderm and epiblast
(B) Extraembryonic somatic mesoderm and cytotrophoblast
(C) Extraembryonic somatic mesoderm and syncytiotrophoblast
(D) Extraembryonic somatic mesoderm, cytotrophoblast, and syncytiotrophoblast
(E) Extraembryonic visceral mesoderm, cytotrophoblast, and syncytiotrophoblast

6. A 16-year-old girl presents on May 10 in obvious emotional distress. On questioning, she relates that on May 1 she experienced sexual intercourse for the first time, without any means of birth control. Most of her anxiety stems from her fear of pregnancy. What should the physician do to alleviate her fear?

(A) Prescribe diazepam and wait to see if she misses her next menstrual period
(B) Use ultrasonography to document pregnancy
(C) Order a laboratory assay for serum hCG
(D) Order a laboratory assay for serum progesterone
(E) Prescribe diethylstilbestrol ("morning-after pill")

7. Carcinoembryonic antigen (CEA) is an oncofetal antigen that is generally associated with which one of the following tumors?

(A) Hepatoma
(B) Germ cell tumor
(C) Squamous cell carcinoma
(D) Colorectal carcinoma
(E) Teratocarcinoma

Questions 8–13

For each of the following statements or words concerning a 14-day-old blastocyst, select the most appropriate structure in the diagram (right).

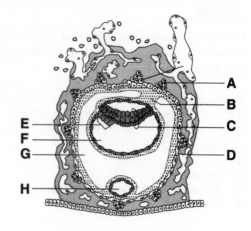

8. Future site of the mouth

9. Forms definitive structures found in the adult

10. Chorion

11. Chorionic cavity

12. Primary chorionic villi

13. Connecting stalk

14. A 42-year-old woman presents with complaints of severe headaches, blurred vision, slurred speech, and loss of muscle coordination. Her last pregnancy 5 years ago resulted in a hydatidiform mole. Laboratory results show a high hCG level. Which of the following conditions is a probable diagnosis?

(A) Vasa previa
(B) Placenta previa
(C) Succenturiate placenta
(D) Choriocarcinoma
(E) Membranous placenta

15. At what location does the amniotic cavity develop?

(A) Between the cytotrophoblast and syncytiotrophoblast
(B) Within the extraembryonic mesoderm
(C) Between the endoderm and mesoderm
(D) Within the hypoblast
(E) Within the epiblast

16. At the end of week 2 of development (day 14), what is the composition of the embryonic disk?

(A) Epiblast only
(B) Epiblast and hypoblast
(C) Ectoderm and endoderm
(D) Ectoderm, mesoderm, endoderm
(E) Epiblast, mesoderm, hypoblast

ANSWERS AND EXPLANATIONS

1. B. The syncytiotrophoblast plays the most active role in invading the endometrium of the mother's uterus. During the invasion, endometrial blood vessels and endometrial glands are eroded, and a lacunar network is formed.

2. E. The extraembryonic mesoderm is derived from the epiblast and is located between the exocoelomic membrane and the cytotrophoblast. The overall effect is to completely separate the embryoblast from the trophoblast with the extraembryonic mesoderm serving as a conduit (connection) between them.

3. A. During week 2 of development, the embryoblast receives its nutrients from endometrial blood vessels, endometrial glands, and decidual cells via diffusion. Diffusion of nutrients does not pose a problem given the small size of the blastocyst during week 2. Although the beginnings of a uteroplacental circulation are established during week 2, no blood vessels have yet formed in the extraembryonic mesoderm to carry nutrients directly to the embryoblast (this occurs in week 3).

4. C. The prochordal plate is a circular, midline thickening of hypoblast cells that are firmly attached to the overlying epiblast cells. The plate eventually develops into a membrane called the oropharyngeal membrane at the site of the future mouth. It is interesting to note that at this early stage of development the cranial versus caudal region of the embryo is established by the prochordal plate. And since the prochordal plate is located in the midline, bilateral symmetry is also established.

5. D. The definitive chorion consists of three components: extraembryonic somatic mesoderm, cytotrophoblast, and syncytiotrophoblast. The chorion defines the chorionic cavity in which the embryoblast is suspended and is vital in the formation of the placenta.

6. C. Human chorionic gonadotropin (hCG) can be assayed in maternal serum at day 8 of development and in urine at day 10. If this teenager is pregnant, the blastocyst would be in week 2 of development (day 10). Laboratory assay of hCG in either the serum or urine can be completed; however, serum hCG might be more reliable. It is important to note that if she is pregnant, she will not miss a menstrual period until May 15 at which time the embryo will be entering week 3 of development.

7. D. Oncofetal antigens are normally expressed during embryonic development, remain unexpressed in normal adult cells, but reexpress on transformation to malignant neoplastic tissue. CEA is associated with colorectal carcinoma.

8. E. The prochordal plate indicates the site of the future mouth. At this early stage of development, the orientation of the embryo in the cranial versus caudal direction is established. The prochordal plate is a thickening of hypoblast cells that are firmly attached to the epiblast cells.

9. C. The bilaminar embryonic disk develops definitive adult structures after gastrulation occurs, in contrast to the trophoblast, which is involved in placental formation.

10. D. The chorion consists of three layers; namely, extraembryonic somatic mesoderm, cytotrophoblast, and syncytiotrophoblast. The chorion is vital in the formation of the placenta.

11. G. The chorion forms the walls of the chorionic cavity in which the conceptus is suspended by the connecting stalk. Note that the inner lining of the chorionic cavity is extraembryonic mesoderm.

12. A. The cytotrophoblast is mitotically active so that local mounds of cells (primary chorionic villi) form that bulge into the surrounding syncytiotrophoblast. As development continues, primary chorionic villi form secondary chorionic villi, and finally tertiary chorionic villi as part of placental formation.

13. B. The extraembryonic mesoderm can be thought of as initially forming in a continuous layer and then splitting as isolated cavities begin to appear everywhere except dorsally near the amniotic cavity and epiblast. When the isolated cavities coalesce, the extraembryonic coelom (or chorion cavity) and connecting stalk are formed.

14. D. After a hydatidiform mole, it is very important to ensure that all the invasive trophoblastic tissue is removed. High levels of hCG are a good indicator of retained trophoblastic tissue because such tissue produces this hormone. In this case, the trophoblastic tissue has developed into a malignant choriocarcinoma and metastasized to the brain, causing her symptoms of headache, blurred vision, and so on.

15. E. The amniotic cavity develops within the epiblast, and it is a cavity that contains the embryo and amniotic fluid.

16. B. The embryoblast consists of the two distinct cell layers (epiblast and hypoblast) at the end of development week 2 (day 14), which forms a bilaminar embryonic disk.

Embryonic Period (Weeks 3–8)

I. General Considerations

By the end of the embryonic period, all major organ systems have begun to develop, although functionality may be minimal. The development of the cardiovascular system is essential particularly because diffusion of nutrients by the early uteroplacental circulation can no longer satisfy the nutritional needs of the rapidly developing embryo. During the embryonic period, folding of the embryo occurs in two distinct planes. **Craniocaudal folding** is caused by the growth of the central nervous system (CNS) and the amnion, whereas **lateral folding** is caused by the growth of the somites, amnion, and other components of the lateral body wall. Both craniocaudal folding and lateral folding change the shape of the embryo from a two-dimensional disk to a three-dimensional cylinder. By the end of week 8, the embryo has a distinct human appearance. During the embryonic period, the basic segmentation of the human embryo in the craniocaudal direction is controlled by the **Hox (homeobox) complex** of genes. The development of each individual organ system is reviewed in upcoming chapters. However, it is important to realize that all organ systems develop simultaneously during the embryonic period.

II. Further Development of the Embryoblast

A. Gastrulation (Figure 4-1) is the process that establishes the three definitive germ layers of embryo (**ectoderm, intraembryonic mesoderm, and endoderm**), thereby forming a **trilaminar embryonic disk** by day 21 of development. These three germ layers give rise to all the tissues and organs of the adult. Gastrulation is first indicated by the formation of the **primitive streak**, caused by a proliferation of epiblast cells. The primitive streak consists of the **primitive groove, primitive node,** and **primitive pit**. Located caudal to the primitive streak is the future site of the anus, known as the **cloacal membrane**, where epiblast and hypoblast cells are fused. The ectoderm, intraembryonic mesoderm, and endoderm of the trilaminar embryonic disk all are derived from the epiblast. The term *intraembryonic mesoderm* describes the germ layer that forms during week 3 (gastrulation) in contrast to the *extraembryonic mesoderm*, which formed during week 2. Intraembryonic mesoderm forms various tissues and organs found in the adult, whereas extraembryonic mesoderm is involved in placenta formation. In this regard, we will not use the term "intraembryonic mesoderm" when discussing tissue and organ development of the adult in later chapters but instead shorten the term to only "mesoderm."

B. Changes involving intraembryonic mesoderm (Figure 4-2)
  1. **Paraxial mesoderm** is a thick plate of mesoderm located on each side of the midline. Paraxial mesoderm becomes organized into segments known as **somitomeres**, which form in a craniocaudal sequence. **Somitomeres 1–7** do not form somites but contribute meso-

25

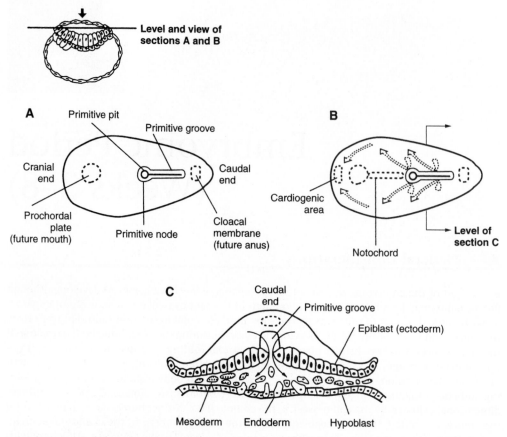

Figure 4-1. Schematic representation of gastrulation. Embryoblast in upper left is for orientation. **(A)** Dorsal view of the epiblast. **(B)** *Dotted arrows* show the migration of cells through the primitive streak during gastrulation. **(C)** Cross section showing the migration of cells that will form the intraembryonic mesoderm and displace the hypoblast to form endoderm. Epiblast cells begin to migrate to the primitive streak and invaginate into a space between the epiblast and hypoblast. Some of these migrating epiblast cells displace the hypoblast to form the definitive endoderm. The remainder of the epiblast cells migrate laterally, cranially, and along the midline to form the definitive intraembryonic mesoderm. After the formation of the endoderm and intraembryonic mesoderm, the epiblast is called the definitive ectoderm.

derm to the pharyngeal arches. The remaining somitomeres further condense in a craniocaudal sequence to form **42–44 pairs of somites**. The first pair of somites forms on day 20, and new somites appear at a rate of 3/day. The somites closest to the caudal end eventually disappear to give a final count of approximately **35 pairs of somites**. The number of somites is one of the criteria for determining age of the embryo. Somites further differentiate into these components:

    a. Sclerotome forms the cartilage and bone components of the vertebral column.

    b. Myotome forms epimeric and hypomeric muscles.

    c. Dermatome forms dermis and subcutaneous area of skin.

2. **Intermediate mesoderm** is a longitudinal dorsal ridge of mesoderm located between the paraxial mesoderm and lateral mesoderm. This ridge forms the **urogenital ridge**, which is involved in the formation of the future kidneys and gonads.

3. **Lateral mesoderm** is a thin plate of mesoderm located along the lateral sides of the embryo. Large spaces develop in the lateral mesoderm and coalesce to form the **intraembryonic coelom**. The intraembryonic coelom divides the lateral mesoderm into two layers:

    a. Intraembryonic somatic mesoderm (also called somatopleure)

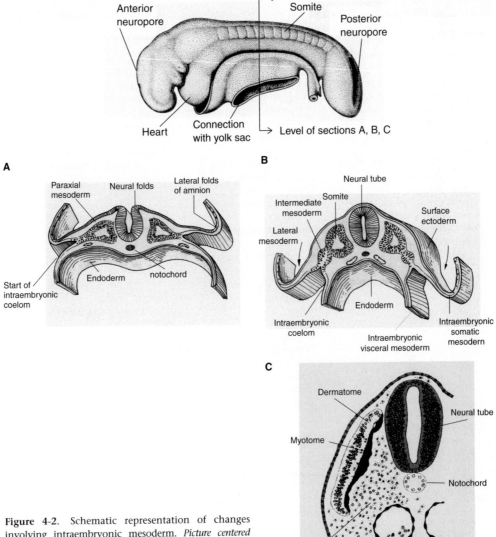

Figure 4-2. Schematic representation of changes involving intraembryonic mesoderm. *Picture centered above* is for orientation. *(A)* Cross section at day 19. *(B)* Cross section at day 21, with *arrows* indicating lateral folding of the embryo. *(C)* Cross section showing differentiation of the somite.

    b. Intraembryonic visceral mesoderm (also called visceropleure or splanchnopleure)

  4. Notochord is a solid cylinder of mesoderm extending in the midline of the trilaminar embryonic disk from the primitive node to the prochordal plate. The notochord has a number of important functions, which include the following:

    a. It induces the overlying ectoderm to differentiate into neuroectoderm to form the neural plate.

    b. It induces the formation of each vertebral body.

    c. It forms the nucleus pulposus of each intervertebral disk.

  5. Cardiogenic region is a horseshoe-shaped region of mesoderm located at the cranial end of the trilaminar embryonic disk rostral to the prochordal plate. This region is involved in the formation of the future heart.

  6. Specific derivatives of mesoderm are indicated in Table 4-1.

TABLE 4–1	*Summary Table of Germ Layer Derivatives*

Ectoderm	Mesoderm	Endoderm
Epidermis, hair, nails, sweat and sebaceous glands	Muscle (smooth, cardiac, skeletal)	Hepatocytes
Utricle, semicircular ducts, vestibular ganglion of CN VIII	Extraocular muscles, ciliary muscle of eye, iris stroma, ciliary body stroma, substantia propria of cornea, corneal endothelium, sclera, choroid	Principal and oxyphil cells of parathyroid
Saccule, cochlear duct (organ of Corti), spiral ganglion of CN VIII		Thyroid follicular cells
		Epithelial reticular cells of thymus
Olfactory placode, CN I	Muscles of tongue (occipital somites)	Acinar and islet cells of pancreas
Ameloblasts (enamel of teeth)	Pharyngeal arch muscles	Acinar cells of submandibular and sublingual glands
Adenohypophysis	Laryngeal cartilages	Epithelial lining of:
Lens of eye	Connective tissue	GI tract
Anterior epithelium of cornea	Dermis and subcutaneous layer of skin	Trachea, bronchi, lungs
Acinar cells of parotid gland	Bone and cartilage	Biliary apparatus
Acinar cells of mammary gland	Dura mater	Urinary bladder, female urethra, most of male urethra
Epithelial lining of:	Endothelium of blood and lymph vessels	
Lower anal canal	RBCs, WBCs, microglia, and Kupffer cells	Inferior two thirds of vagina
Distal part of male urethra	Spleen	Auditory tube, middle ear cavity
External auditory meatus	Kidney	Crypts of palatine tonsils
	Adrenal cortex	
	Testes, epididymis, ductus deferens, seminal vesicle, ejaculatory duct	
	Ovary, uterus, uterine tubes, superior third of vagina	

Neuroectoderm
All neurons within brain and spinal cord (CNS)
Retina, iris epithelium, ciliary body epithelium, optic nerve (CN II), optic chiasm, optic tract, dilator and sphincter pupillae muscles
Astrocytes, oligodendrocytes, ependymocytes, tanycytes, choroid plexus cells
Neurohypophysis
Pineal gland

Neural crest
Ganglia (dorsal root, cranial, autonomic)
Schwann cells
Odontoblasts (dentin of teeth)
Pia and arachnoid
Chromaffin cells (adrenal medulla)
Parafollicular (C) cells of thyroid
Melanocytes
Aorticopulmonary septum
Pharyngeal arch skeletal components
Bones of neurocranium

CN = cranial nerve; GI = gastrointestinal; RBCs = red blood cells; WBCs = white blood cells.

C. Changes involving ectoderm   The major change involving a specific portion of ectoderm is its induction by the underlying notochord to differentiate into neuroectoderm and neural crest cells, thereby forming the future nervous system. Specific derivatives of ectoderm are indicated in Table 4-1.

D. Changes involving endoderm   Specific derivatives of endoderm are indicated in Table 4-1.

III.   Vasculogenesis

Vasculogenesis (de novo blood vessel formation) occurs in two general locations.

A. In extraembryonic mesoderm   Vasculogenesis occurs first within extraembryonic visceral mesoderm around the yolk sac on day 17. By day 21, vasculogenesis extends into extraembryonic somatic mesoderm located around the connecting stalk to form the **umbilical vessels** and in secondary villi to form **tertiary chorionic villi**. Angiogenesis occurs by means of a process in which extraembryonic mesoderm differentiates into **angioblasts**, which form clusters known as **angiogenic cell clusters**. The angioblasts located at the periphery of angiogenic cell clusters give rise to **endothelial cells,** which fuse with each other to form small blood vessels.

B. In intraembryonic mesoderm   Blood vessels form within the embryo by the same mechanism as in extraembryonic mesoderm. Eventually, blood vessels formed in the extraembryonic mesoderm become continuous with blood vessels within the embryo, thereby establishing a blood vascular system between the embryo and placenta.

IV.   Hematopoiesis (Figure 4-3)

Hematopoiesis (blood cell formation) first occurs within the extraembryonic visceral mesoderm around the yolk sac during week 3 of development. During this process, angioblasts within the cen-

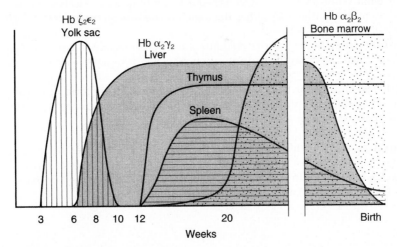

Figure 4-3.   A schematic diagram showing the contribution of various organs to hematopoiesis during development. During the period of yolk sac hematopoiesis, the earliest embryonic form of hemoglobin is synthesized called hemoglobin $\zeta_2\epsilon_2$. During the period of liver hematopoiesis, the fetal **form** of hemoglobin (HbF) is synthesized called hemoglobin $\alpha_2\gamma_2$ During the period of bone marrow hematopoiesis (about week 30), the adult form of hemoglobin (HbA) is synthesized called hemoglobin $\alpha_2\beta_2$, which gradually replaces hemoglobin $\alpha_2\gamma_2$. Hemoglobin $\alpha_2\gamma_2$ is the predominant form of hemoglobin during pregnancy because it has a higher affinity for oxygen than the adult form of hemoglobin and thereby "pulls" oxygen from the maternal blood into fetal blood.

ter of angiogenic cell clusters give rise to primitive blood cells. Beginning at week 5, hematopoiesis is taken over by a sequence of embryonic organs: **liver, spleen, thymus,** and **bone marrow.**

V. Clinical Considerations

A. Sacrococcygeal teratoma (ST; Figure 4-4) is a tumor that arises from remnants of the primitive streak, which normally degenerates and disappears. ST is derived from pluripotent cells of the primitive streak and often contains various types of tissue (e.g., bone, nerve, and hair). ST occurs more commonly in female infants and usually becomes malignant during infancy (must be removed by age 6 months).

B. Caudal dysplasia (sirenomelia) refers to a constellation of syndromes ranging from minor lesions of lower vertebrae to complete fusion of the lower limbs. Caudal dysplasia is caused by abnormal gastrulation, in which the migration of mesoderm is disturbed. It can be associated with various cranial anomalies:
1. **VATER,** which includes vertebral defects, anal atresia, tracheoesophageal fistula, and renal defects
2. **VACTERL,** which is similar to VATER but also includes cardiovascular defects and upper limb defects

C. Chordoma (CD) is either a benign or malignant tumor that arises from remnants of the notochord. CD may be found either intracranially or in the sacral region and occurs more commonly in men late in adult life (age 50).

D. First missed menstrual period is usually the first indication of pregnancy. Week 3 of embryonic development coincides with the first missed menstrual period. Note that at this time the embryo has already undergone 2 weeks of development. It is crucial that the woman become aware of a pregnancy as soon as possible because the embryonic period is a period of high susceptibility to teratogens.

E. Thalassemia syndromes are a heterogeneous group of genetic defects characterized by the lack of or decreased synthesis of either the α-globin chain (**α-thalassemia**) or β-globin chain (**β-thalassemia**) of hemoglobin $\alpha_2\beta_2$.
1. **Hydrops fetalis** is the most severe form of α-thalassemia and causes severe pallor, generalized edema, and massive hepatosplenomegaly and invariably leads to intrauterine fetal death.
2. **β-Thalassemia major (Cooley's anemia)** is the most severe form of β-thalassemia and causes a severe, transfusion-dependent anemia. It is most common in Mediterranean countries and parts of Africa and Southeast Asia.

F. Hydroxyurea (a cytotoxic drug) has been shown to promote fetal hemoglobin (HbF) production by the re-activation of γ-chain synthesis. Hydroxyurea has been especially useful in the treatment of **sickle cell disease** in which the presence of HbF counteracts the low oxygen affinity of sickle cell hemoglobin (HbS) and inhibits the sickling process.

A   B

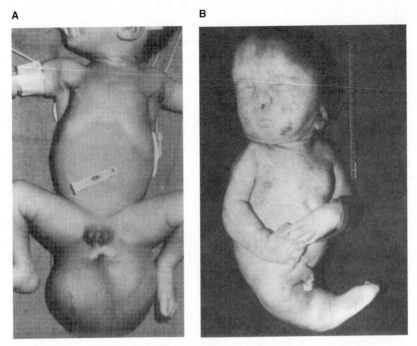

Figure 4-4.   **(A)** Sacrococcygeal teratoma. **(B)** Caudal dysplasia (sirenomelia).

STUDY QUESTIONS FOR CHAPTER 4

*Directions: Each of the numbered items or incomplete statements in this section is followed by answers or by completions of the statement. Select the **one** lettered answer or completion that is **best** in each case.*

1. Which germ layers are present at the end of week 3 of development (day 21)?

(A) Epiblast only
(B) Epiblast and hypoblast
(C) Ectoderm and endoderm
(D) Ectoderm, mesoderm, and endoderm
(E) Epiblast, mesoderm, and hypoblast

2. Which process establishes the three definitive germ layers?

(A) Neurulation
(B) Gastrulation
(C) Craniocaudal folding
(D) Lateral folding
(E) Angiogenesis

3. The first indication of gastrulation in the embryo is

(A) formation of the primitive streak
(B) formation of the notochord
(C) formation of the neural tube
(D) formation of extraembryonic mesoderm
(E) formation of tertiary chorionic villi

4. Somites may differentiate into which of the following?

(A) Urogenital ridge
(B) Kidneys
(C) Notochord
(D) Epimeric and hypomeric muscles
(E) Epithelial lining of the GI tract

5. Intermediate mesoderm gives rise to the

(A) neural tube
(B) heart
(C) kidneys and gonads
(D) somites
(E) notochord

6. The developing embryo has a distinct human appearance by the end of

(A) week 4
(B) week 5
(C) week 6
(D) week 7
(E) week 8

7. The lateral mesoderm is divided into two distinct layers by the formation of the

(A) extraembryonic coelom
(B) intraembryonic coelom
(C) cardiogenic region
(D) notochord
(E) yolk sac

8. Very often the first indication that a woman has that she is pregnant is a missed menstrual period. In which week of embryonic development does a woman experience her first missed menstrual period?

(A) Start of week 3
(B) Start of week 4
(C) Start of week 5
(D) Start of week 8
(E) End of week 8

9. A female newborn was found to have a large midline tumor in the lower sacral area, which was diagnosed as a sacrococcygeal tumor. Which of the following courses of treatment is recommended for this child?

(A) Immediate chemotherapy and radiation treatment
(B) Surgical removal of the tumor by age 6 months
(C) Surgical removal of the tumor at age 4–5 years
(D) Surgical removal of the tumor at age 13–15 years
(E) No treatment because this tumor normally regresses with age

10. A woman has her pregnancy suddenly terminated because of intrauterine fetal death. At autopsy, the fetus shows severe pallor, generalized edema, and hepatosplenomegaly. Which of the following would you suspect?

(A) VATER
(B) β-Thalassemia minor
(C) β-Thalassemia major
(D) Hydrops fetalis
(E) VACTERL

11. The specialized group of mesenchymal cells that aggregate to form blood islands centrally and primitive blood vessels peripherally are called

(A) fibroblasts
(B) cardiac progenitor cells
(C) angioblasts
(D) myoblasts
(E) osteoblasts

12. The epiblast is capable of forming which of the following germ layers?

(A) Ectoderm only
(B) Ectoderm and mesoderm only
(C) Ectoderm and endoderm only
(D) Ectoderm, mesoderm, endoderm
(E) Mesoderm and endoderm only

13. A male newborn has a hemangioma on the left frontotemporal region of his face and scalp. The cells forming the hemangioma are derived from which of the following cell layers?

(A) Ectoderm only
(B) Mesoderm only
(C) Endoderm only
(D) Ectoderm and mesoderm
(E) Endoderm and mesoderm

14. Which structure is derived from the same embryonic primordium as the dorsal root ganglia?

(A) Gonads
(B) Kidney
(C) Pineal gland
(D) Liver
(E) Adrenal medulla

15. Which structure is derived from the same embryonic primordium as the kidney?

(A) Gonads
(B) Epidermis
(C) Pineal gland
(D) Liver
(E) Adrenal medulla

ANSWERS AND EXPLANATIONS

1. **D.** During week 3 of development, the process of gastrulation occurs. This establishes the three primary germ layers (ectoderm, intraembryonic mesoderm, and endoderm). The origin of all tissues and organs of the adult can be traced to one of these germ layers since these tissues and organs "germinate" from these germ layers.

2. **B.** Gastrulation establishes the three primary germ layers during week 3 of development. Neurulation is the process by which neuroectoderm forms the neural plate, which eventually folds to form the neural tube.

3. **A.** The formation of the primitive streak on the dorsal surface of the bilaminar embryonic disk is the first indication of gastrulation.

4. **D.** Approximately 35 pairs of somites form; they are derived from a specific subdivision of intraembryonic mesoderm called paraxial mesoderm. Somites differentiate into the components called sclerotome (cartilage and bone of the vertebral column), myotome (epimeric and hypomeric muscle), and dermatome (dermis and subcutaneous area of skin).

5. **C.** Intermediate mesoderm is a subdivision of intraembryonic mesoderm that forms a longitudinal dorsal ridge called the urogenital ridge from which the kidneys and gonads develop.

6. **E.** The embryo starts the embryonic period as a two-dimensional disk and ends as a three-dimensional cylinder. This dramatic change in geometry is caused by formation of all the major organ systems. As the organ systems gradually develop during the embryonic period, the embryo appears more and more human-like; it has a distinct human appearance at the end of week 8.

7. **B.** The lateral mesoderm is a subdivision of intraembryonic mesoderm and initially is a solid plate of mesoderm. The intraembryonic coelom forms in the middle of the lateral mesoderm, thereby dividing it into the intraembryonic somatic mesoderm and intraembryonic visceral mesoderm.

8. **A.** Assuming a regular 28-day menstrual cycle, a woman who starts menses on February 1, for example, will ovulate on February 14, and the secondary oocyte is fertilized within 24 hours. So, the zygote undergoes week 1 of development from February 15 to 21. Week 2 of development is from February 22 to 28. On March 1, the woman should enter her next menstrual cycle, but because she is pregnant, she will not menstruate. Therefore, this first missed menstrual period corresponds with the start of week 3 of embryonic development. The embryonic period (weeks 3–8) is a time of high susceptibility to teratogens.

9. **B.** The preponderance of sacrococcygeal tumors is found in female newborns. Since these tumors develop from pluripotent cells of primitive streak origin, malignancy is of great concern, and the tumor should be surgically removed by age 6 months. Occasionally, these tumors may recur after surgery, demonstrating malignant properties.

10. **D.** Hydrops fetalis is the most severe form of α-thalassemia, which is a direct result of the lack of or decreased synthesis of the α-globin chain of hemoglobin $\alpha_2\beta_2$.

11. **B.** The angioblasts are the mesenchymal cells that form blood vessels in embryonic development as well as embryonic blood cells.

12. **D.** The epiblast is capable of forming all three germ layers (ectoderm, mesoderm, and endoderm) during gastrulation. Epiblast cells migrate to the primitive streak and invaginate into a space between the epiblast and hypoblast. Some of these epiblast cells displace the hypoblast to

form the definitive endoderm. Migrating epiblast cells also form the intraembryonic mesoderm. The remaining epiblast cells form the ectoderm.

13. B. A hemangioma is a vascular tumor that can be present at birth in which the abnormal proliferation of blood vessels leads to a mass resembling a neoplasm. Hemangiomas are mesodermal in origin as they are formed by embryonic blood cells and the vascular endothelium formed by angioblasts.

14. E. Both the chromaffin cells of the adrenal medulla and the dorsal root ganglia are derived from the neural crest cells.

15. A. Both the kidneys and the gonads are derived from intermediate mesoderm. This longitudinal dorsal ridge of mesoderm forms the urogenital ridge, which is involved with the formation of the future kidneys and gonads.

Cardiovascular System

I. Formation of Heart Tube (Figure 5-1)

Lateral plate mesoderm (at the cephalic area of the embryo) splits into a somatic layer and splanchnic layer, thus forming the **pericardial cavity**. Precardiac mesoderm is preferentially distributed to the splanchnic layer and is now called **heart-forming regions (HFRs)**. As lateral folding of the embryo occurs, the HFRs fuse in the midline to form a continuous sheet of mesoderm. Hypertrophied foregut endoderm secretes **vascular endothelial growth factor (VEGF)**, which induces the sheet of mesoderm to form discontinuous vascular channels that eventually get remodeled into a single **endocardial tube (endocardium)**. Mesoderm around the endocardium forms the **myocardium**, which secretes a layer of extracellular matrix proteins called **cardiac jelly**. Mesoderm migrating into the cardiac region from the coelomic wall near the liver forms the **epicardium**.

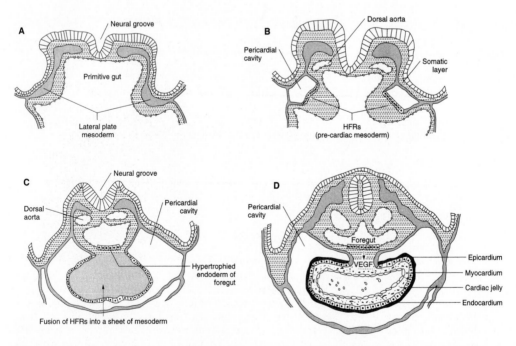

Figure 5-1. A schematic diagram depicting cross sections of an embryo at the level of the developing heart. **(A)** Formation of lateral plate mesoderm. **(B)** Splitting of lateral plate mesoderm. **(C)** Fusion of heart-forming regions (HFRs) in the midline into a sheet of mesoderm. **(D)** Vascular endothelial growth factor (VEGF) induction of single endocardial tube.

II.   Primitive Heart Tube Dilatations (Figure 5-2)

Five dilatations soon become apparent along the length of the tube: **truncus arteriosus, bulbus cordis, primitive ventricle, primitive atrium**, and **sinus venosus**. These five dilatations develop into the adult structures of the heart.

III.   Dextral Looping (see Figure 5-2)

In the primitive heart tube, venous blood flows through the left ventricle *prior to* the right ventricle. This situation must be corrected because in the normal adult heart venous blood flows into the right ventricle. Dextral looping is the key event in this correction such that the location of the atrioventricular canal and the conoventricular canal become properly aligned.

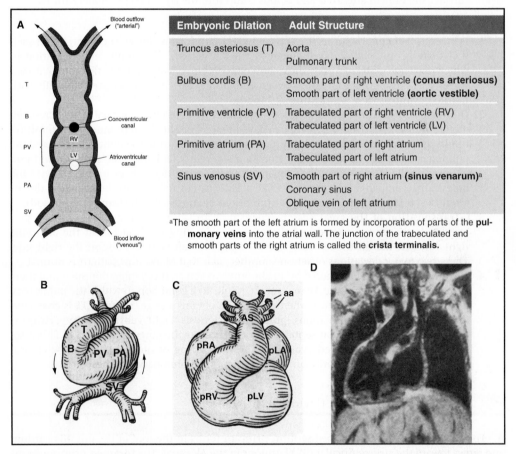

Embryonic Dilation	Adult Structure
Truncus asteriosus (T)	Aorta Pulmonary trunk
Bulbus cordis (B)	Smooth part of right ventricle **(conus arteriosus)** Smooth part of left ventricle **(aortic vestibule)**
Primitive ventricle (PV)	Trabeculated part of right ventricle (RV) Trabeculated part of left ventricle (LV)
Primitive atrium (PA)	Trabeculated part of right atrium Trabeculated part of left atrium
Sinus venosus (SV)	Smooth part of right atrium **(sinus venarum)**[a] Coronary sinus Oblique vein of left atrium

[a]The smooth part of the left atrium is formed by incorporation of parts of the **pulmonary veins** into the atrial wall. The junction of the trabeculated and smooth parts of the right atrium is called the **crista terminalis.**

Figure 5-2.   A schematic diagram depicting the primitive heart tube and its five dilatations and a table indicating adult structures. **(A)** 22 days. Note the location of the atrioventricular canal and conoventricular canal. *Arrows* show the direction of blood flow from the "venous" blood inflow at the sinus venosus to the "arterial" blood outflow at the truncus arteriosus. Note that "venous" blood inflow enters the left ventricle (LV) before it enters the right ventricle (RV). **(B)** 26 days. Note that the straight heart tube begins dextral looping (*curved arrows*). *T* = truncus arteriosus; *B* = bulbus cordis; *PV* = primitive ventricle; *PA* = primitive atrium; *SV* = sinus venosus. **(C)** 30–35 days. Dextral looping is complete, and the four primitive heart chambers are apparent. *aa* = aortic arches; *AS* = aortic sac; *pRA* = primitive right atrium; *pRV* = primitive right ventricle; *pLA* = primitive left atrium; *pLV* = primitive left ventricle. **(D)** Coronal MRI of a cyanotic infant with asplenia (heart in right hemithorax with apex pointing to the right), demonstrating dextrocardia and midline liver.

A. Early looping seems to be inherently programmed within the myocardial cells.

B. Convergence begins to bring the atrioventricular canal and the conoventricular canal into proper alignment.

C. Wedging causes the conoventricular canal to nestle between the tricuspid and mitral valves and occurs concurrently with the formation of the aorticopulmonary (AP) septum.

D. Repositioning causes the atrioventricular canal to straddle both the right and left ventricles.

IV.   The Aorticopulmonary (AP) Septum (Figure 5-3)

A. Formation   Neural crest cells migrate from the hindbrain region through pharyngeal arches 3, 4, and 6 and invade both the **truncal ridges** and **bulbar ridges.** The truncal and bulbar ridges grow and twist around each other in a spiral fashion and eventually fuse to form the AP septum. The AP septum divides the truncus arteriosus and bulbus cordis into the aorta and pulmonary trunk.

B. Clinical considerations
   1. **Persistent truncus arteriosus (PTA)** is caused by abnormal neural crest cell migration such that there is *partial* development of the AP septum. PTA results in a condition in which one large vessel leaves the heart and receives blood from both the right and left ventricles. PTA is usually accompanied by a membranous VSD and is associated clinically with **marked cyanosis (R → L shunting of blood).**
   2. **D-Transposition of the great arteries (complete)** is caused by abnormal neural crest cell migration such that there is *nonspiral* development of the AP septum. D-Transposition results in a condition in which the aorta arises abnormally from the right ventricle and the pulmonary trunk arises abnormally from the left ventricle; hence, the systemic and pulmonary circulations are *completely* separated from each other. It is incompatible with life unless an accompanying shunt exists like a VSD, patent foramen ovale, or patent ductus arteriosus. It is associated clinically with **marked cyanosis (R → L shunting of blood).**
   3. **L-Transposition of the great vessels (corrected).** In L-Transposition, the aorta and pulmonary trunk are transposed and the ventricles are "inverted" such that the anatomic right ventricle lies on the left side and the anatomic left ventricle lies on the right side. These two major deviations offset one another such that blood flow pattern is normal.
   4. **Tetralogy of Fallot (TF)** is caused by an abnormal neural crest cell migration such that there is *skewed* development of the AP septum. TF results in a condition in which the pulmonary trunk obtains a small diameter, whereas the aorta obtains a large diameter. TF is characterized by four classic malformations: **p̲ulmonary stenosis, r̲ight ventricular hypertrophy, o̲verriding aorta, v̲entricular septal defect (VSD).** Note the mnemonic PROVE. TF is associated clinically with **marked cyanosis (R → L shunting of blood)** whereby the clinical consequences depend primarily on the severity of the pulmonary stenosis.

V.   The Atrial Septum (Figure 5-4)

A. Formation   The crescent-shaped **septum primum** forms in the roof of the primitive atrium and grows toward the atrioventricular (AV) cushions in the AV canal. The **foramen primum** forms between the free edge of the septum primum and the AV cushions; it is closed when the septum primum fuses with the AV cushions. The **foramen secundum** forms in the center of the septum primum. The crescent-shaped septum secundum forms to the right of the septum primum. The **foramen ovale** is the opening between the upper and lower limbs of the septum secundum. During embryonic life, blood is shunted from the right atrium to the left atrium via the foramen ovale. Immediately after birth, functional closure of the foramen ovale is facilitated both by a **decrease in right atrial pressure** from occlusion of placental circulation and by an **increase in left atrial pressure** due to increased pulmonary venous return. Later in life, the septum primum and septum secundum anatomically fuse to complete the formation of the atrial septum.

B. Clinical considerations: atrial septal defects (ASDs)
1. **Foramen secundum defect** is caused by excessive resorption of septum primum, septum secundum, or both. This results in a condition in which there is an opening between the right and left atria. Some defects can be tolerated for a long time, with clinical symptoms manifesting as late as age 30. It is the most common clinically significant ASD.
2. **Common atrium (cor triloculare biventriculare)** is caused by the complete failure of septum primum and septum secundum to develop. This results in a condition in which there is formation of only one atrium.
3. **Probe patency of the foramen ovale** is caused by incomplete anatomic fusion of septum primum and septum secundum. It is present in approximately 25% of the population and is usually of no clinical importance.
4. **Premature closure of foramen ovale** is closure of foramen ovale during prenatal life. It results in hypertrophy of the right side of the heart and underdevelopment of the left side of the heart.

VI.   The Atrioventricular (AV) Septum (Figure 5-5)

A. Formation   The **dorsal AV cushion** and **ventral AV cushion** approach each other and fuse to form the AV septum. The AV septum partitions the AV canal into the right AV canal and left AV canal.

B. Clinical considerations
1. **Persistent common AV canal** is caused by failure of fusion of the dorsal and ventral AV cushions. It results in a condition in which the common AV canal is never partitioned into the right and left AV canals so that a large hole can be found in the center of the heart. Consequently, the tricuspid and bicuspid valves are represented by one valve common to both sides of the heart. Two common hemodynamic abnormalities are found:
   a. L→R shunt of blood from the left atrium to the right atrium causing an enlarged right atrium and right ventricle
   b. Mitral valve regurgitation causing an enlarged left atrium and left ventricle
2. **Ebstein's anomaly** is caused by the failure of the posterior and septal leaflets of the tricuspid valve to attach normally to the annulus fibrosus but are instead displaced inferiorly into the right ventricle. It results in a condition in which the right ventricle is divided into a large, upper, "atrialized" portion and a small, lower, functional portion. Owing to the small, functional portion of the right ventricle, there is reduced amount of blood available to the pulmonary trunk. It is usually associated with an ASD.
3. **Foramen primum defect** is caused by a failure of the AV septum to fuse with the septum primum. It results in a condition in which the foramen primum is never closed and is generally accompanied by an abnormal mitral valve.
4. **Tricuspid atresia (hypoplastic right heart)** is caused by an insufficient amount of AV cushion tissue available for the formation of the tricuspid valve. It results in a condition in which there is complete agenesis of the tricuspid valve so that no communication between the right atrium and right ventricle exists. It is associated clinically with **marked cyanosis** and is always accompanied by the following:
   a. Patent foramen ovale
   b. Interventricular septum defect
   c. Overdeveloped left ventricle
   d. Underdeveloped right ventricle

VII.   The Interventricular (IV) Septum (Figure 5-6)

A. Formation   The muscular IV septum develops in the midline on the floor of the primitive ventricle and grows toward the fused AV cushions. The IV foramen is located between the free edge of the muscular IV septum and the fused AV cushions. This foramen is closed by the membranous IV septum, which forms by the proliferation and fusion of tissue from three sources: the right bulbar ridge, left bulbar ridge, and AV cushions.

B. Clinical considerations: septal defects (VSDs)

1. **Membranous VSD** is caused by faulty fusion of the **right bulbar ridge, left bulbar ridge, and AV cushions.** It results in a condition in which an opening between the right and left ventricles allows free flow of blood. A large VSD is initially associated with a L→R shunting of blood, increased pulmonary blood flow, and pulmonary hypertension. One of the secondary effects of a large VSD and its associated pulmonary hypertension is proliferation of the tunica intima and tunica media of pulmonary muscular arteries and arterioles, resulting in a narrowing of their lumen. Ultimately, pulmonary resistance may become higher than systemic resistance and cause R→L shunting of blood and cyanosis. At this stage, the characteristic of the patient has been termed the **Eisenmenger complex.** This is the most common type of VSD.

2. **Muscular VSD** is caused by single or multiple perforations in the muscular IV septum.

3. **Common ventricle (cor triloculare biatriatum)** is caused by failure of the membranous and muscular IV septa to form.

VIII. The Conduction System of the Heart

At week 5, cardiac myocytes in the sinus venosus region of the primitive heart tube begin to undergo spontaneous electrical depolarizations at a *faster rate* than cardiac myocytes in other regions. As dextral looping occurs, the sinus venous becomes incorporated into the right atrium, and these fast-rate depolarizing cardiac myocytes become the **sinoatrial (SA) node** and the **atrioventricular (AV) node.** In the adult, the cardiac myocytes of the SA and AV nodes remain committed to the fast rate of electrical depolarizations rather than developing contractile properties. As the atria and ventricles become electrically isolated by the formation of the **fibrous skeleton** of the heart, the **AV node** provides the *only* pathway for depolarizations to flow from the atria to the ventricles. The **AV bundle** or **bundle of His** develops from a ringlike cluster of cells found at the AV junction that specifically expresses the homeobox gene, **msx-2.** The **intramural network of Purkinje myocytes** has a distinct embryologic origin (versus the bundle of His) in that Purkinje myocytes develop from already contractile cardiac myocytes within the myocardium and can therefore be considered as **modified cardiac myocytes.**

IX. Coronary Arteries

Progenitor stem cells from the liver migrate into the primitive heart tube and take residence beneath the epicardium. These progenitor stem cells form vascular channels that grow toward the truncus arteriosus (future aorta) and form a **peritruncal capillary ring.** Only two of these capillaries survive, and these become the proximal portions of the right and left coronary arteries.

X. Development of the Arterial System (Figure 5-7)

A. General pattern In the head and neck region, the arterial pattern develops mainly from six pairs of arteries (called **aortic arches**) that course through the pharyngeal arches. The aortic arch arteries undergo a complex remodeling process that results in the adult arterial pattern. In the rest of the body, the arterial pattern develops mainly from the **right and left dorsal aortae.** The right and left dorsal aortae fuse to form the **dorsal aorta,** which then sprouts **posterolateral arteries, lateral arteries,** and **ventral arteries (vitelline** and **umbilical).**

(text continues on page 45)

A. Formation of the AP Septum

1   2   3

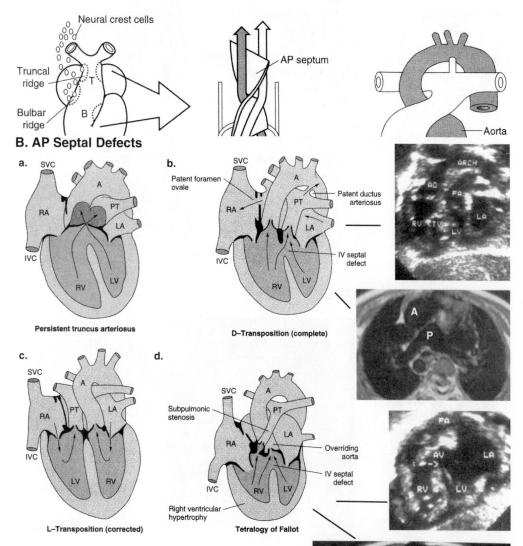

Figure 5-3. **(A)** Formation of the AP septum (*1, 2, 3*). **(B)** AP septal defects. *(a)* Persistent truncus arteriosus. *(b)* D-transposition of the great arteries (complete). Echocardiogram (*subxiphoid view*) is shown. *AO* = aorta; *ARCH* = aortic arch; *LA* = left atrium; *LV* = left ventricle; *PA* = pulmonary artery; *RV* = right ventricle; *TV* = tricuspid valve. MRI is shown. Note that the ascending aorta (*A*) is abnormally positioned anterior to the pulmonary artery (*P*). Normally, at the level of the semilunar valves, the ascending aorta is positioned posterior and to the right of the pulmonary artery. *(c)* L-transposition of the great arteries. *(d)* Tetralogy of Fallot. Echocardiogram (*subxiphoid view*) is shown. The deviation of the AP septum is shown above the *arrow*. → = IV septal defect; : = subpulmonic stenosis; *AV* = aortic valve; *LA* = left atrium; *LV* = left ventricle; *RV* = right ventricle; *PA* = pulmonary artery. MRI is shown. Note the small right pulmonary artery (*R*) and larger but still diminutive left pulmonary artery (*L*). Note also the very large diameter of the aortic arch (*A*). There is also a prominent bronchial artery (*arrow*) branching from the descending aorta (*a*). *Arrows* indicate direction of blood flow. *T* = truncus arteriosus; *B* = bulbus cordis; *AP* = aorticopulmonary; *A* = aorta; *IV* = interventricular; *IVC* = inferior vena cava; *LA* = left atrium; *LV* = left ventricle; *PT* = pulmonary trunk; *RA* = right atrium; *RV* = right ventricle; *SVC* = superior vena cava.

A. Formation of the Atrial Septum

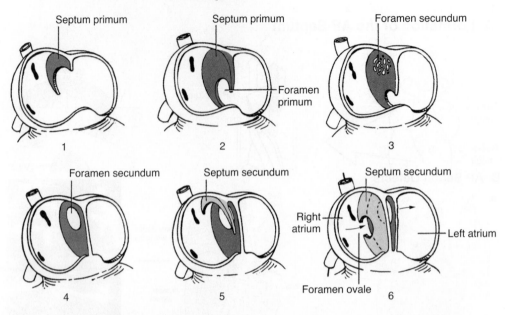

B. Atrial Septal Defects (ASDs)

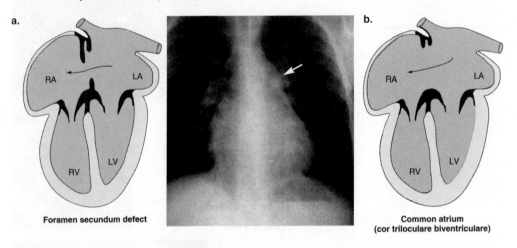

Figure 5-4. **(A)** Formation of the atrial septum (*1, 2, 3, 4, 5, 6*). The *arrows in #6* indicate the direction of blood flow across the fully developed septum, from the right atrium to the left atrium. **(B)** Atrial septal defects (ASDs). *(a)* Foramen secundum defect. AP radiograph of a foramen secundum defect shows cardiomegaly due to enlargement of the right atrium and right ventricle (left atria and ventricle are generally normal-sized), enlargement of pulmonary artery (*arrow*), and increased pulmonary vascularity. The enlarged pulmonary arteries prevent the aorta from forming the normal left border of the heart (i.e., the aortic knob is small). *(b)* Common atrium. *Arrows* indicate direction of blood flow. *LA* = left atrium; *LV* = left ventricle; *RA* = right atrium; *RV* = right ventricle.

A. Formation of the AV Septum

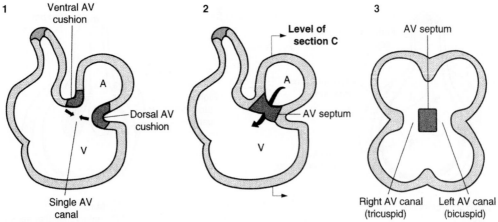

1   Ventral AV cushion

Dorsal AV cushion

Single AV canal

A

V

2   Level of section C

A

V

AV septum

3   AV septum

Right AV canal (tricuspid)   Left AV canal (bicuspid)

B. AV Septal Defects

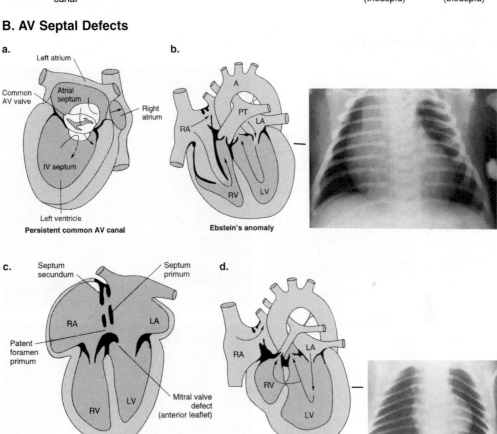

a.

Left atrium

Common AV valve

Atrial septum

Right atrium

IV septum

Left ventricle

Persistent common AV canal

b.

A

PT

LA

RA

RV   LV

Ebstein's anomaly

c.

Septum secundum   Septum primum

RA   LA

Patent foramen primum

RV   LV

Mitral valve defect (anterior leaflet)

Foramen primum defect

d.

RA   LA

RV

LV

Tricuspid atresia

Figure 5-5.   **(A)** Formation of the atrioventricular (AV) septum (*1, 2, 3*), which partitions the atrioventricular canal. **(B)** AV septal defects. *(a)* Persistent common AV canal. *(b)* Ebstein's anomaly. AP radiograph shows massive cardiomegaly due to enlargement of the right atrium. The left cardiac contour is also abnormal because of displacement of the right ventricular outflow tract. *(c)* Foramen primum defect. *(d)* Tricuspid atresia. AP radiograph shows a normal-sized heart with a convex left cardiac contour. *Arrows* indicate direction of blood flow. *A* = aorta; *V* = ventricle; *LA* = left atrium; *LV* = left ventricle; *PT* = pulmonary trunk; *RA* = right atrium; *RV* = right ventricle.

A. Formation of IV Septum

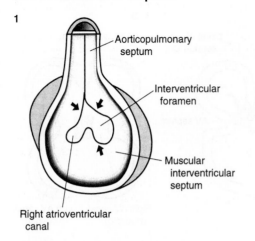

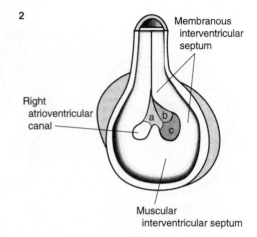

B. IV Septal Defects (VSDs)

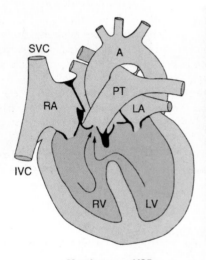

Membranous VSD

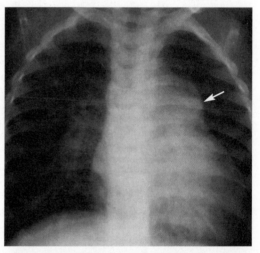

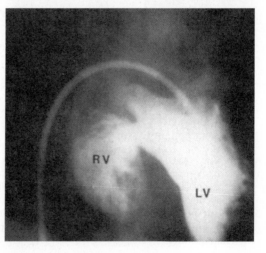

Figure 5-6. (A) Formation of the interventricular (IV) septum (*1, 2*), which partitions the primitive ventricle. *Shaded portion (a, b, c)* in *2* indicates the three sources of the membranous interventricular septum. *a* = right bulbar ridge; *b* = left bulbar ridge; *c* = AV cushions. (B) IV septal defects (VSDs). A membranous VSD is shown. *A* = aorta; *LA* = left atrium; *LV* = left ventricle; *RA* = right atrium; *RV* = right ventricle; *PT* = pulmonary trunk; *IVC* = inferior vena cava; *SVC* = superior vena cava. AP radiograph demonstrates cardiomegaly and a marked enlargement of the main pulmonary artery (*arrow*). Left ventriculography in the LAO position demonstrates flow of contrast material from the LV through a membranous VSD into the RV. *Arrows* indicate direction of blood flow.

B. Clinical considerations Most anomalies of the great arteries occur as a result of persistence of parts of the aortic arch system that normally regress and regression of parts that normally persist.

1. **Abnormal origin of the right subclavian artery** occurs when the right aortic arch 4 and the right dorsal aorta cranial to the seventh intersegmental artery abnormally regress. As development continues, the right subclavian artery comes to lie on the left side just inferior to the left subclavian artery. The artery must cross the midline posterior to the trachea and esophagus to supply the right arm. This anomaly may constrict the trachea or esophagus. However, it is generally not clinically significant.

2. **Double aortic arch** occurs when an abnormal right aortic arch develops in addition to a left aortic arch owing to persistence of the distal portion of the right dorsal aorta. This forms a vascular ring around the trachea and esophagus, which causes difficulties in breathing and swallowing.

3. **Right aortic arch** occurs when the entire right dorsal aorta abnormally persists and part of the left dorsal aorta regresses. The right aortic arch may pass anterior or posterior (retroesophageal right arch) to the esophagus and trachea. A retroesophageal right arch may cause difficulties in swallowing or breathing.

4. **Patent ductus arteriosus** occurs when the ductus arteriosus, a connection between the left pulmonary artery and aorta, fails to close. Normally, the ductus arteriosus functionally closes within a few hours after birth via smooth muscle contraction to ultimately form the **ligamentum arteriosum**. A patent ductus arteriosus causes a L→R shunting of oxygen-rich blood from the aorta back into the pulmonary circulation. This can be treated with prostaglandin synthesis inhibitors (e.g., indomethacin), which promote closure. It is very common in premature infants and maternal rubella infection. Clinical signs include a harsh, machine-like, continuous murmur in the upper left parasternal area.

5. **Postductal coarctation** of the aorta occurs when the aorta is abnormally constricted. A postductal coarctation is found distal to the origin of the left subclavian artery and inferior to the ductus arteriosus. It is clinically associated with increased blood pressure in the upper extremities, lack of pulse in the femoral artery, high risk of both cerebral hemorrhage and bacterial endocarditis, and Turner syndrome. Less commonly, a **preductal coarctation** may occur in which the constriction is located superior to the ductus arteriosus.

XI. Development of the Venous System (Figure 5-8)

A. General pattern The general pattern develops mainly from three pairs of veins: **vitelline, umbilical,** and **cardinal** that empty blood into the sinus venosus. These veins undergo remodeling due to a L→R shunting of venous blood to the right atrium.

B. Clinical considerations Most anomalies of the venous system occur as a result of persistence of the veins on the left side of the body that normally regress during the L→R shunting of blood.

1. **Double inferior vena cava** occurs when the left supracardinal vein persists, thereby forming an additional inferior vena cava below the level of the kidneys.

2. **Left superior vena cava** occurs when the left anterior cardinal vein persists, forming a superior vena cava on the left side. The right anterior cardinal vein abnormally regresses.

3. **Double superior vena cava** occurs when the left anterior cardinal vein persists, forming a superior vena cava on the left side. The right anterior cardinal vein also forms a superior vena cava on the right side.

4. **Absence of the hepatic portion of the inferior vena cava** occurs when the right vitelline vein fails to form a segment of the inferior vena cava. Consequently, blood from the lower part of the body reaches the right atrium via the azygos vein, hemiazygos vein, and superior vena cava.

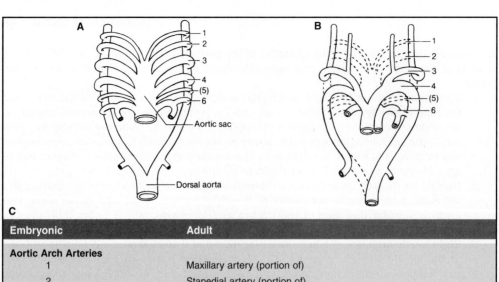

C

Embryonic	Adult
Aortic Arch Arteries	
1	Maxillary artery (portion of)
2	Stapedial artery (portion of)
3	R & L common carotid arteries (portion of)
	R & L internal carotid arteries
4	Right subclavian artery (portion of)
	Arch of the aorta (portion of)
5	Regresses in the human
6[a]	R & L pulmonary arteries (portion of)
	Ductus arteriosus
Dorsal Aorta	
Posterolateral arteries	Arteries to the upper and lower extremities, intercostal, lumbar, and lateral sacral arteries
Lateral arteries	Renal, suprarenal, and gonadal arteries
Ventral arteries	
Vitelline	Celiac, superior mesenteric, and inferior mesenteric arteries
Umbilical	Internal iliac (portion of)and superior vesical arteries
	Medial umbilical ligaments

[a]Early in development, the recurrent laryngeal nerves hook around aortic arch 6. On the right side, the distal part of aortic arch 6 regresses, and the right recurrent laryngeal nerve moves up to hook around the right subclavian artery. On the left side, aortic arch 6 persists as the ductus arteriosus (or ligamentum arteriosus in the adult); the left recurrent laryngeal nerve remains hooked around the ductus arteriosus.

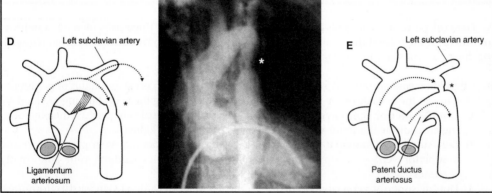

Figure 5-7. (A, B) Development and fate of the aortic arches during the remodeling process. Note the portions of the aortic arches that degenerate during the remodeling process (*dotted lines*). (C) Table shows the correspondence of embryonic arteries to their derivative adult counterparts. (D) Postductal coarctation. Blood reaches lower part of the body via collateral circulation through the left subclavian, intercostal, and internal thoracic arteries. Angiogram of a postductal coarctation is shown. Note the well-developed collateral blood vessels. (E) Preductal coarctation. Blood reaches lower part of the body through a patent ductus arteriosus. Asterisk (*) indicates point of constriction. *Dotted arrows* indicate direction of blood flow. Prostaglandin treatment is required to maintain the patent ductus arteriosus until surgery.

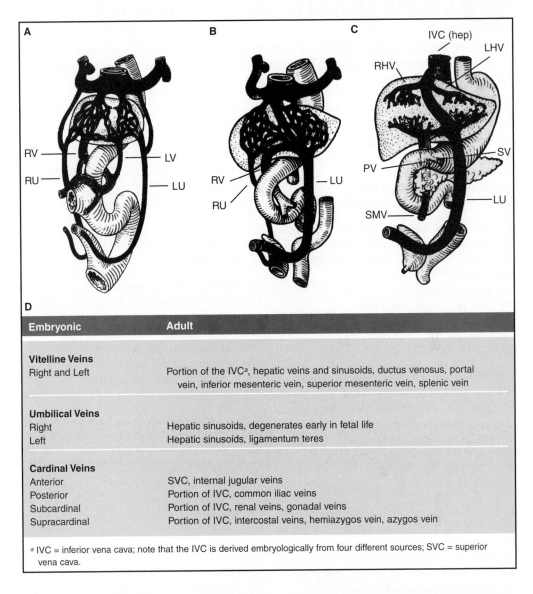

Embryonic	Adult
Vitelline Veins	
Right and Left	Portion of the IVC[a], hepatic veins and sinusoids, ductus venosus, portal vein, inferior mesenteric vein, superior mesenteric vein, splenic vein
Umbilical Veins	
Right	Hepatic sinusoids, degenerates early in fetal life
Left	Hepatic sinusoids, ligamentum teres
Cardinal Veins	
Anterior	SVC, internal jugular veins
Posterior	Portion of IVC, common iliac veins
Subcardinal	Portion of IVC, renal veins, gonadal veins
Supracardinal	Portion of IVC, intercostal veins, hemiazygos vein, azygos vein

[a] IVC = inferior vena cava; note that the IVC is derived embryologically from four different sources; SVC = superior vena cava.

Figure 5-8. Development of the vitelline and umbilical veins. (**A**) Week 5. (**B**) Month 2. (**C**) Month 3. Both the vitelline and umbilical veins contribute to the hepatic sinusoidal network within the liver. Owing to the L→R shunting of venous blood, the right vitelline vein enlarges, while the proximal part of the left vitelline vein disappears. Note that the right umbilical vein degenerates early in fetal life, whereas the left umbilical vein enlarges to carry oxygenated blood from the placenta to the fetus. (**D**) Table shows the correspondence of the embryonic veins to their adult counterparts. *IVC (hep)* = inferior vena cava; *LHV* = left hepatic vein; *LU* = left umbilical; *LV* = left ventricle; *PV* = primitive ventricle; *RHV* = right hepatic vein; *RU* = right umbilical; *RV* = right ventricle; *SMV* = superior mesenteric vein; *SV* = sinus venosus.

STUDY QUESTIONS FOR CHAPTER 5

*Directions: Each of the numbered items or incomplete statements in this section is followed by answers or by completions of the statement. Select the **one** lettered answer or completion that is **best** in each case.*

1. The most common interventricular septal defect (VSD) seen clinically is

(A) persistent truncus arteriosus
(B) membranous VSD
(C) common ventricle
(D) foramen secundum defect
(E) premature closure of foramen ovale

2. Which of the following clinical signs would be most obvious on examination of a patient with either tetralogy of Fallot or transposition of the great vessels?

(A) Sweaty palms
(B) Lack of femoral artery pulse
(C) Pulmonary hypertension
(D) Cyanosis
(E) Diffuse red rash

3. Which of the following congenital cardiovascular malformations is most commonly associated with maternal rubella infection?

(A) Isolated dextrocardia
(B) Patent ductus arteriosus
(C) Persistent truncus arteriosus
(D) Coarctation of the aorta
(E) Double aortic arch

4. The most common atrial septal defect (ASD) seen clinically is

(A) common atrium
(B) foramen secundum defect
(C) premature closure of the foramen ovale
(D) persistent truncus arteriosus
(E) probe patency of the foramen ovale

5. The ventral surface of the adult heart as seen on gross examination or radiography is composed primarily of the

(A) left atrium
(B) left ventricle
(C) inferior vena cava
(D) bulbus cordis
(E) right ventricle

6. The left recurrent laryngeal nerve recurs around the

(A) left primary bronchus
(B) left subclavian artery
(C) left subclavian vein

(D) ductus arteriosus
(E) left common carotid artery

7. Which of the three primary germ layers forms the histologically definitive endocardium of the adult heart?

(A) Ectoderm
(B) Endoderm
(C) Mesoderm
(D) Epiblast
(E) Hypoblast

8. Which of the following is responsible for the proper alignment of the atrioventricular canal and the conoventricular canal?

(A) Lateral folding of the embryo
(B) Craniocaudal folding of the embryo
(C) Programmed cell migration
(D) Formation of the AP septum
(E) Dextral looping

9. The hepatic sinusoids that can be observed histologically in an adult liver are derived from the

(A) supracardinal veins
(B) anterior cardinal veins
(C) posterior cardinal veins
(D) vitelline veins
(E) subcardinal veins

10. Which of the following arterial malformations is very common in premature infants?

(A) Patent ductus arteriosus
(B) Coarctation of the aorta
(C) Right aortic arch
(D) Double aortic arch
(E) Abnormal origin of the right subclavian artery

11. A physician monitoring a newborn infant's heart sounds using a stethoscope hears the characteristic murmur of a patent ductus arteriosus. How soon after birth should this murmur normally disappear?

(A) 1–2 months
(B) 1–2 weeks
(C) 1–2 days
(D) 1–2 hours
(E) Immediately

12. How soon after birth does the foramen ovale close?

(A) 1–2 months
(B) 1–2 weeks
(C) 1–2 days
(D) 1–2 hours
(E) Immediately

13. A 9-year-old boy presents with complaints of numbness and tingling in both feet. Examination reveals no pulse in the femoral artery, increased blood pressure in the arteries of the upper extremity, and enlarged intercostal veins. Which of the following abnormalities would be suspected?

(A) Double aortic arch
(B) Tetralogy of Fallot
(C) Postductal coarctation of the aorta
(D) Right aortic arch
(E) Abnormal origin of the right subclavian artery

14. The coronary sinus is derived from which of the following?

(A) Truncus arteriosus
(B) Bulbus cordis
(C) Primitive ventricle
(D) Primitive atrium
(E) Sinus venosus

15. The conus arteriosus is derived from which of the following?

(A) Truncus arteriosus
(B) Bulbus cordis
(C) Primitive ventricle
(D) Primitive atrium
(E) Sinus venosus

16. The proximal part of the aorta is derived from which of the following?

(A) Truncus arteriosus
(B) Bulbus cordis
(C) Primitive ventricle
(D) Primitive atrium
(E) Sinus venosus

17. The trabeculated part of the right ventricle is derived from which of the following?

(A) Truncus arteriosus
(B) Bulbus cordis
(C) Primitive ventricle
(D) Primitive atrium
(E) Sinus venosus

18. Tricuspid atresia is a cardiac malformation that involves which of the following septa?

(A) Aorticopulmonary septum
(B) Atrial septum
(C) Atrioventricular septum
(D) Interventricular septum

19. A muscular VSD is a cardiac malformation that involves which of the following septa?

(A) Aorticopulmonary septum
(B) Atrial septum
(C) Atrioventricular septum
(D) Interventricular septum

20. Tetralogy of Fallot is a cardiac malformation that involves which of the following septa?

(A) Aorticopulmonary septum
(B) Atrial septum
(C) Atrioventricular septum
(D) Interventricular septum

21. D-transposition of the great arteries is a cardiac malformation that involves which of the following septa?

(A) Aorticopulmonary septum
(B) Atrial septum
(C) Atrioventricular septum
(D) Interventricular septum

22. An insufficient amount of AV cushion material will result in which of the following?

(A) Persistent truncus arteriosus
(B) Ebstein's anomaly
(C) Transposition of the great arteries
(D) Common ventricle
(E) Tricuspid atresia

23. A partial development of the AP septum results in which of the following?

(A) Persistent truncus arteriosus
(B) Ebstein's anomaly
(C) Transposition of the great arteries
(D) Common ventricle
(E) Tricuspid atresia

24. A failure of the tricuspid leaflets to attach to the annulus fibrosus results in which of the following?

(A) Persistent truncus arteriosus
(B) Ebstein's anomaly
(C) Transposition of the great arteries
(D) Common ventricle
(E) Tricuspid atresia

25. A faulty fusion of the right and left bulbar ridges and AV cushion results in which of the following?

(A) Persistent truncus arteriosus
(B) Ebstein's anomaly
(C) Transposition of the great arteries
(D) Common ventricle
(E) Membranous VSD

26. The superior mesenteric artery is derived from which of the following?

(A) Posterolateral arteries
(B) Lateral arteries
(C) Ventral arteries

27. The arteries to the upper extremity are derived from which of the following?

(A) Posterolateral arteries
(B) Lateral arteries
(C) Ventral arteries

28. The gonadal arteries are derived from which of the following?

(A) Posterolateral arteries
(B) Lateral arteries
(C) Ventral arteries

29. The proximal part of the internal carotid artery is derived from which of the following?

(A) Aortic arch 1
(B) Aortic arch 2
(C) Aortic arch 3
(D) Aortic arch 4
(E) Aortic arch 6

30. A portion of the arch of the aorta is derived from which of the following?

(A) Aortic arch 1
(B) Aortic arch 2
(C) Aortic arch 3
(D) Aortic arch 4
(E) Aortic arch 6

31. The proximal part of the right subclavian artery is derived from which of the following?

(A) Aortic arch 1
(B) Aortic arch 2
(C) Aortic arch 3
(D) Aortic arch 4
(E) Aortic arch 6

32. The portal vein is derived from which of the following?

(A) Vitelline veins
(B) Umbilical veins
(C) Anterior cardinal veins
(D) Posterior cardinal veins
(E) Subcardinal veins

33. The renal veins are derived from which of the following?

(A) Vitelline veins
(B) Umbilical veins
(C) Anterior cardinal veins
(D) Posterior cardinal veins
(E) Subcardinal veins

34. The superior mesenteric vein is derived from which of the following?

(A) Vitelline veins
(B) Umbilical veins
(C) Anterior cardinal veins
(D) Posterior cardinal veins
(E) Subcardinal veins

35. Closure of the foramen primum results from fusion of which of the following structures?

(A) Septum secundum and the fused atrioventricular cushions
(B) Septum secundum and the septum primum
(C) Septum primum and the fused atrioventricular cushions
(D) Septum primum and the septum spurium
(E) Septum primum and the sinoatrial valves

36. A 3-day-old male delivered at 32 weeks of gestation is experiencing respiratory distress syndrome. The physician detects a heart murmur characteristic of a patent ductus arteriosis, a diagnosis that is confirmed with an echocardiogram. Which embryonic structure is involved in this diagnosis?

(A) Left third aortic arch
(B) Right third aortic arch
(C) Left sixth aortic arch
(D) Umbilical arteries
(E) Vitelline arteries

ANSWERS AND EXPLANATIONS

1. B. The most common of all cardiac congenital malformations seen clinically are membranous VSDs. The membranous interventricular septum forms by the proliferation and fusion of tissue from three different sources: the right and left bulbar ridges and the atrioventricular (AV) cushions. Because of this complex formation, the probability of defects is very high.

2. D. Marked cyanosis is a distinct clinical sign in both tetralogy of Fallot and transposition of the great vessels. Any congenital cardiac malformation that allows right-to-left shunting of blood is sometimes called cyanotic heart disease. Right-to-left shunting allows poorly oxygenated blood from the right side of the heart to mix with highly oxygenated blood on the left side of the heart. This causes decreased oxygen tension to peripheral tissues, leading to a characteristic blue tinge (cyanosis) and bulbous thickening of the fingers and toes (clubbing).

3. B. Patent ductus arteriosus (PDA) is the most common congenital cardiac malformation associated with rubella infection of the mother. It is unclear how the rubella virus acts to cause PDA.

4. B. The most common ASD is foramen secundum defect, which is caused by excessive resorption of the septum primum or the septum secundum. This results in an opening between the atria (patent foramen ovale). Some of these defects may remain undiagnosed and may be tolerated for a long time (up to age 30 before the person presents clinically).

5. E. During embryologic formation of the heart, the arterial and venous ends of the heart tube are fixed in place. As further growth continues, the heart tube folds to the right. This greatly contributes to the ventral surface of the adult heart being comprised primarily of the right ventricle. The definitive anatomic orientation of the adult heart within the thorax is not at all similar to the strong image we have in our minds of the classic Valentine's Day heart.

6. D. The left recurrent laryngeal nerve recurs around the ductus arteriosus (ligamentum arteriosus in the adult). Early in embryologic development, both the right and left recurrent laryngeal nerves hook (recur) around aortic arch 6. The left aortic arch 6 persists as the ductus arteriosus.

7. C. The entire cardiovascular system is of mesodermal origin.

8. E. Dextral looping aligns these two canals through early looping, convergence, wedging, and repositioning. This is especially important in correcting the unusual blood flow pattern in the primitive heart tube where venous blood flows into the left ventricle prior to the right ventricle.

9. D. Because of the location of the vitelline veins and the tremendous growth of the developing liver (hepatic diverticulum), the vitelline veins are surrounded by the liver and give rise to the hepatic sinusoids. The umbilical veins also contribute to the hepatic sinusoidal network.

10. A. Patent ductus arteriosus is very common in premature infants. Infants with birth weight less than 1750 grams typically have a PDA during the first 24 hours postnatally. PDA is more common in female infants than in male infants.

11. D. The ductus arteriosus functionally closes within a few hours (1–2) after birth via smooth muscle contraction of the tunica media. Before birth, the patency of the ductus arteriosus is controlled by the low oxygen content of the blood flowing through it, which in turn stimulates production of prostaglandins, which cause smooth muscle to relax. After birth, the high oxygen content of the blood due to lung ventilation inhibits production of prostaglandins, causing smooth muscle contraction. Premature infants can be treated with prostaglandin synthesis inhibitors (such as indomethacin) to promote closure of the ductus arteriosus.

12. E. The foramen ovale functionally closes almost immediately after birth as pressure in the right atrium decreases and pressure in the left atrium increases, thereby pushing the septum primum against the septum secundum. Anatomic fusion occurs much later in life; over 25% of the population have probe patency of the foramen ovale, in which anatomic fusion does not occur.

13. C. No pulse in the femoral artery, increased blood pressure in the arteries of the upper extremity, enlarged intercostal veins, and numbness and tingling in both feet are clinical symptoms indicative of postductal coarctation of the aorta. Because of the constriction of the aorta, the blood supply to the lower extremity is compromised.

14. E. The coronary sinus is derived from the sinus venosus.

15. B. The smooth part of the right ventricle, known as the conus arteriosus, is derived from the bulbus cordis.

16. A. The proximal part of the aorta is derived from the truncus arteriosus.

17. C. The trabeculated part of the right ventricle is derived from the primitive ventricle.

18. C. Tricuspid atresia involves the atrioventricular septum.

19. D. Muscular VSD is caused by perforations in the muscular interventricular septum.

20. A. Tetralogy of Fallot involves the aorticopulmonary septum.

21. A. D-transposition involves the aorticopulmonary septum.

22. E. Insufficient amount of AV cushion material causes tricuspid atresia.

23. A. Partial development of the AP septum causes persistent truncus arteriosus.

24. B. Failure of fusion of the tricuspid leaflets with the annulus fibrosus results in Ebstein's anomaly.

25. E. Faulty fusion of the right and left bulbar ridges and AV cushions causes membranous VSD.

26. C. The superior mesenteric artery is derived from ventral branches of the dorsal aorta, specifically the vitelline arteries.

27. A. Arteries to the upper extremity are derived from posterolateral branches of the dorsal aorta.

28. B. The gonadal arteries are derived from lateral branches of the dorsal aorta.

29. C. The proximal part of the internal carotid artery is derived from aortic arch 3.

30. D. Part of the arch of the aorta is derived from aortic arch 4.

31. D. The proximal part of the right subclavian artery is derived from aortic arch 4.

32. A. The portal vein is derived from the right vitelline vein.

33. E. The renal veins are derived from the subcardinal veins.

34. A. The superior mesenteric vein is derived from the vitelline veins.

35. C. The foramen primum forms between the free edge of the septum primum and the atrioventricular (AV) cushions. It is closed when the septum primum fuses with the atrioventricular (AV) cushions.

36. C. Patent ductus arteriosus (PDA) is a condition in which the ductus arteriosus, a blood vessel that allows blood to bypass the baby's lungs before birth, fails to normally close after birth. The ductus arteriosus is derived from the distal portion of the left sixth aortic arch.

Placenta and Amniotic Fluid

I.　Formation of the Placenta (Figure 6-1)

The placenta is formed as the endometrium of the uterus is invaded by the developing embryo and as the trophoblast forms the villous chorion. Villous chorion formation goes through three stages: **primary chorionic villi**, **secondary chorionic villi**, and **tertiary chorionic villi**.

II.　Placental Components: Decidua Basalis and Villous Chorion (Figure 6-2)

The human placenta is hemomonochorial and discoid-shaped.

A.　The maternal component of the placenta consists of the **decidua basalis**, which is derived from the endometrium of the uterus located between the blastocyst and the myometrium. The decidua basalis and **decidua parietalis** (which includes all portions of the endometrium other than the site of implantation) are shed as part of the afterbirth. The **decidua capsularis**, the portion of endometrium that covers the blastocyst and separates it from the uterine cavity, becomes attenuated and degenerates at week 22 of development because of a reduced blood supply. The term decidua means "falling off," "shed," or "sloughed off." The **maternal surface** of the placenta is characterized by 8 to 10 compartments called **cotyledons** (imparting a **cobblestone appearance**), which are separated by decidual (placental) septa. The maternal surface is **dark red in color and oozes blood** owing to torn maternal blood vessels.

B.　The fetal component of the placenta consists of **tertiary chorionic villi** derived from both the trophoblast and the extraembryonic mesoderm, which collectively become known as the **villous chorion**. The villous chorion develops most prolifically at the site of the decidua basalis. The villous chorion is in contrast to an area of no villus development known as the **smooth chorion** (which is related to the decidua capsularis). The **fetal surface** of the placenta is characterized by the well-vascularized chorionic plate containing the chorionic (fetal) blood vessels. The fetal surface has a **smooth, shiny, light-blue or blue-pink appearance** (because the amnion covers the fetal surface), and five to eight large chorionic (fetal) blood vessels should be apparent.

III.　Placental Membrane (Figure 6-3)

The placental membrane separates maternal blood from fetal blood. A common misperception is that the placental membrane acts as a strict "barrier." However, a wide variety of substances freely cross the placental membrane. Some substances that cross can be either beneficial or harmful. Other substances do not cross the placental membrane. The composition of the placental membrane changes during pregnancy.

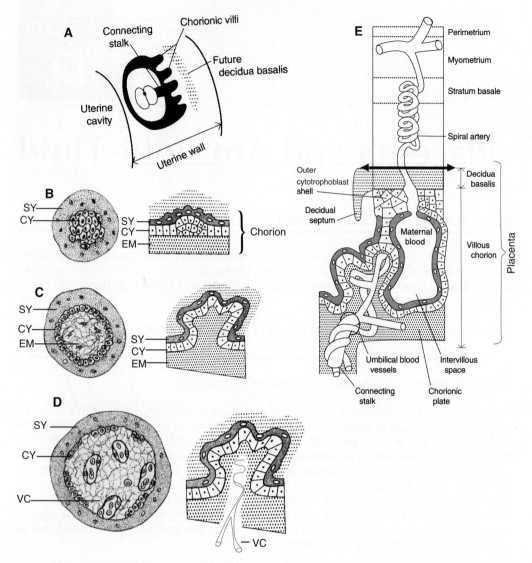

Figure 6-1.   Diagram of the various stages of villous chorion formation as it relates to placental development. **(A)** A week 2 embryo completely embedded in the wall of the uterus. **(B)** Primary chorionic villus during week 2. A primary villus consists of a core of cytotrophoblastic cells surrounded by syncytiotrophoblast. **(C)** Secondary chorionic villus during the start of week 3. A secondary villus consists of a core of extraembryonic mesoderm surrounded by cytotrophoblastic cells and syncytiotrophoblast. **(D)** Tertiary chorionic villus at the end of week 3. A tertiary villus consists of a core of villous (fetal) capillaries surrounded by cytotrophoblastic cells and syncytiotrophoblast. **(E)** The villous chorion (consisting of tertiary chorionic villi) and decidua basalis are the two components of the definitive placenta. Note that the cytotrophoblast penetrates the syncytiotrophoblast to make contact with the decidua basalis and form the outer cytotrophoblast shell. The *thick double-headed arrow* indicates the plane of separation when the placenta is shed during the afterbirth. (Note: The stratum basale is not part of the placenta.) *CY* = cytotrophoblast; *EM* = extraembryonic mesoderm; *SY* = syncytiotrophoblast; *VC* = villous capillaries

A. In early pregnancy, the placental membrane has four layers: **syncytiotrophoblast, cytotrophoblast (Langhans cells), connective tissue,** and **endothelium of fetal capillaries.** Hofbauer cells (large, sometimes pigmented, elliptical cells found in connective tissue) are most numerous in early pregnancy and have characteristics similar to those of macrophages.

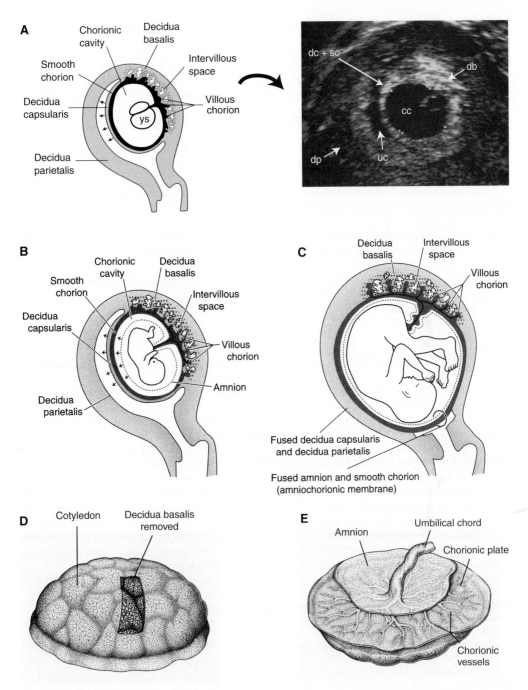

Figure 6-2.   Diagram showing the relationship of the fetus, uterus, and placenta. **(A)** Week 4. Sonogram shows the decidua basalis (*db*), decidua parietalis (*dp*), and decidua capsularis and smooth chorion (*dc+sc*). Note the location of the uterine cavity (*uc*) and chorionic cavity (*cc*). Within the chorionic cavity, the yolk sac can be observed. **(B)** Early fetal period. *Outer arrows* indicate that as the fetus grows within the uterine wall, the decidua capsularis expands and fuses with the decidua parietalis, thereby obliterating the uterine cavity. *Inner arrows* indicate that as the fetus grows, the amnion expands toward the smooth chorion, thereby obliterating the chorionic cavity. **(C)** Late fetal period. The uterine cavity and chorionic cavity are obliterated. The fused amnion and smooth chorion form the amniochorionic membrane ("bag of waters"), which passes over the cervical opening. **(D)** Maternal surface of the placenta. **(E)** Fetal surface of the placenta.

B. In late pregnancy, the placental membrane has two layers: the **syncytiotrophoblast** and **endothelium of fetal capillaries**.

IV. Placenta as Endocrine Organ

The placenta produces both protein and steroid hormones as indicated below.

A. Human chorionic gonadotropin (hCG) is a glycoprotein hormone that stimulates the production of progesterone by the corpus luteum.

B. Human placental lactogen (hPL) is a protein hormone that induces lipolysis, thus elevating free fatty acid levels in the mother; it is considered to be the "growth hormone" of the fetus.

C. Estrone, estradiol (most potent), and **estriol** are steroid hormones produced by the placenta, but little is known about their specific functions in either mother or fetus.

D. Progesterone is a steroid hormone that maintains the endometrium during pregnancy, is used by the fetal adrenal cortex as a precursor for glucocorticoid and mineralocorticoid synthesis, and is used by the fetal testes as a precursor of testosterone synthesis.

V. Umbilical Cord

A patent opening called the **primitive umbilical ring** exists on the ventral surface of the developing embryo through which three structures pass: the **yolk sac (vitelline duct), connecting stalk,** and **allantois.** The allantois is not functional in humans and degenerates to form the **median umbilical ligament** in the adult. As the amnion expands, it pushes the vitelline duct, connecting stalk, and allantois together to form the **primitive umbilical cord.** At week 6, the gut tube connected to the yolk sac herniates **(physiologic umbilical herniation)** into the extraembryonic coelom; the herniation is reduced by week 11. The gut tube eventually returns to the abdominal cavity, whereas the yolk sac (vitelline duct) and allantois degenerate. The definitive umbilical cord at term is pearl-white, 1 to 2 cm in diameter, 50 to 60 cm long, and eccentrically positioned. It contains the **right and left umbilical arteries, left umbilical vein,** and **mucous connective tissue (Wharton's jelly).** Physical inspection of the umbilicus in a newborn may reveal a light-gray shiny sac indicating an **omphalocele,** fecal (meconium) discharge indicating an **ileal (Meckel's) diverticulum,** or a urine discharge indicating a **urachal fistula.**

VI. Circulatory System of the Fetus (Figure 6-4)

Fetal circulation involves three shunts: **ductus venosus, ductus arteriosus,** and **foramen ovale.**

Figure 6-3. The placental membrane. **(A)** In early pregnancy. **(B)** In late pregnancy. Langhans cells are cytotrophoblastic cells that serve as stem cells for the syncytiotrophoblast. **(C)** Light micrograph of a tertiary chorionic villous showing the placental membrane in an early pregnancy. Note the location of maternal and fetal blood. **(D)** Electron microscopy of a tertiary chorionic villous showing the placental membrane in a late pregnancy. Note the location of maternal and fetal blood and the microvillous border (*mv*) of the syncytiotrophoblast cells. *CT* = connective tissue; *CY* = cytotrophoblast; *FE* = fetal endothelium; *HC* = Hofbauer cell; *RBC* = red blood cell; *SY* = syncytiotrophoblast; *VC* = villous (fetal) capillaries; *arrowhead* = group of syncytiotrophoblast nuclei. **(E)** Table of substances that cross and that do not cross the placental membrane. Substances cross the placenta by simple diffusion, facilitated diffusion (e.g., glucose), active transport (e.g., many amino acids), receptor-mediated endocytosis (e.g., IgG and IgA), and pinocytosis (e.g., large proteins).

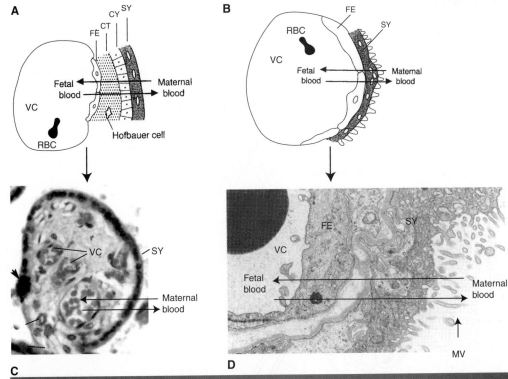

A

FE CT CY SY

Fetal blood ← → Maternal blood

VC

RBC

Hofbauer cell

B

FE

RBC

VC SY

Fetal blood ← → Maternal blood

C

VC SY

Maternal blood

D

FE SY

VC

Fetal blood ← → Maternal blood

MV

SUBSTANCES THAT CROSS OR DO NOT CROSS THE PLACENTAL MEMBRANE

BENEFICIAL SUBSTANCES THAT CROSS THE PLACENTAL MEMBRANE

- O_2, CO_2
- Glucose. L-form amino acids, free fatty acids, vitamins
- H_2O, Na^+, Cl^-, K^+, I^-, Ca^{2+}, PO_4^{2+}
- Urea, uric acid, bilirubin
- Fetal and maternal RBCs
- Maternal serum proteins, α-fetoprotein, transferrin ñ Fe^{2+} complex, LDL, prolactin
- Steroid hormones (unconjugated)
- IgG, IgA

HARMFUL SUBSTANCES THAT CROSS THE PLACENTAL MEMBRANE

- Virusesó e.g., rubella, cytomegalovirus, herpes simplex type 2, varicella zoster, Coxsackie, variola, measles, poliomyelitis

- Category X Drugs (absolute contraindication in pregnancy)ó e.g., thalidomide, aminopterin, methotrexate, busulfan (Myleran), chlorambucil (Leukeran), cyclophosphamide (Cytoxan), phenytoin (Dilantin), triazolam (Halcion), estazolam (ProSom), warfarin (Coumadin), isotretinoin (Accutane), clomiphene (Clomid), diethylstilbestrol (DES), ethisterone, norethisterone, megestrol (Megace), oral contraceptives (Ovcon, Levlen, Norinyl), nicotine, alcohol, ACE inhibitors (Captopril, enalapril)

- Category D Drugs (definite evidence of risk to fetus)ó e.g., tetracycline (Achromycin), doxycycline (Vibramycin), streptomycin, Amikacin, tobramycin (Nebcin), phenobarbital (Donnatal), pentobarbital (Nembutal), valproic acid (Depakene), diazepam (Valium), chlordiazepoxide (Librium), alprazolam (Xanax), lorazepam (Ativan), lithium, hydrochlorothiazide (Diuril)

- Carbon monoxide
- Organic mercury, lead, polychlorinated biphenyls (PCBs), potassium iodide,
- Cocaine, heroin
- *Toxoplasma gondii, Treponema pallidum, Listeria monocytogenes*
- Rubella virus vaccine
- Anti-Rh antibodies

SUBSTANCES THAT DO NOT CROSS THE PLACENTAL MEMBRANE

- Maternally-derived cholesterol, triglycerides, and phospholipids
- Protein hormones (e.g., insulin)
- Drugs (e.g., succinylcholine, curare, heparin, methyldopa, drugs similar to amino acids)
- IgD, IgE, IgM
- Bacteria in general

E

57

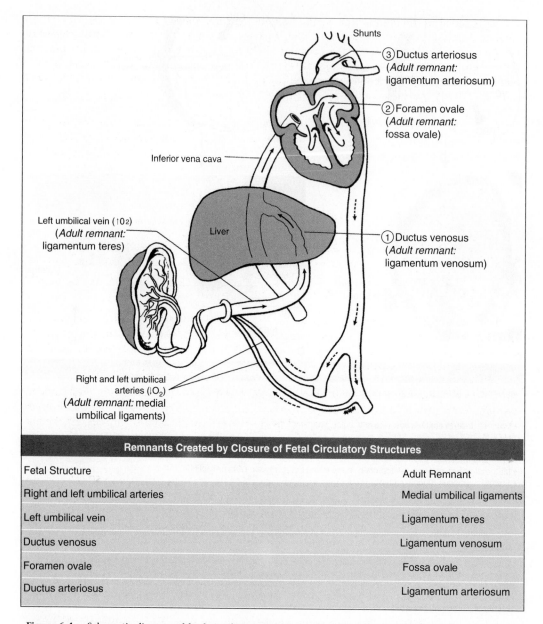

Figure 6-4.   Schematic diagram of fetal circulation and remnants of fetal circulatory structures.

A.   Highly oxygenated and nutrient-enriched blood returns to the fetus from the placenta via the **left umbilical vein**. (Note: Highly oxygenated blood is carried by the left umbilical vein, not by an artery as in the adult.) Some blood percolates through the hepatic sinusoids; most of the blood bypasses the sinusoids by passing through the **ductus venosus** and enters the inferior vena cava (IVC). From the IVC, blood enters the right atrium, where most of the blood bypasses the right ventricle through the **foramen ovale** to enter the left atrium. From the left atrium, blood enters the left ventricle and is delivered to fetal tissues via the aorta.

B.   Poorly oxygenated and nutrient-poor fetal blood is sent back to the placenta via **right and left umbilical arteries**.

C. Some blood in the right atrium enters the right ventricle; blood in the right ventricle enters the pulmonary trunk, but most of the blood bypasses the lungs through the **ductus arteriosus**. Fetal lungs receive only a minimal amount of blood for growth and development; the blood is returned to the left ventricle via pulmonary veins. Fetal lungs are not capable of performing their adult respiratory function because they are functionally immature and the fetus is underwater (amniotic fluid). The placenta provides respiratory function.

D. Circulatory system changes at birth are facilitated by a **decrease in right atrial pressure** from occlusion of placental circulation and by an **increase in left atrial pressure** due to increased pulmonary venous return. Changes include closure of the right and left umbilical arteries, left umbilical vein, ductus venosus, ductus arteriosus, and foramen ovale.

VII. Amniotic Fluid

The amniotic fluid is maternally derived water that contains electrolytes, carbohydrates, amino acids, lipids, proteins (hormones, enzymes, α-fetoprotein), urea, creatinine, lactate, pyruvate, desquamated fetal cells, fetal urine, fetal feces (meconium), and fetal lung liquid (useful for lecithin/sphingomyelin ratio measurement for lung maturity).

A. **Production of amniotic fluid** Amniotic fluid is constantly produced during pregnancy by **direct transfer** from maternal circulation in response to osmotic and hydrostatic forces and by **excretion of fetal urine by the kidneys** into the amniotic sac. Kidney defects (e.g., bilateral kidney agenesis) result in **oligohydramnios**.

B. **Resorption of amniotic fluid** Amniotic fluid is constantly resorbed during pregnancy by the following sequence of events: the fetus swallows amniotic fluid, amniotic fluid is absorbed into fetal blood through the gastrointestinal tract, excess amniotic fluid is removed via the placenta and passed into maternal blood. Swallowing defects (e.g., esophageal atresia) or absorption defects (e.g., duodenal atresia) result in **polyhydramnios**.

C. **The amount of amniotic fluid** is gradually increased during pregnancy from **50 mL at week 12** to **1000 mL at term**. The rate of water exchange within the amniotic sac at term is 400–500 mL/hr, with a net flow of 125–200 mL/hr moving from the amniotic fluid into the maternal blood. The near-term fetus excretes about 500 mL of urine daily, which is mostly water because the placenta exchanges metabolic wastes. The fetus swallows about 400 mL of amniotic fluid daily.

VIII. Twinning (Figure 6-5)

A. **Dizygotic (fraternal) twins** result from the fertilization of two different secondary oocytes by two different sperm. The resulting two zygotes form two blastocysts, each of which implants separately into the endometrium of the uterus. Hence, these twins are no more genetically alike than siblings born at different times. Dizygotic twins and 35% of monozygotic twins have **two placentas, two amniotic sacs,** and **two chorions (i.e., a diamnionic-dichorionic membrane)**.

B. **Monozygotic (identical) twins** result from the fertilization of one secondary oocyte by one sperm. The resulting zygote forms a blastocyst in which the inner cell mass (embryoblast) splits into two. Hence, these twins are genetically identical. In 65% of cases, monozygotic (identical) twins have **one placenta, two amniotic sacs, and one chorion (i.e., a diamnionic-monochorionic membrane)**.

C. **Conjoined (Siamese) twins** form exactly like monozygotic twins except that the inner cell mass (embryoblast) does not completely split. Hence, two embryos form, but they are joined by tissue bridges at various regions of the body (e.g., head, thorax, or pelvis).

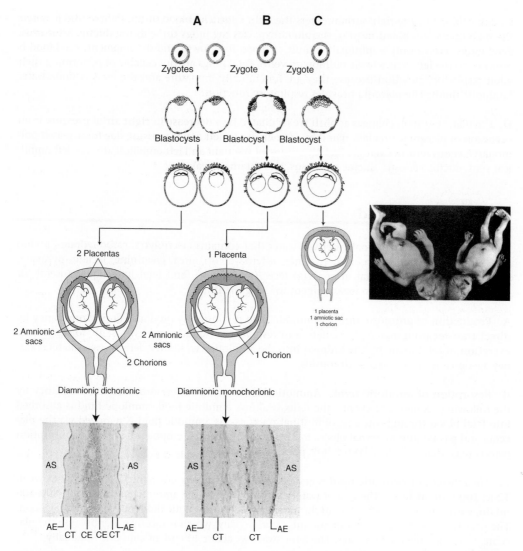

Figure 6-5. Diagram of twinning. **(A)** Dizygotic twins. Note that dizygotic twins and 35% of monozygotic twins have two placentas, two amniotic sacs, and two chorions (diamnionic-dichorionic membrane; remember: 222). Light micrograph shows the histologic arrangement of the placental components in dizygotic twins and 35% of monozygotic twins. Note the two amniotic sacs (*AS*), two layers of simple cuboidal epithelium of the amnion (*AE*), and two chorions consisting of connective tissue (*CT*) and chorionic epithelium (*CE*). The gross appearance of a diamnionic-dichorionic membrane is opaque with some remnants of blood vessels. **(B)** Monozygotic twins. In 65% of cases, monozygotic (identical) twins have one placenta, two amniotic sacs, and one chorion (diamnionic-monochorionic membrane; remember: 121). Light micrograph shows the histologic arrangement of the placental components in 65% of monozygotic (identical) twins. Note the two amniotic sacs (*AS*), two layers of simple cuboidal epithelium of the amnion (*AE*), and surrounding connective tissue (*CT*). Also, note the absence of the intervening cellular chorionic layer as seen in A. The gross appearance of a diamnionic-monochorionic membrane is transparent. **(C)** Conjoined twins. Twins here are conjoined at the head (i.e., craniopagus) with lower limb deformities.

IX.   Clinical Considerations (Figure 6-6)

A. Velamentous placenta is a placenta in which the umbilical (fetal) blood vessels abnormally travel through the amniochorionic membrane before reaching the placenta proper. If these blood vessels cross the internal os, a serious condition called **vasa previa** exists. In vasa previa, if one of the umbilical (fetal) blood vessels ruptures during pregnancy, labor, or during delivery, the fetus will bleed to death.

B. Circumvallate placenta is a placenta peripheral cuplike attachment of the amnion on the fetal surface of the placenta.

C. Bipartite or tripartite placenta is a placenta made up of two or three connected lobes.

D. Duplex or triplex placenta is a placenta made up of two or three separate lobes.

E. Succenturiate placenta is a placenta consisting of small accessory lobes completely separate from the main placenta. Care must be taken to assure that the accessory lobes are eliminated in the afterbirth.

F. Membranous placenta is a thin placenta that forms over the greater part of the uterine cavity. Care must be taken to ensure that all the placenta is eliminated during the afterbirth; this may require curettage.

G. Placenta previa occurs when the placenta attaches in the lower part of the uterus, **covering the internal os.** The placenta normally implants in the posterior superior wall of the uterus. Uterine (maternal) blood vessels rupture during the later part of pregnancy as the uterus gradually dilates. The mother may bleed to death, and the fetus will also be placed in jeopardy because of the compromised blood supply. Because the placenta blocks the cervical opening, delivery is usually accomplished by cesarean section. This condition is clinically associated with **repeated episodes of bright red vaginal bleeding**.

H. Placental abruption occurs when a normally implanted placenta prematurely separates from the uterus before delivery of the fetus. It is associated with maternal hypertension.

I. Placental accreta occurs when there is abnormal adherence of the chorionic villi to the uterine wall with partial or complete absence of the decidua basalis.

J. Placental percreta occurs when the chorionic villi penetrate the myometrium to reach the perimetrium.

K. Premature rupture of the amniochorionic membrane is the most common cause of premature labor and oligohydramnios. It is commonly referred to as "breaking of the waters."

L. Amniotic band syndrome occurs when bands of amniotic membrane encircle and constrict various parts of the fetus, causing limb amputations and craniofacial anomalies.

M. Presence of a single umbilical artery (SUA) within the cord is an abnormal condition that is associated with poor intrauterine fetal growth, prematurity, and cardiovascular anomalies. (Normally two umbilical arteries are present.)

N. Umbilical cord knots The umbilical cord frequently forms loops producing a **false knot**, which is of no clinical significance. However, in some cases, **true knots** are formed, which may cause fetal death due to fetal anoxia.

O. Erythroblastosis fetalis   The **Rh factor** in red blood cells (RBCs) is clinically important in pregnancy. If the mother is Rh-negative, she will produce Rh antibodies if the fetus is Rh-positive. This situation will not affect the first pregnancy, but will affect the second pregnancy with an Rh-positive fetus. In the second pregnancy with a Rh-positive fetus, a hemolytic condition of RBCs occurs known as **Rh-hemolytic disease of newborn (erythroblastosis fetalis)**. This causes destruction of fetal RBCs, which leads to the release of large amounts of **bilirubin** (a breakdown product of hemoglobin). This causes fetal brain damage due to a condition called **kernicterus**, which is a pathologic deposition of bilirubin in the basal ganglia. **Severe hemolytic disease** whereby the fetus is severely anemic and demonstrates total body edema (i.e., **hydrops fetalis**) may lead to death. In these cases, an intrauterine transfusion is indicated.

There are two main treatments for erythroblastosis fetalis as indicated below.

1. **Intravascular transfusion (IVT).** IVT of red blood cells (RBCs) is indicated for treatment of severe fetal anemia in preterm fetuses in the following conditions: **RBC alloimmunization** (the most prevalent antibodies are anti-D, anti-K1, and anti-c); **parvovirus infection,** which is caused by the arrest of bone marrow precursors; **chronic fetomaternal hemorrhage,** which presents with a perception by the mother of decreased fetal movements; and **inherited RBC disorders** (e.g., α-thalassemia, congenital dyserythropoietic anemia). The access site for IVT is the **umbilical vein at the umbilical cord insertion** into the placenta (using the umbilical arteries is associated with fetal bradycardia) or the **intrahepatic part of the umbilical vein.** IVTs are performed between **18 and 35 weeks of gestation.** IVTs prior to 18 weeks of gestation are rarely successful because of the small size of anatomic structures and limited visualization. IVTs after 35 weeks of gestation are not done because IVT-related morbidity is greater than morbidity associated with delivery.

2. **Rh_0 (D) immune globulin (RhOGAM, MICROGAM)** is a human immunoglobulin (IgG) preparation that contains antibodies against Rh factor and prevents a maternal antibody response to Rh+ cells that may enter the maternal bloodstream of an Rh− mother. This drug is administered to Rh− mothers within 72 hours after the birth of an Rh+ baby to prevent erythroblastosis fetalis during subsequent pregnancies. **Rh_0 (D) immune globulin (RhoGAM, MICRhoGAM)** is a human immunoglobulin (IgG) preparation that contains antibodies against Rh factor and prevents a maternal antibody response to Rh-positive cells that may enter the maternal bloodstream of a Rh-negative mother. This drug is administered to Rh-negative mothers within 72 hours after the birth of an Rh-positive baby to prevent erythroblastosis fetalis during subsequent pregnancies.

P. Oligohydramnios occurs when there is a low amount of amniotic fluid (**<400 mL in late pregnancy**). Oligohydramnios may be associated with the inability of the fetus to excrete urine into the amniotic sac owing to **renal agenesis.** This results in many fetal deformities (**Potter syndrome**) and **hypoplastic lungs** due to increased pressure on the fetal thorax.

Q. Polyhydramnios occurs when there is a high amount of amniotic fluid (**>2000 mL in late pregnancy**). Polyhydramnios may be associated with the inability of the fetus to swallow because of **anencephaly** or **esophageal atresia.** Polyhydramnios is commonly associated with **maternal diabetes.**

R. α-Fetoprotein (AFP) is "fetal albumin" that is produced by fetal hepatocytes. AFP is routinely assayed in amniotic fluid and maternal serum between **weeks 14 and 18** of gestation. AFP levels change with gestational age so that proper interpretation of AFP levels is dependent on an accurate gestational age.

1. **Elevated AFP levels** are associated with **neural tube defects** (e.g., **spina bifida or anencephaly**), **omphalocele** (allows fetal serum to leak into the amniotic fluid), **esophageal and duodenal atresia** (which interfere with fetal swallowing).
2. Reduced AFP levels are associated with **Down syndrome.**

S. Preeclampsia and eclampsia   Preeclampsia is a complication of pregnancy characterized by hypertension, edema, and/or proteinuria. Severe preeclampsia is the sudden development of **maternal hypertension (>160/110 mm Hg), edema (hands and/or face), and proteinuria (>5 g/24 hr)** usually after week 32 of gestation (third trimester). Eclampsia includes the additional symptom of convulsions. The pathophysiology of preeclampsia involves a **generalized arteriolar constriction** that impacts the brain (seizures and stroke), kidneys (oliguria and renal failure), liver (edema), and small blood vessels (thrombocytopenia and disseminated intravascular coagulation). Treatment of severe preeclampsia involves **magnesium sulfate** (for seizure prophylaxis) and **hydralazine** (blood pressure control); once the patient is stabilized, delivery of the fetus should ensue immediately. Risk factors include nulliparity, diabetes, hypertension, renal disease, twin gestation, or hydatidiform mole (produces first trimester preeclampsia).

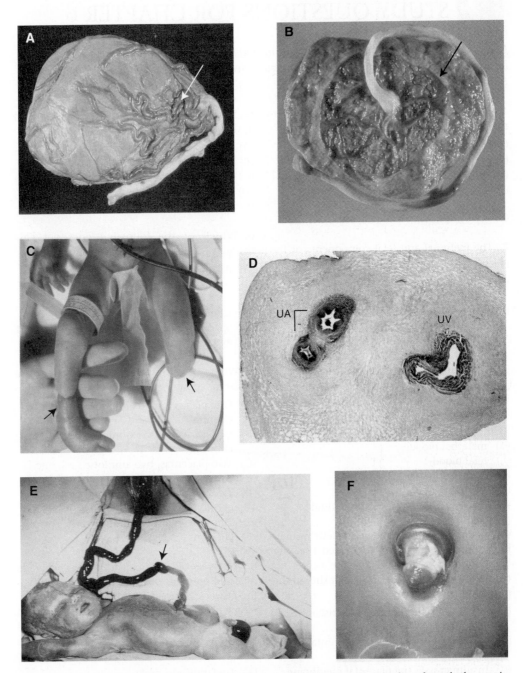

Figure 6-6.   (A) Velamentous placenta shows umbilical (fetal) blood vessels traveling through the amnio-chorionic membrane (*arrow*). (B) Circumvallate placenta shows a peripheral cuplike attachment of the amnion (*arrow*). (C) Amniotic band syndrome shows a constriction of the right leg and amputation of the left leg (*arrows*). (D) Light micrograph of a normal umbilical cord shows the two umbilical arteries (*UA*) and one umbilical vein (*UV*). (E) A true knot (*arrow*) of the umbilical cord is shown, which caused fetal death. (F) Abnormal pattern of umbilical cord drying caused by persistent fetal ducts, either the vitelline duct (indicating an ileal or Meckel's diverticulum) or urachus (indicating a urachal fistula).

STUDY QUESTIONS FOR CHAPTER 6

*Directions: Each of the numbered items or incomplete statements in this section is followed by answers or by completions of the statement. Select the **one** lettered answer or completion that is **best** in each case.*

1. During the later stages of pregnancy, maternal blood is separated from fetal blood by

(A) syncytiotrophoblast only
(B) cytotrophoblast only
(C) syncytiotrophoblast and cytotrophoblast
(D) syncytiotrophoblast and fetal endothelium
(E) cytotrophoblast and fetal endothelium

2. The maternal and fetal components of the placenta are

(A) decidua basalis and secondary chorionic villi
(B) decidua capsularis and secondary chorionic villi
(C) decidua parietalis and tertiary chorionic villi
(D) decidua capsularis and villous chorion
(E) decidua basalis and villous chorion

3. The intervillous space of the placenta contains

(A) maternal blood
(B) fetal blood
(C) maternal and fetal blood
(D) amniotic fluid
(E) maternal blood and amniotic fluid

4. A young insulin-dependent diabetic woman in her first pregnancy is concerned that her daily injection of insulin will cause a congenital malformation in her baby. What should the physician tell her?

(A) Insulin is highly teratogenic; discontinue treatment
(B) Insulin does not cross the placental membrane
(C) Insulin crosses the placental membrane but is degraded rapidly
(D) Insulin will benefit her baby by increasing glucose metabolism
(E) Insulin crosses the placental membrane but is not teratogenic

5. What is a normal amount of amniotic fluid at term?

(A) 50 mL
(B) 500 mL
(C) 1000 mL
(D) 1500 mL
(E) 2000 mL

6. Which of the following does *not* pass through the primitive umbilical ring?

(A) Allantois
(B) Amnion
(C) Yolk sac
(D) Connecting stalk
(E) Space connecting the intraembryonic and extraembryonic coeloms

7. Which of the following best describes the placental components of dizygotic twins?

(A) One placenta, two amniotic sacs, one chorion
(B) One placenta, two amniotic sacs, two chorions
(C) Two placentas, two amniotic sacs, one chorion
(D) Two placentas, two amniotic sacs, two chorions
(E) One placenta, two amniotic sacs, two chorions

8. A 26-year-old pregnant woman experiences repeated episodes of bright red vaginal bleeding at week 28, week 32, and week 34 of pregnancy. The bleeding spontaneously subsided each time. Using ultrasound, the placenta is located in the lower right portion of the uterus over the internal os. What is the diagnosis?

(A) Hydatidiform mole
(B) Vasa previa
(C) Placenta previa
(D) Placental abruption
(E) Premature rupture of the amniochorionic membrane

9. A 19-year-old woman in week 32 of a complication-free pregnancy is rushed to the emergency department because of profuse vaginal bleeding. The bleeding subsides, but afterwards no fetal heart sounds can be heard, indicating intrauterine fetal death. The woman goes into labor and delivers a stillborn infant. On examination of the afterbirth, a velamentous placenta is detected. Although not much can be done at this point, what is the diagnosis?

(A) Placenta previa
(B) Vasa previa
(C) Hydatidiform mole
(D) Premature rupture of the amniochorionic membrane
(E) Amniotic band syndrome

10. A 32-year-old pregnant woman at 30 weeks of gestation comes to her physician because of excess weight gain in a 2-week period. Ultrasonography reveals polyhydramnios. Which fetal abnormality is most likely responsible for the polyhydramnios?

(A) Bilateral kidney agenesis
(B) Umbilical cord knots
(C) Velamentous placenta
(D) Hypoplastic lungs
(E) Esophageal atresia

11. A 25-year-old pregnant woman at 17 weeks of gestation comes to her OB/GYN for a normal examination. During routine blood tests, her serum α-fetoprotein (AFP) concentration is markedly decreased for her gestational age. Which abnormality will the physician need to rule out based upon these low AFP levels?

(A) Spina bifida
(B) Anencephaly
(C) Omphalocele
(D) Down syndrome
(E) Esophageal atresia

 ANSWERS AND EXPLANATIONS

1. D. During the later stages of pregnancy, the placental membrane becomes very thin and consists of two layers, the syncytiotrophoblast and fetal endothelium.

2. E. The placenta is a unique organ in that it is a composite of tissue from two different sources, the mother and the fetus. The maternal component is the decidua basalis, and the fetal component is the villous chorion.

3. A. The intervillous space contains only maternal blood as the spiral arteries of the endometrium penetrate the outer cytotrophoblast shell.

4. B. Insulin, like all protein hormones, does not cross the placental membrane in significant amounts.

5. C. The normal amount of amniotic fluid at term is 1000 mL. However, the amount of amniotic fluid at various stages of pregnancy can be indicative of congenital malformations. Oligohydramnios (400 mL in late pregnancy) may be indicative of renal agenesis. Polyhydramnios (2000 mL in late pregnancy) may be indicative of either anencephaly or esophageal atresia.

6. B. The amnion does not pass through the primitive umbilical ring. As craniocaudal folding occurs, the amnion becomes the outer covering of the umbilical cord.

7. D. Dizygotic twins and 35% of monozygotic twins have two placentas, two amniotic sacs, and two chorions (i.e., 222).

8. C. A placenta implanted in the lower part of the uterus near the internal os is called placenta previa. The repeated episodes of bright red vaginal bleeding are caused by the gradual dilation of the uterus in the later stages of pregnancy. As the uterus dilates, spiral arteries and veins supplying the placenta are ruptured. The mother may bleed to death, and the fetus is placed in jeopardy because of the compromised maternal blood flow.

9. B. A velamentous placenta occurs when umbilical blood vessels abnormally travel through the amniochorionic membrane before reaching the placenta proper. If the vessels cross the internal os, a serious condition called vasa previa exists. As the fetus grows during pregnancy and the amniochorionic membrane stretches, the umbilical vessels may rupture. When that happens, the fetus will bleed to death. The mother is in no danger of bleeding to death in vasa previa because only the umbilical vessels rupture.

10. E. Polyhydramnios is associated with the inability of the fetus to swallow because of esophageal atresia or anencephaly. Polyhydramnios can also result from absorption defects such as duodenal atresia. The inability of the embryo to swallow the amniotic fluid means the fluid cannot be absorbed into the fetal blood and removed by the placenta and passed into the maternal blood.

11. D. Reduced AFP levels are associated with Down syndrome. All of the other defects (neural tube defects such as spina bifida and anencephaly, omphalocele, and esophageal atresias) are associated with elevated AFP levels.

Nervous System

I. Overview

A. The **central nervous system (CNS)** is formed in week 3 of development as the **neural plate**. The neural plate consisting of **neuroectoderm** becomes the **neural tube**, which gives rise to the brain and spinal cord.

B. The **peripheral nervous system (PNS)** is derived from three sources:
1. **Neural crest cells**; see III, Neural Crest Cells.
2. **Neural tube** gives rise to all preganglionic autonomic fibers and all fibers that innervate skeletal muscles.
3. **Mesoderm** gives rise to the dura mater and to connective tissue investments of peripheral nerve fibers (endoneurium, perineurium, and epineurium).

II. Development of the Neural Tube (Figure 7-1)

Neurulation refers to the formation and closure of the neural tube. Bone morphogenetic protein (BMP-4), noggin (an inductor protein), chordin (an inductor protein), fibroblast growth factor (FGF-8), and neural cell adhesion molecule (N-CAM) appear to play a role in neurulation. The events of neurulation occur as follows:

A. The **notochord** induces the overlying ectoderm to differentiate into **neuroectoderm** and form the neural plate. The notochord forms the **nucleus pulposus** of the intervertebral disk in the adult.

B. The neural plate folds to give rise to the neural tube, which is open at both ends at the **anterior** and **posterior neuropores.** The anterior and posterior neuropores connect the lumen of the neural tube to the amniotic cavity.
1. The **anterior neuropore** closes during week 4 (day 25) and becomes the **lamina terminalis.** Failure of the anterior neuropore to close results in upper neural tube defects (NTDs; e.g., anencephaly).
2. The **posterior neuropore** closes during week 4 (day 27). Failure of the posterior neuropore to close results in lower NTDs (e.g., spina bifida with myeloschisis).

C. As the neural plate folds, some cells differentiate into **neural crest cells.**

D. The rostral part of the neural tube becomes the adult **brain.**

E. The caudal part of the neural tube becomes the adult **spinal cord.**

F. The lumen of the neural tube gives rise to the **ventricular system** of the brain and **central canal** of the spinal cord.

III. Neural Crest Cells (see Figure 7-1)

The neural crest cells differentiate from cells located along the lateral border of the neural plate, which is mediated by **BMP-4** and **BMP-7**. The differentiation of neural crest cells is marked by the expression of *slug* (a zinc-finger transcription factor), which characterizes cells that break away from the neuroepithelium of the neural plate and migrate into the extracellular matrix as mesenchymal cells. Neural crest cells experience an extracellular environment rich in extracellular matrix molecules. Molecules that promote cell migration are **fibronectin, laminin,** and **Type IV collagen.** Molecules that restrict cell migration are **chondroitin sulfate–rich proteoglycans.** Neural crest cells undergo a prolific migration throughout the embryo (both the cranial region and trunk region) and ultimately differentiate into a wide array of adult cells and structures (see also Table 4-1).

A. **Cranial neural crest cells**   There is a remarkable relationship between the origin of cranial neural crest cells from the rhombencephalon (hindbrain) and their final migration into pharyngeal arches (see Table 12-1). The rhombencephalon is divided into eight segments called **rhombomeres (R1–R8).** Cranial neural crest cells from R1 and R2 migrate into pharyngeal arch 1 (which also receives neural crest cells from the midbrain area). Cranial neural crest cells from R4 migrate into pharyngeal arch 2. Cranial neural crest cells from R6 and R7 migrate into pharyngeal arch 3. This pattern seems to be controlled by the expression of the *Hoxb* gene complex and OTX2. Cranial neural crest cells differentiate into the following adult cells and structures: **pharyngeal arch skeletal and connective tissue components; bones of neurocranium; pia and arachnoid; parafollicular (C) cells of thyroid; aorticopulmonary septum; odontoblasts (dentin of teeth); sensory ganglia of cranial nerves CN V, CN VII, CN IX, and CN X; and ciliary (CN III), pterygopalatine (CN VII), submandibular (CN VII), and otic (CN IX) parasympathetic ganglia.**

B. Trunk neural crest cells extend from somite 6 to the most caudal somites and migrate in a dorsolateral, ventral, and ventrolateral direction throughout the embryo. Trunk neural crest cells differentiate into the following adult cells and structures: **melanocytes, Schwann cells, chromaffin cells of adrenal medulla, dorsal root ganglia, sympathetic chain ganglia, prevertebral sympathetic ganglia, enteric parasympathetic ganglia of the gut (Meissner and Auerbach; CN X), and abdominal/pelvic cavity parasympathetic ganglia.**

C. **Clinical considerations**
   1. **Neurocristopathy** is a term used to describe any disease related to maldevelopment of neural crest cells.
   2. **Medullary carcinoma of thyroid (MC).** MC is an endocrine neoplasm of the parafollicular (C) cells of neural crest origin that secrete calcitonin. The carcinoma cells are usually arranged in cell nests surrounded by bands of stroma containing amyloid.
   3. **Schwannoma.** A schwannoma is a benign tumor of Schwann cells of neural crest origin. These tumors are well-circumscribed, encapsulated masses that may or not be attached to the nerve. The most common location within the cranial vault is at the cerebellopontine angle near the vestibular branch of CN VIII (often referred to as an acoustic neuroma). Clinical signs include tinnitus and hearing loss. CN V (trigeminal nerve) is also commonly affected.
   4. **Neurofibromatosis Type 1 (NF1; von Recklinghausen disease).** NF1 is a relatively common autosomal dominant disorder due to a mutation in the **NF1 gene** that is located on chromosome 17q11.2 and codes for the protein neurofibromin. Neurofibromin downregulates **p21 Ras oncoprotein** so that the NF1 gene belongs to the family of tumor-suppressor genes. The key features of NF include multiple neural tumors (called neurofibromas), which are widely dispersed over the body and reveal proliferation of all elements of a peripheral nerve including neurites, fibroblasts, and Schwann cells of neural crest origin; numerous pigmented skin lesions (called café-au-lait spots) probably associated with melanocytes of neural crest origin; and pigmented iris hamartomas (called Lisch nodules).

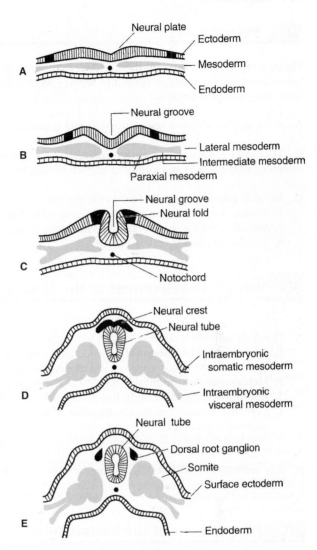

Figure 7-1. Schematic diagrams of transverse sections of embryos at various stages. (A) Neural plate stage. (B) Early neural groove stage. (C) Late neural groove stage. (D) Early neural tube and neural crest stage. (E) Neural tube and dorsal root ganglion stage.

5. **CHARGE association.** The CHARGE association is understandable only if the wide distribution of neural crest cell derivatives is appreciated. The cause of CHARGE is unknown but seems to involve an insult during the second month of gestation probably involving the neural crest cells. The key features of CHARGE include **c**oloboma of the retina, lens, or choroid; **h**eart defects (e.g., tetralogy of Fallot, ventricular septal defect, patent ductus arteriosus); **a**tresia choanae; **r**etardation of growth; **g**enital abnormalities in male infants (e.g., cryptorchidism, microphallus); **e**ar abnormalities or deafness.

6. **Waardenburg syndrome (WS).** WS is an autosomal dominant disorder due to a mutation in either the ***PAX3* gene**, which is located on chromosome 2q35 (for Type I WS), or ***MITF* gene**, which is located on chromosome 3p12.3-p14.1 (for Type II WS). The key features of WS include lateral displacement of lacrimal puncta, a broad nasal root, heterochromia of the iris, congenital deafness, and piebaldism including a white forelock and a triangular area of hypopigmentation.

7. **Hirschsprung disease.** See Chapter 10 IV.B.

8. **Cleft cleft palate and lip.** See Chapter 12 VIII.G, H.

9. **DiGeorge syndrome.** See Chapter 12 VIII.I and Chapter 24 II.C.

10. **Pheochromocytoma.** See Chapter 13 IX.C.

11. **Neuroblastoma.** See Chapter 13 IX.C.

IV. Placodes

Placodes are localized thickenings of surface **ectoderm**. They give rise to cells that migrate into underlying mesoderm and develop into sensory receptive organs of cranial nerves (CN I and CN VIII) and the lens of the eye.

A. The **lens placode** gives rise to the **lens** and is induced by the optic vesicles.

B. The **nasal (olfactory) placodes** differentiate into neurosensory cells that give rise to the **olfactory nerve (CN I)** and induce formation of olfactory bulbs.

C. The **otic placodes** give rise to the **otic vesicle**, which forms the following:
1. Utricle, semicircular ducts, and vestibular ganglion of CN VIII
2. Saccule, cochlear duct (organ of Corti), spiral ganglion of CN VIII
3. Vestibulocochlear nerve (CN VIII)

V. Vesicle Development of the Neural Tube (Figure 7-2)

A. The three primary brain vesicles and two associated flexures develop during week 4.
1. **Prosencephalon (forebrain)** is associated with the appearance of the optic vesicles and gives rise to the telencephalon and diencephalon.
2. **Mesencephalon (midbrain)** remains as the mesencephalon.
3. **Rhombencephalon (hindbrain)** gives rise to the metencephalon and myelencephalon.
4. **Cephalic flexure (midbrain flexure)** is located between the prosencephalon and the rhombencephalon.
5. **Cervical flexure** is located between the rhombencephalon and the future spinal cord.

B. Five **secondary brain vesicles** become visible in week 6 of development and form various adult derivatives of the brain.

VI. Histogenesis of the Neural Tube

The cells of the neural tube are neuroectodermal (or neuroepithelial) cells that give rise to the following cell types:

A. **Neuroblasts** form all neurons found in the CNS.

B. **Glioblasts (spongioblasts)** are, for the most part, formed after cessation of neuroblast formation. Radial glial cells are an exception and develop before neurogenesis is complete. Glioblasts form the supporting cells of the CNS and include the following:
1. **Astroglia (astrocytes)** have the following characteristics and functions: project foot processes to capillaries that contribute to the blood-brain barrier, play a role in the metabolism of neurotransmitters (e.g., glutamate, GABA, serotonin), buffer the [K+] of the CNS extracellular space, form the external and internal glial-limiting membrane in the CNS, form glial scars in a damaged area of the CNS (i.e., astrogliosis), undergo hypertrophy and hyperplasia in reaction to CNS injury, and contain the **glial fibrillary acidic protein (GFAP)** and **glutamine synthetase**, which are good markers for astrocytes.
2. **Radial glial cells** are of astrocytic lineage, are GFAP-positive, and provide guidance for migrating neuroblasts.
3. **Oligodendroglia (oligodendrocytes)** produce the myelin in the CNS. A single oligodendrocyte can myelinate several (up to 30) axons.

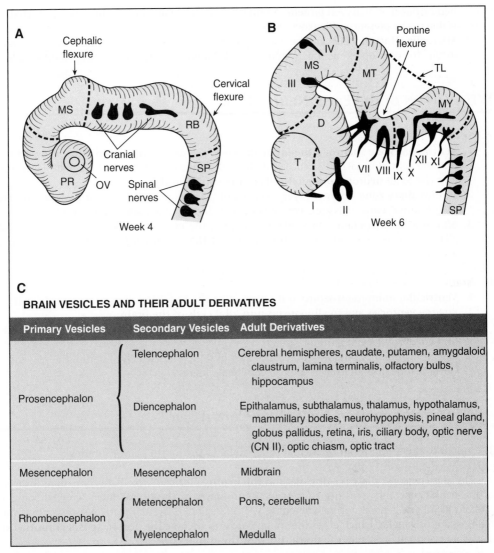

Figure 7-2. Schematic illustrations of the developing brain vesicles. **(A)** Three-vesicle stage of the brain in a 4-week-old embryo. Divisions are indicated by *dotted lines*. *MS* = mesencephalon; *OV* = optic vesicle; *PR* = prosencephalon; *RB* = rhombencephalon; *SP* = spinal cord. **(B)** Five-vesicle stage of the brain in a 6-week-old embryo. Divisions are indicated by *dotted lines*. Cranial nerves (CN) are indicated by *Roman numerals*. CN VI is not shown because it exits the brain stem from the ventral surface. *D* = diencephalon; *MS* = mesencephalon; *MT* = metencephalon; *MY* = myelencephalon; *SP* = spinal cord; *T* = telencephalon; *TL* = tela choroidea. **(C)** Table indicating the brain vesicles and their adult derivatives.

4. **Ependymocytes** line the central canal and ventricles of the brain. These cells are not joined by tight junctions so that exchange between the cerebrospinal fluid (CSF) and CNS extracellular fluid occurs freely.

5. **Tanycytes** are modified ependymal cells that mediate transport between CSF in the ventricles and the neuropil. These cells usually project to hypothalamic nuclei that regulate the release of gonadotropic hormones from the adenohypophysis.

6. **Choroid plexus cells** are a continuation of the ependymal layer that is reflected over the choroid plexus villi and **secrete CSF** by selective transport of molecules from blood. These cells are joined by tight junctions that are the basis of the **blood–CSF barrier.** CSF is normally clear. A yellow color (xanthochromia) indicates previous bleeding (subarachnoid

hemorrhage) or increased protein. A pinkish color is usually due to a bloody tap. Turbidity is due to the presence of leukocytes.

7. **Microglia (Hortega cells)** are the macrophages of the CNS. They arise from monocytes and invade the developing nervous system in week 3 along with the developing blood vessels.

VII. Layers of the Early Neural Tube

A. **Spinal cord**
1. **Ventricular zone (neuroepithelial layer)** gives rise to a layer of ependymal cells, which line the central canal. The neuroepithelial cells migrate into the intermediate layer and give rise to all **neurons and glial cells of the spinal cord.**
2. **Intermediate zone (mantle layer)** consists of neurons and glial cells of the **gray matter of the spinal cord.** This zone contains the developing **alar plate** and **basal plate.**
3. **Marginal zone** contains nerve fibers (axons) of the neuroblasts of the mantle layer and glial cells. This zone forms the **white matter of the spinal cord** through myelination of axons.

B. **Brain**
1. **Ventricular zone (neuroepithelial layer)** gives rise to a layer of ependymal cells, which line the ventricles and to all **neurons and glial cells of the brain.**
2. **Intermediate zone (mantle layer)**, along with the ventricular layer, gives rise to the **cerebral cortex** and **basal ganglia.**
3. **Marginal zone** becomes the molecular layer of the cortex, which underlies the pia.
4. **Cortex** is the **gray matter** of the cerebral hemispheres.

VIII. Development of the Spinal Cord (Figure 7-3)

The spinal cord develops from the neural tube caudal to the fourth pair of somites.

A.   The **alar (sensory) plate** is a **dorsolateral thickening** of the intermediate zone (mantle layer) of the neural tube and gives rise to **sensory neuroblasts of the dorsal horn** (general somatic afferent [GSA] and general visceral afferent [GVA] cell regions). The alar plate receives axons from the dorsal root ganglia, which enter the spinal cord and become the **dorsal (sensory) roots.** The alar plate eventually becomes the **dorsal horn of the spinal cord.**

B.   The **basal (motor) plate** is a **ventrolateral thickening** of the intermediate zone (mantle layer) of the neural tube and gives rise to **motor neuroblasts of the ventral and lateral horns** (general somatic efferent [GSE] and general visceral efferent [GVE] cell regions). The basal plate projects axons from motor neuroblasts, which exit the spinal cord and become the **ventral (motor) roots.** The basal plate eventually becomes the **ventral horn of the spinal cord.**

C.   The **sulcus limitans (SL)** is a **longitudinal groove** in the lateral wall of the neural tube that appears during week 4 of development and separates the alar and basal plates. The SL disappears in the adult spinal cord, but is retained in the rhomboid fossa of the brain stem. The SL extends from the spinal cord to the rostral midbrain.

D.   The **roof plate** is the nonneural roof of the central canal, which connects the two alar plates.

E.   The **floor plate** is the nonneural floor of the central canal, which connects the two basal plates. The floor plate contains the ventral white commissure.

F.   The **caudal eminence** arises from the primitive streak and blends with the neural tube. It gives rise to **sacral** and **coccygeal segments of the spinal cord.**

G. Myelination of the spinal cord begins during month 4 in the ventral (motor) roots. **Oligodendrocytes** accomplish myelination in the **CNS**, and **Schwann cells** accomplish myelination in the **PNS**. Myelination of the corticospinal tracts is not completed until the end of 2 years of age (i.e., when the corticospinal tracts become myelinated and functional). Myelination of the **association neocortex** extends to 30 years of age.

H. Positional changes of the spinal cord   **At week 8** of development, the spinal cord extends the length of the vertebral canal. **At birth**, the **conus medullaris** extends to the level of the third lumbar vertebra **(L-3)**. **In adults**, the conus medullaris terminates at **L1-L2 interspace.** Disparate growth (between the vertebral column and the spinal cord) results in the formation of the **cauda equina**, consisting of dorsal and ventral roots, which descends below the level of the conus medullaris. Disparate growth results in the nonneural **filum terminale**, which anchors the spinal cord to the coccyx.

IX.   Development of Myelencephalon (Figure 7-4)

The myelencephalon develops from the rhombencephalon and gives rise to the medulla oblongata.

A. Alar plate sensory neuroblasts give rise to the following:
  1. **Dorsal column nuclei**, which consist of the gracile and cuneate nuclei
  2. **Inferior olivary nuclei**, which are cerebellar relay nuclei
  3. **Solitary nucleus**, which forms the GVA (taste) and special visceral afferent (SVA) column
  4. **Spinal trigeminal nucleus**, which forms the GSA column
  5. **Cochlear and vestibular nuclei**, which form the special somatic afferent (SSA) column and lie in the medullopontine junction

B. Basal plate motor neuroblasts give rise to the following:
  1. **Hypoglossal nucleus**, which forms the GSE column
  2. **Nucleus ambiguus**, which forms the special visceral efferent (SVE) column (CN IX, CN X, and CN XI)
  3. **Dorsal motor nucleus of the vagus nerve (CN X)** and the **inferior salivatory nucleus of the glossopharyngeal nerve (CN IX)**, which form the GVE column

C. The **roof plate** forms the roof of the fourth ventricle. The roof plate is called the **tela choroidea**, which is a monolayer of ependymal cells covered with pia mater. The tela choroidea is invaginated by pial blood vessels to form the **choroid plexus** of the fourth ventricle.

X.   Development of Metencephalon (see Figure 7-5A)

The metencephalon develops from the rhombencephalon and gives rise to the **pons** and **cerebellum**.

A. Pons (Figure 7-5A)
  1. **Alar plate sensory neuroblasts** give rise to the following:
     a. **Solitary nucleus**, which forms the SVA column (taste) of CN VII
     b. **Vestibular and cochlear nuclei**, which form the SSA column of CN VIII
     c. **Spinal and principal trigeminal nuclei**, which form the GSA column of CN V
     d. **Pontine nuclei**, which consist of cerebellar relay nuclei (pontine gray)
  2. **Basal plate motor neuroblasts** give rise to the following:
     a. **Abducens nucleus**, which forms the GSE column
     b. **Facial and motor trigeminal nuclei**, which form the special visceral efferent SVE column
     c. **Superior salivatory nucleus**, which forms the GVE column of CN VII

3. The **base of pons** contains pontine nuclei from the alar plate; from the corticobulbar, corticospinal, and corticopontine fibers from the cerebral cortex; and from pontocerebellar fibers.

B. Cerebellum (see Figure 7-5*A*) is formed by the **rhombic lips**, which are the two thickened alar plates of the mantle layer. The rostral part of the cerebellum is derived from the caudal mesencephalon. The cerebellar plates give rise to the following:

1. **Vermis** is formed by midline growth.
2. **Cerebellar hemispheres** are formed by lateral growth.
3. **Three-layered cerebellar cortex (molecular layer, Purkinje cell layer, and granular or internal layer)** and **four pairs of cerebellar nuclei** are formed by cell migration from the ventricular zone into the marginal layer.
4. **External granular layer (EGL)** is a germinal (proliferative) layer on the surface of the cerebellum, which is present from week 8 of development to 2 years of age. The EGL gives rise only to granule cells and not to basket (inner stellate) or stellate (outer stellate) neurons, as has long been thought. Persistent cell nests may give rise to a **medulloblastoma**. The EGL is sensitive to antiviral agents, which block the synthesis of DNA.
5. **Folia and fissures** are formed by differential cortical growth.

XI. Development of Mesencephalon (see Figure 7-5*B*)

The mesencephalon remains unchanged during primary to secondary vesicle formation and gives rise to the **midbrain.**

A. Alar plate sensory neuroblasts form the cell layers of the superior colliculi and the nuclei of the inferior colliculi.

B. Basal plate motor neuroblasts give rise to the following:

1. **Oculomotor (CN III)** and **trochlear nuclei (CN IV)**, which form the GSE column
2. **Edinger-Westphal nucleus of CN III**, which forms the most rostral cell group of the GVE column
3. **Substantia nigra**
4. **Red nucleus**

C. Basis pedunculi (crus cerebri) contain corticobulbar, corticospinal, and corticopontine fibers, derived from the cerebral cortex of the telencephalon.

XII. Development of Diencephalon, Optic Structures, and Hypophysis (see Figure 7-5*C, D*)

A. Diencephalon (see Figure 7-5*C*)   The diencephalon develops from the prosencephalon within the walls of the primitive third ventricle. It gives rise to the **epithalamus, thalamus, hypothalamus,** and **subthalamus.**

1. **Epithalamus** develops from the embryonic roof plate and dorsal parts of alar plates. It gives rise to the **pineal body (epiphysis), tela choroidea,** and **choroid plexus** of the third ventricle.
2. **Thalamus** is an alar plate derivative, which gives rise to the **thalamic nuclei.**
3. **Hypothalamus** develops from the alar plate and floor plate. It gives rise to **hypothalamic nuclei, mammillary bodies,** and **neurohypophysis.**
4. **Subthalamus** is an alar plate derivative and includes the subthalamic nucleus. The subthalamus gives rise to neuroblasts that migrate into the telencephalic white matter to become the **globus pallidus (pallidum),** which is a basal ganglion.

B. **Optic vesicles, cups, and stalks** are derivatives of the diencephalon. They give rise to the **retina, iris, ciliary body, optic nerve (CN II), optic chiasm,** and **optic tract** (see Chapter 9).

C. **Hypophysis (pituitary gland)** (see Figure 7-5*D*) The hypophysis is attached to the hypothalamus by the pituitary stalk and consists of two lobes.
1. **Anterior lobe (adenohypophysis)** develops from **Rathke's pouch,** which is an ectodermal diverticulum of the primitive mouth cavity (stomodeum). Remnants of Rathke's pouch may give rise to a **craniopharyngioma.**
2. **Posterior lobe (neurohypophysis)** develops from a ventral evagination of the hypothalamus. The posterior lobe includes the **median eminence, infundibular stem,** and **pars nervosa.**

XIII. Development of Telencephalon (Figure 7-6)

The telencephalon develops from the prosencephalon. The telencephalon gives rise to the **cerebral hemispheres, caudate, putamen, amygdaloid, claustrum, lamina terminalis, olfactory bulbs,** and **hippocampus.**

A. **Cerebral hemispheres** (see Figure 7-6) develop as bilateral evaginations of the lateral walls of the prosencephalic vesicle and contain the **cerebral cortex, cerebral white matter, basal ganglia,** and **lateral ventricles.** The cerebral hemispheres are interconnected by three commissures: the **corpus callosum, anterior commissure,** and **hippocampal (fornical) commissure.** Continuous hemispheric growth gives rise to **frontal, parietal, occipital,** and **temporal lobes,** which overlie the insula and dorsal brain stem.

B. **Cerebral cortex (pallium)** is formed by neuroblasts that migrate from the ventricular and intermediate layers to form a stratified subpial zone called the **gray matter.** The cerebral cortex is classified as **neocortex** and **allocortex.**
1. **Neocortex (isocortex)** is a six-layered cortex that represents 90% of the cortical mantle.
2. **Allocortex** is a three-layered cortex that represents 10% of the cortical mantle. The allocortex is subdivided into the **archicortex,** which includes the hippocampal formation, and the **paleocortex,** which includes the olfactory cortex.

C. **Corpus striatum (striatal eminence)** appears in week 5 of development in the floor of the telencephalic vesicle (see Figure 7-5*C*). The corpus striatum gives rise to the basal ganglia: the **caudate nucleus, putamen, amygdaloid nucleus,** and **claustrum.** It is divided into the caudate nucleus and the lentiform nucleus by corticofugal and corticopetal fibers, which make up the internal capsule. The neurons of the globus pallidus (also a basal ganglion) have their origin in the subthalamus, and these neurons migrate into the telencephalic white matter and become the medial segments of the lentiform nucleus.

D. **Commissures** are fiber bundles that interconnect the hemispheres and cross the midline via the embryonic lamina terminalis (commissural plate).
1. **Anterior commissure** interconnects the olfactory structures and the middle and inferior temporal gyri.
2. **Hippocampal (fornical) commissure** interconnects the two hippocampi.
3. **Corpus callosum** appears between weeks 12 and 22 of development. The corpus callosum is the largest commissure of the brain and interconnects homologous neocortical areas of the two cerebral hemispheres. The corpus callosum does not project commissural fibers from the visual cortex (area 17) or the hand area of the motor or sensory strips (areas 4 and 3, 1, 2).

E. **Gyri and fissures** In month 4, no gyri or sulci are present; that is, the brain is smooth or **lissencephalic.** In month 8, all major sulci are present; that is, the brain is convoluted or **gyrencephalic.**

(*text continues on page 79*)

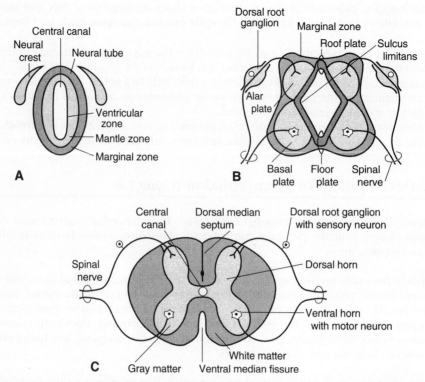

Figure 7-3.   Schematic illustration of three successive stages (A, B, C) in the development of the spinal cord. Note that the neural crest gives rise to the dorsal root ganglion and that the alar and basal plates give rise to the dorsal and ventral horns, respectively.

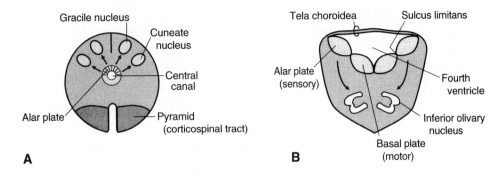

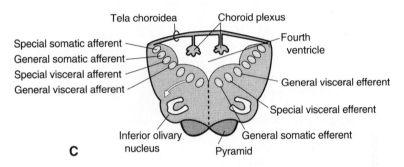

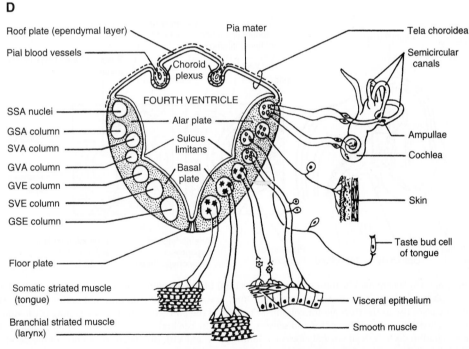

Figure 7-4. Schematic illustrations of the development of the medulla. **(A)** Transverse section of the caudal medulla, showing the development of the gracile and cuneate nuclei from the alar plates. **(B)** Schematic sketch through the rostral (open) medulla, showing the relationships of the alar and basal plates. The inferior olivary nucleus is derived from the alar plate. **(C)** A later stage of B shows the four sensory modalities of the alar plate and the three motor modalities of the basal plate. The *white arrow* indicates the lateral migration of the special visceral efferent column (CN IX, X, and XI). The pyramids consist of motor fibers of the corticospinal tracts. **(D)** Schematic diagram of the brain stem, illustrating the cell columns derived from alar and basal plates. The seven cranial nerve modalities are shown. *GSA* = general somatic afferent; *GSE* = general somatic efferent; *GVA* = general visceral afferent; *GVE* = general visceral efferent; *SSA* = special somatic afferent; *SVA* = special visceral afferent; *SVE* = special visceral efferent.

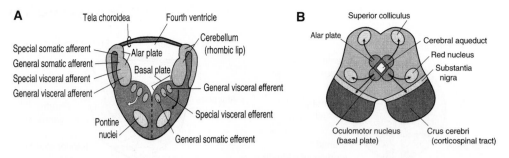

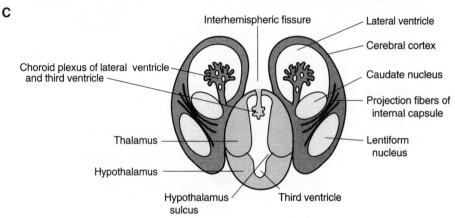

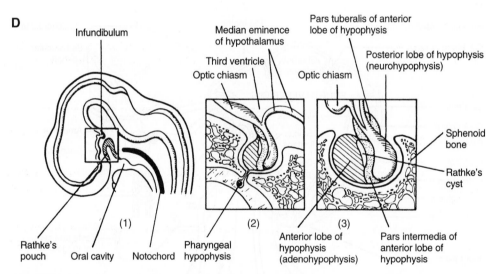

Figure 7-5. **(A)** Schematic illustration (transverse section) of the development of the pons and cerebellum. The alar plate (rhombic lip) gives rise to the cerebellum, four sensory cell columns, and pontine nuclei. The basal plate gives rise to the three motor columns. The base of the pons contains the descending corticospinal tracts, which originate from the motor and sensory strips of the cerebral cortex. The *white arrow* indicates the lateral migration of the special visceral efferent column (CN V and VII). **(B)** Transverse section of the development of the midbrain. The alar plate gives rise to the layers of the superior colliculus and nuclei of the inferior colliculus. The basal plate gives rise to the oculomotor and trochlear nuclei, substantia nigra, and red nucleus. The cerebral peduncles contain the descending corticospinal tracts. **(C)** Transverse section of the development of the forebrain. The cerebral cortex and basal ganglia are shown. The internal capsule divides the corpus striatum into the caudate nucleus and the lentiform nucleus. The alar plate of the diencephalon gives rise to the thalamus and hypothalamus. **(D)** Schematic drawings illustrating the development of the hypophysis (pituitary gland). (*1*) Midsagittal section through a 6-week-old embryo, showing Rathke's pouch as a dorsal outpocketing of the oral cavity and the infundibulum as a thickening in the floor of the hypothalamus. (*2* and *3*). Development at week 11 and week 16, respectively. The anterior lobe, pars tuberalis, and pars intermedia are derived from Rathke's pouch.

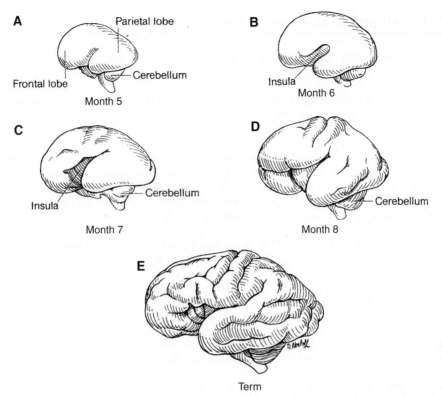

Figure 7-6. Development of the cerebral cortex from month 5 until term. Note change in the cerebral cortex from a smooth surface or lissencephalic structure to a convoluted surface or gyrencephalic structure.

XIV. Development of Sympathetic Nervous System

The sympathetic nervous system originates from the basal plate of the neural tube and neural crest cells.

A. The basal plate of the neural tube gives rise to **preganglionic sympathetic neurons within the intermediolateral cell column** of the spinal cord, which form white communicating rami found between T1 and L3.

B. The neural crest cells give rise to **postganglionic sympathetic neurons within the sympathetic chain ganglia, prevertebral sympathetic ganglia** (e.g., celiac ganglia), and **chromaffin cells of adrenal medulla.**

XV. Development of Parasympathetic Nervous System

The parasympathetic nervous system originates from the basal plate of the neural tube and neural crest cells.

A. The basal plate of the neural tube gives rise to **preganglionic parasympathetic neurons within the nuclei of the midbrain (CN III), pons (CN VII), medulla (CN IX, X), and spinal cord at S2 to S4.**

B. The neural crest cells give rise to **postganglionic parasympathetic neurons within the ciliary ganglion (CN III), pterygopalatine ganglion (CN VII), submandibular ganglion (CN VII), otic ganglion (CN IX), enteric ganglia of the gut (Meissner and Auerbach; CN X), and abdominal/pelvic cavity parasympathetic ganglia.**

XVI. Development of Cranial Nerves

A. Olfactory nerve (CN I) is derived from the **nasal (olfactory) placode** and mediates smell (olfaction). CN I is capable of regeneration.

B. Optic nerve (CN II) is derived from the **ganglion cells of the retina** (which is a diverticulum of the diencephalon) and mediates vision. CN II is not capable of regeneration after transection. CN II is not a true cranial nerve, but a tract of the diencephalon.

C. Oculomotor nerve (CN III) is derived from the **basal plate of the rostral midbrain** and mediates eye movements by innervation of the medial rectus muscle, superior rectus muscle, inferior rectus muscle, and inferior oblique muscle, upper eyelid movement by innervation of the levator palpebrae muscle, pupillary constriction by innervation of sphincter pupillae muscle of the iris, and accommodation by innervation of the ciliary muscle.

D. Trochlear nerve (CN IV) is derived from the **basal plate of the caudal midbrain** and mediates eye movements by innervation of the superior oblique muscle.

E. Trigeminal nerve (CN V)   The motor division of CN V is derived from the **basal plate of the rostral pons.** The sensory division of CN V is derived from the cranial **neural crest cells.** CN V mediates the sensory and motor innervation of pharyngeal arch 1 derivatives.

F. Abducens nerve (CN VI) is derived from the **basal plate of the caudal pons** and mediates eye movements by innervation of the lateral rectus muscle.

G. Facial nerve (CN VII)   The motor division of CN VII is derived from the **basal plate of the pons.** The sensory division of CN VII is derived from the cranial **neural crest cells.** CN VII mediates the sensory and motor innervation of pharyngeal arch 2 derivatives.

H. Vestibulocochlear nerve (CN VIII) is derived from the **otic placode.** The vestibular division of CN VIII mediates balance and equilibrium. The cochlear division of CN VIII mediates hearing.

I. Glossopharyngeal nerve (CN IX)   The motor division of CN IX is derived from the **basal plate of the medulla.** The sensory division of CN IX is derived from the cranial **neural crest cells.** CN IX mediates the sensory and motor innervation of pharyngeal arch 3 derivatives.

J. Vagal nerve (CN X)   The motor division of CN X is derived from the **basal plate of the medulla.** The sensory division of CN X is derived from the cranial **neural crest cells.** CN X mediates the sensory and motor innervation of pharyngeal arches 4 and 6 derivatives.

K. Accessory nerve (CN XI) is derived from the **basal plate of the spinal segments C-1 to C-6.** CN XI innervates the sternocleidomastoid and trapezius muscles.

L. Hypoglossal nerve (CN XII) is derived from the **basal plate of the medulla.** CN XIII innervates the intrinsic and extrinsic muscles of the tongue.

XVII. Development of Choroid Plexus

The choroid plexus develops from the **roof plates of the rhombencephalon and diencephalon,** and within the **choroid fissure of the telencephalon.** It consists of modified ependymal cells and a vascular pia mater (tela choroidea). The choroid plexus produces 500 mL of CSF per day. The CSF is returned to the venous system via the **arachnoid (granulations)** villi of the venous dural sinuses (e.g., superior sagittal sinus).

XVIII. Congenital Malformations of the Central Nervous System

A. Variations of spina bifida (Figure 7-7). Spina bifida occurs when the **bony vertebral arches** fail to form properly, thereby creating a vertebral defect usually in the **lumbosacral region.**

1. **Spina bifida occulta** is evidenced by a tuft of hair in the lumbosacral region. It is the least severe variation and occurs in 10% of the population.
2. **Spina bifida with meningocele** occurs when the meninges protrude through a vertebral defect and form a sac filled with CSF. The spinal cord remains in its normal position.
3. **Spina bifida with meningomyelocele** occurs when the meninges and spinal cord protrude through a vertebral defect and form a sac filled with CSF.
4. **Spina bifida with rachischisis** occurs when the posterior neuropore of the neural tube fails to close during week 4 of development. This condition is the most severe type of spina bifida causing paralysis from the level of the defect caudally and presents clinically as an open neural tube that lies on the surface of the back. This spina bifida variation also falls into a classification called **neural tube defects (NTDs). Lower NTDs** (i.e., spina bifida with rachischisis) result from a failure of the **posterior neuropore** to close during week 4 of development; these usually occur in the lumbosacral region. **Upper NTDs** (e.g., anencephaly) result from failure of the **anterior neuropore** to close during week 4 of development. NTDs can be diagnosed prenatally by detecting elevated levels of α-**fetoprotein** in the amniotic fluid. About 75% of all NTDs can be prevented if all women capable of becoming pregnant consume **folic acid** (dose: 0.4 mg of folic acid/day).

B. Variations of cranium bifida (Figure 7-8*A–D*) Cranium bifida occurs when the **bony skull** fails to form properly, thereby creating a skull defect usually in the **occipital region.**

1. **Cranium bifida with meningocele** occurs when the meninges protrude through the skull defect and form a sac filled with CSF.
2. **Cranium bifida** with **meningoencephalocele** occurs when the meninges and brain protrude through the skull defect and form a sac filled with CSF. This defect usually comes to medical attention within the infant's first few days or weeks of life. The outcome is poor (i.e., 75% of the infants die or are severely retarded).
3. **Cranium bifida with meningohydroencephalocele** occurs when the meninges, brain, and a portion of the ventricle protrude through the skull defect.
4. **Anencephaly (meroanencephaly)** is a type of upper NTD that occurs when the **anterior neuropore** fails to close during week 4 of development. This results in failure of the brain to develop (however, a rudimentary brain is present), failure of the lamina terminalis to form, and failure of the bony cranial vault to form. Anencephaly is incompatible with extrauterine life. If not stillborn, infants with anencephaly survive from only a few hours to a few weeks. Anencephaly is the most common serious birth defect seen in stillborn fetuses. Anencephaly is easily diagnosed by ultrasound, and a therapeutic abortion is usually performed at the mother's request.

C. Arnold-Chiari malformation (Figure 7-8*D*) occurs when the caudal vermis and tonsils of the cerebellum and the medulla oblongata herniate through the foramen magnum. Clinical signs are caused by compression of the medulla oblongata and stretching of CN IX, CN X, and CN XII and include spastic dysphonia, difficulty in swallowing, laryngeal stridor (vibrating sound heard during respiration as a result of obstructed airways), diminished gag reflex, apnea, and vocal cord paralysis. This malformation is commonly associated with a **lumbar meningomyelocele, platybasia** (bone malformation of base of skull) along with malformation of the occipitovertebral joint, and **obstructive hydrocephalus** (due to obliteration of the foramen of Magendie and foramina of Luschka of the fourth ventricle; however, about 50% of cases demonstrate **aqueductal stenosis**).

D. Hydrocephalus (Figure 7-9) is a dilation of the ventricles due to an excess of CSF that may result from either a blockage of CSF circulation or, rarely, an overproduction of CSF (e.g., due to a choroid plexus papilloma). There are two general categories of hydrocephalus:

1. **Communicating (or nonobstructive) hydrocephalus.** In this type of hydrocephalus, there is free communication between the ventricles and the subarachnoid space. The blockage of CSF in this type of hydrocephalus is usually in the subarachnoid space or arachnoid granulations and results in the enlargement of all the ventricular cavities as well as the subarachnoid space.

2. **Noncommunicating (or obstructive) hydrocephalus.** In this type of hydrocephalus, there is a lack of communication between the ventricles and the subarachnoid space. The blockage of CSF in this type of hydrocephalus is in the foramen of Monro, cerebral aqueduct, or foramen of Magendie/foramina of Luschka. Noncommunicating hydrocephalus results in the enlargement of only those ventricular cavities proximal to the blockage. There are two types of **congenital hydrocephalus**, both of which produce a noncommunicating (obstructive) hydrocephalus.

   a. **Congenital aqueductal stenosis** is the most common cause of congenital hydrocephalus. This type may be transmitted by an X-linked trait, or it may be caused by cytomegalovirus or toxoplasmosis.

   b. **Dandy-Walker syndrome** appears to be associated with atresia of the foramen of Magendie and foramina of Luschka (although it remains controversial). This syndrome is usually associated with dilation of the fourth ventricle, posterior fossa cyst, agenesis of the cerebellar vermis, small cerebellar hemispheres, occipital meningocele, and frequently agenesis of the splenium of the corpus callosum.

E. Porencephaly (encephaloclastic porencephaly) (Figure 7-10*A*) is the presence of one or more fluid-filled cystic cavities within the brain that may communicate with the ventricles, but do not extend to the cerebral cortical surface. The cysts are lined by ependyma and have smooth or irregular walls. These cysts form as a result of brain destruction early in gestation before the brain is capable of a glial response to form a scar.

F. Hydranencephaly (Figure 7-10*B, C*) is the presence of a huge, fluid-filled cystic cavity that completely replaces the cerebral hemispheres. The cyst is lined by glial and meningeal elements. This cystic cavity forms as a result of **occlusion of the internal carotid arteries** in utero causing widespread destruction of the cerebral cortex (the brain stem and cerebellum are usually spared, since vertebrobasilar circulation is not affected). Other causes include toxoplasmosis, rubella, cytomegalovirus, and herpesvirus.

G. Schizencephaly (Figure 7-10*D*) is the presence of a cerebral cortical cleft of brain tissue that extends from the ventricles to the cerebral cortical surface. The cleft is lined by cortical brain tissue and is fluid filled (i.e., a fluid-filled cleft). The cleft forms as a result of abnormal neuronal migration during embryologic formation of the brain.

H. Holoprosencephaly (arrhinencephaly) (Figure 7-10*E, F*) occurs when the prosencephalon fails to cleave down the midline such that the telencephalon contains a single ventricle. It is characterized by the absence of olfactory bulbs and tracts (arrhinencephaly) and is often seen in trisomy 13 (Patau syndrome), trisomy 18 (Edwards syndrome), short arm deletion of chromosome 18, and Meckel syndrome. Because the fetal face develops at the same time as the brain, facial anomalies (e.g., cyclopia, cleft lip, cleft palate) are commonly seen with holoprosencephaly. Holoprosencephaly is the most severe manifestation of **fetal alcohol syndrome** resulting from alcohol abuse during pregnancy (especially in the first 4 weeks of pregnancy). There are three types of holoprosencephaly:

1. **Alobar prosencephaly** (most severe form) occurs when there is complete absence of cleavage of the prosencephalon. Affected infants are stillborn or die shortly after birth and have cyclopia, single rudimentary proboscis, cleft lip, cleft palate, hypotelorism, and micrognathia. Sonographic findings include a single, horseshoe-shaped ventricle

(monoventricle), fused thalami, and a pancake-like mantle of undifferentiated cerebral cortical tissue.

2. **Semilobar prosencephaly** (intermediate form) occurs when there is absence of cleavage of the prosencephalon anteriorly but partial cleavage of the prosencephalon posteriorly.

3. **Lobar prosencephaly** (least severe form) occurs when there is absence of cleavage of the prosencephalon anteriorly but cleavage of the prosencephalon posteriorly.

I.   **Tethered spinal cord (filum terminale syndrome)** (Figure 7-10*G*) occurs when a thick, short filum terminale forms. The result is weakness and sensory deficits in the lower extremity and a neurogenic bladder. Tethered spinal cord is frequently associated with lipomatous tumors or meningomyeloceles. Deficits usually improve after transection.

J.   **Chordoma** is a tumor that arises from remnants of the notochord.

XIX. Selected Photographs, Sonograms, and Radiographs of Various Congenital Malformations

A. **Variations of spina bifida** (Figure 7-7)

B. **Variations of cranium bifida, anencephaly, and Arnold-Chiari malformation** (Figure 7-8)

C. **Communicating hydrocephalus, congenital aqueductal stenosis, and Dandy-Walker syndrome** (Figure 7-9)

D. **Porencephaly, hydranencephaly, schizencephaly, holoprosencephaly, and tethered spinal cord** (Figure 7-10)

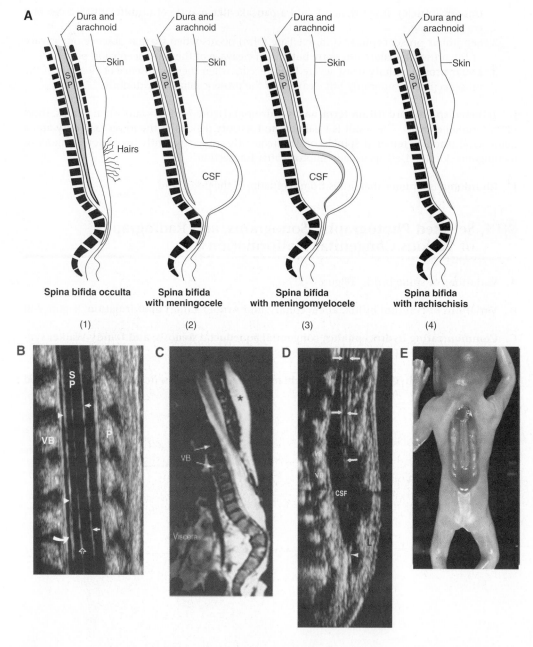

Figure 7-7. **(A)** Schematic drawings illustrating the various types of spina bifida. (*1*) Spina bifida occulta. (*2*) Spina bifida with meningocele. (*3*) Spina bifida with meningomyelocele. (*4*) Spina bifida with rachischisis. **(B)** Sonogram of a normal spinal cord in lower thoracic and upper lumbar region. Note the vertebral bodies (*VB*), spinous processes (*P*), spinal cord (*SP*) with its anterior median fissure (*open arrow*), posterior surface of the spinal cord (*arrows*), anterior surface of the spinal cord (*arrowheads*), and subarachnoid space containing cerebrospinal fluid (*curved arrow*). **(C)** Spina bifida occulta. Note the presence of the bony vertebral bodies (*VB*) along the entire length of the vertebral column. However, the bony spinous processes terminate much higher (*) because the vertebral arches fail to form properly. This creates a bony vertebral defect. The spinal cord is intact. **(D)** Spina bifida with meningomyelocele. Note the spinal cord (*arrows*), cerebrospinal fluid (*CSF*)-filled sac, a small subcutaneous lipoma (*L*), and the filum terminale (*arrowhead*). **(E)** Spina bifida with rachischisis. Photograph of a newborn infant shows the open neural tube on the back.

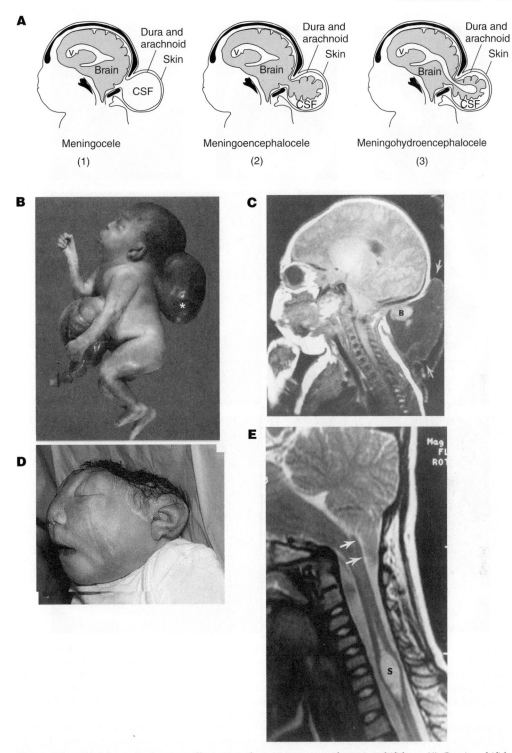

Figure 7-8. (**A**) Schematic drawings illustrating the various types of cranium bifidum. (*1*) Cranium bifida with meningocele. (*2*) Cranium bifida with meningoencephalocele. (*3*) Cranium bifida with meningohydroencephalocele. (**B**) Photograph of a fetus with an occipital encephalocele (*). (**C**) MRI of a meningoencephalocele demonstrates a large encephalocele (*arrows*) extending through an occipital bone defect that contains brain tissue (*B*). (**D**) Photograph of a newborn infant with anencephaly. (**E**) MRI of the Arnold-Chiari malformation. Note the herniation of the brain stem and cerebellum (*arrows*) through foramen magnum. Note the presence of a syrinx (*S*) in the cervical spinal cord.

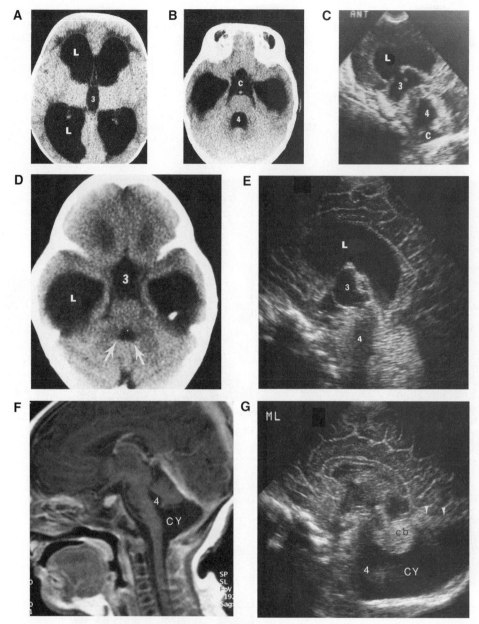

Figure 7-9. **(A to C)** Communicating hydrocephalus. **(A)** CT scan shows dilated lateral ventricles (*L*) and a dilated third ventricle (*3*). **(B)** CT scan (lower level) shows a dilated fourth ventricle (*4*) and the cisterna magna (*C*). **(C)** Sonogram shows the dilated lateral ventricle (*L*) communicating through a dilated foramen of Monro with a dilated third ventricle (*3*) and dilated fourth ventricle (*4*). The cisterna magna (*C*) is also shown. **(D, E)** Congenital aqueductal stenosis. **(D)** CT scan shows dilated lateral ventricles (*L*), dilated third ventricle (*3*), but normal-size fourth ventricle (*arrows*). Therefore, obstruction at the cerebral aqueduct is presumed. **(E)** Sonogram shows dilated lateral ventricles (*L*), dilated third ventricle (*3*), but normal-size fourth ventricle (*4*). Therefore, obstruction at the cerebral aqueduct is presumed. **(F, G)** Dandy-Walker syndrome. **(F)** MRI shows a dilated fourth ventricle (*4*) communicating with a posterior fossa cyst (*CY*) along with small cerebellar hemispheres. **(G)** Sonogram shows a massively dilated fourth ventricle (*4*) communicating with a large retrocerebellar fluid-filled cyst (*CY*) along with an elevated tentorium (*arrowheads*). Rudimentary cerebellar hemisphere (*cb*) can be observed.

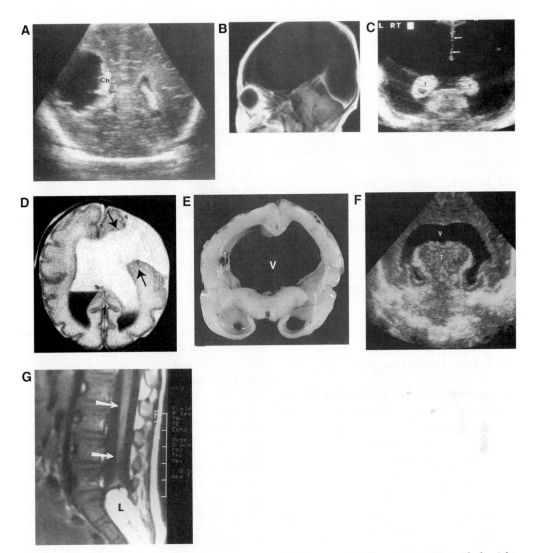

Figure 7-10. (A) Porencephaly. Sonogram shows a fluid-filled cystic cavity (*) communicating with the right lateral ventricle. *Ch* = choroid plexus. (B, C) Hydranencephaly. (B) MRI shows a huge, fluid-filled cystic cavity within the supratentorial compartment (*) that replaces the cerebral hemispheres. Note that the brain stem and cerebellum remain intact. (C) Coronal sonogram shows a huge, fluid-filled cystic cavity (*). Note that the thalami (*T*), cerebellar vermis (*V*), and falx cerebri (*arrows*) are normal. Compare this to holoprosencephaly. (D) Schizencephaly. MRI shows a cleft of brain tissue in the left cerebral hemisphere (*arrows*). This cleft is fluid filled and communicates with the lateral ventricles. (E, F) Holoprosencephaly. (E) Photograph of a gross specimen showing the failure of the prosencephalon to cleave down the midline. Note the single ventricle (*V*) surrounded by a mantle of cerebral cortical tissue, fused thalami (*T*), and absence of the falx cerebri. Compare this with hydranencephaly. (F) Sonogram shows a single, horseshoe-shaped ventricle (*V*) and fused thalami (*T*). (G) Tethered spinal cord. MRI shows a low-positioned spinal cord (*arrows*) attached to an intraspinal lipoma (*L*).

STUDY QUESTIONS FOR CHAPTER 7

Directions: *Each of the numbered items or incomplete statements in this section is followed by answers or by completions of the statement. Select the **one** lettered answer or completion that is **best** in each case.*

1. Which one of the following basal ganglia is derived from the diencephalon?

(A) Amygdaloid nucleus
(B) Head of the caudate nucleus
(C) Tail of the caudate nucleus
(D) Globus pallidus
(E) Putamen

2. When are the axons of the corticospinal tracts fully myelinated?

(A) In the late embryonic period
(B) In the mid-fetal period
(C) At birth
(D) By the end of the first postnatal year
(E) By the end of the second postnatal year

3. Which of the following represents the general somatic efferent (GSE) column of the pons?

(A) Abducens nucleus
(B) Nucleus ambiguus
(C) Hypoglossal nucleus
(D) Inferior olivary nucleus
(E) Inferior salivatory nucleus

4. Which of the following represents the general visceral efferent (GVE) column of the pons?

(A) Cerebellum
(B) Spinal trigeminal nucleus
(C) Principal trigeminal nucleus
(D) Superior salivatory nucleus
(E) Pontine nuclei

5. The external granular layer of the cerebellum gives rise to which of the following?

(A) Outer stellate cells
(B) Purkinje cells
(C) Granule cells
(D) Basket cells
(E) Giant cells of Betz

6. Which of the following statements best describes the pathogenesis of hydranencephaly?

(A) Results from failure of midline cleavage of the embryonic forebrain
(B) Results from atresia of the outlet foramina of the fourth ventricle
(C) Results from blockage of the cerebral aqueduct

(D) Results from internal carotid artery occlusion
(E) Results from failure of the anterior neuropore to close

7. The anterior and posterior neuropores close during which week of embryonic development?

(A) Week 2
(B) Week 3
(C) Week 4
(D) Week 5
(E) Week 6

8. At birth, the conus medullaris is found at which vertebral level?

(A) T-12
(B) L-1
(C) L-3
(D) S-1
(E) S-4

9. Which of the following structures is derived from the telencephalon?

(A) Pineal gland
(B) Hypothalamus
(C) Hippocampus
(D) Optic nerve (CN II)
(E) Globus pallidus

10. Which of the following conditions results from failure of the anterior neuropore to close?

(A) Hydrocephalus
(B) Anencephaly
(C) Mongolism
(D) Craniosynostosis
(E) Meningoencephalocele

11. Which of the following structures is derived from the diencephalon?

(A) Caudate nucleus
(B) Cerebellum
(C) Olfactory bulbs
(D) Neurohypophysis
(E) Adenohypophysis

12. Caudal herniation of the cerebellar tonsils and medulla through the foramen magnum is called

(A) Dandy-Walker syndrome
(B) Down syndrome

(C) Arnold-Chiari syndrome

(D) cranium bifidum

(E) myeloschisis

13. The flexure that develops between the metencephalon and the myelencephalon is called the

(A) cephalic flexure

(B) mesencephalic flexure

(C) pontine flexure

(D) cerebellar flexure

(E) cervical flexure

14. Which of the following statements best describes the sulcus limitans?

(A) It is found in the interpeduncular fossa

(B) It is located between the alar and basal plates

(C) It separates the medulla from the pons

(D) It separates the hypothalamus from the thalamus

(E) It separates the neocortex from the allocortex

15. Myelinated preganglionic sympathetic neurons have their cell bodies in

(A) Clarke's column

(B) substantia gelatinosa

(C) intermediolateral cell column

(D) intermediomedial cell column

16. The choroid plexus of the fourth ventricle is derived from the

(A) alar plate

(B) basal plate

(C) floor plate

(D) rhombic lip

(E) roof plate

17. Tanycytes are found principally in the

(A) area postrema

(B) cerebral aqueduct

(C) lateral ventricles

(D) third ventricle

(E) fourth ventricle

18. Which of the following most accurately describes the herniation of meninges and brain tissue through a defect in occipital bone?

(A) Cranium bifidum with meningoencephalocele

(B) Cranium bifidum with meningohydroencephalocele

(C) Cranium bifidum with meningocele

(D) Arnold-Chiari syndrome

(E) Dandy-Walker syndrome

19. Which of the following is the most common cause of congenital hydrocephalus?

(A) Cranium bifidum with meningoencephalocele

(B) Cranium bifidum with meningohydroencephalocele

(C) Aqueductal stenosis

(D) Arnold-Chiari syndrome

(E) Dandy-Walker syndrome

20. Which of the following is associated with atresia of the foramen of Magendie and foramina of Luschka?

(A) Cranium bifidum with meningoencephalocele

(B) Cranium bifidum with meningohydroencephalocele

(C) Aqueductal stenosis

(D) Arnold-Chiari syndrome

(E) Dandy-Walker syndrome

21. Which of the following is associated with platybasia and malformation of the occipitovertebral joint?

(A) Cranium bifidum with meningoencephalocele

(B) Cranium bifidum with meningohydroencephalocele

(C) Aqueductal stenosis

(D) Arnold-Chiari syndrome

(E) Dandy-Walker syndrome

22. A 22-year-old pregnant woman at 20 weeks of gestation comes to her OB/GYN for a normal examination. During routine blood tests, her serum α-fetoprotein (AFP) concentration is markedly increased for her gestational age. Ultrasonography reveals spina bifida in the fetus. At what week of gestation did this defect most likely occur?

(A) 1 to 2

(B) 4 to 6

(C) 9 to 11

(D) 12 to 15

(E) 16 to 19

23. Which structure is derived from the cranial neural crest cells?

(A) Lens of eye

(B) Pia mater

(C) Dura mater

(D) Pineal gland

(E) Olfactory placode, CN I

ANSWERS AND EXPLANATIONS

1. D. The globus pallidus has its origin from the diencephalon. Neuroblasts from the subthalamus migrate into the telencephalic white matter to form the globus pallidus.

2. E. Axons of the corticospinal tracts are fully myelinated by the end of the second postnatal year; Babinski's sign (extensor plantar reflex) is usually not elicitable before myelination of the corticospinal tracts.

3. A. The abducens nucleus represents the general somatic efferent (GSE) column of the pons.

4. D. The superior salivatory nucleus represents the GVE column of the pons. All somatic and visceral motor nuclei are derived from the basal plate. The cerebellum and pontine nuclei and the sensory nuclei of cranial nerves are derivatives of the alar plate.

5. C. New evidence documents that the external granular layer gives rise only to the granule cells of the internal granular layer and not to the basket (inner stellate) or stellate (outer stellate) neurons, as has long been thought. The giant cells of Betz are found in the cerebral cortex.

6. D. Hydranencephaly consists of huge intracerebral cavitation resulting from infarction in the territory of the internal carotid artery.

7. C. The anterior and posterior neuropores close during week 4 of development, the anterior on day 25, the posterior on day 27. Failure of the anterior neuropore to close results in anencephaly; failure of the posterior neuropore to close results in myeloschisis.

8. C. At birth, the conus medullaris extends to L-3, and in the adult it extends to the L1–L2 interspace. At 8 weeks, the spinal cord extends the entire length of the vertebral canal.

9. C. The hippocampus develops from the telencephalon. The pineal gland, hypothalamus, CN II, and globus pallidus are derived from the diencephalon.

10. B. Failure of the anterior neuropore to close results in anencephaly. The brain fails to develop; no cranial vault is formed.

11. D. The neurohypophysis develops from the diencephalon. The adenohypophysis (pars distalis, pars tuberalis, and pars intermedia) develops from Rathke's pouch, an ectodermal diverticulum of the stomodeum. The caudate nucleus and olfactory bulbs develop from the telencephalon. The cerebellum develops from the metencephalon.

12. C. Arnold-Chiari syndrome is a cerebellomedullary malformation in which the caudal vermis and medulla herniate through the foramen magnum, resulting in communicating hydrocephalus. Arnold-Chiari syndrome is frequently associated with spina bifida.

13. C. The pontine flexure develops between the metencephalon (pons) and the myelencephalon (medulla). The pontine flexure results in lateral expansion of the walls of the metencephalon and myelencephalon, stretching of the roof of the fourth ventricle, and widening of the floor of the fourth ventricle (rhomboid fossa).

14. B. The sulcus limitans separates the sensory alar from the motor basal plates. It is found in the developing spinal cord and on the surface of the adult rhomboid fossa of the fourth ventricle. The bulbopontine sulcus (inferior pontine sulcus) separates the medulla from the pons. The hypothalamic sulcus separates the thalamus from the hypothalamus. The rhinal sulcus separates the neocortex from the allocortex.

15. **C.** Myelinated preganglionic sympathetic neurons have their cell bodies in the intermediolateral cell column of the lateral horn; this cell column extends from C-8 to L-1. Myelinated preganglionic parasympathetic neurons have their cell bodies in the sacral autonomic nucleus, from S-2 to S-4.

16. **E.** The roof plate and its pial covering give rise to the choroid plexus, which invaginates into the fourth ventricle. The alar plate gives rise to sensory neurons; the basal plate gives rise to motor neurons; the floor plate contains decussating fibers; the rhombic lips give rise to the cerebellum.

17. **D.** Tanycytes are modified ependymal cells, found principally in the third ventricle. Tanycytes transport substances from the CSF to the hypophyseal portal system.

18. **A.** Cranium bifidum with meningoencephalocele consists of the herniation of meninges and brain tissue through a defect in occipital bone.

19. **C.** The most common cause of congenital hydrocephalus is aqueductal stenosis.

20. **E.** Dandy-Walker syndrome is congenital hydrocephalus associated with atresia of the outlet foramina of Magendie and Luschka. It is associated with agenesis of the cerebellar vermis and agenesis of the splenium of the corpus callosum.

21. **D.** Arnold-Chiari syndrome, a common congenital malformation, is frequently associated with platybasia and malformation of the occipitovertebral joint; other anomalies frequently seen are beaking of the tectum, aqueductal stenosis, kinking and herniation of the medulla, and herniation of the cerebellar vermis through the foramen magnum. Meningomyelocele (spina bifida) is a common component of the syndrome.

22. **B.** The posterior neuropore closes during week 4 (day 27). Failure of the posterior neuropore to close results in lower neural tube defects, such as spina bifida.

23. **B.** The pia mater is the only listed structure that is derived from the cranial neural crest cells. For a summary of germ cell derivatives refer to Table 4-1.

Ear

I. Overview

The ear is the organ of **balance** and **hearing**. The ear consists of an **internal**, a **middle**, and an **external ear**.

II. The Internal Ear (Figure 8-1)

The ear develops in week 4 from a thickening of the surface **ectoderm** called the **otic placode**. The otic placode invaginates into the connective tissue (mesenchyme) adjacent to the rhombencephalon and becomes the **otic vesicle**. The otic vesicle divides into **utricular** and **saccular portions**.

A. **Utricular portion** of the otic vesicle gives rise to the following:
 1. **Utricle** contains the sensory hair cells and otoliths of the macula utriculi. The utricle responds to **linear acceleration** and the **force of gravity**.
 2. **Semicircular ducts** contain the sensory hair cells of the cristae ampullares. They respond to **angular acceleration**.
 3. **Vestibular ganglion of CN VIII** lies at the base of the internal auditory meatus.
 4. **Endolymphatic duct and sac** is a membranous duct that connects the saccule to the utricle and terminates in a blind sac beneath the dura. The endolymphatic sac absorbs endolymph.

B. **Saccular portion** of the otic vesicle gives rise to the following:
 1. **Saccule** contains the sensory hair cells and otoliths of the macula sacculi. The saccule responds to **linear acceleration** and the **force of gravity**.
 2. **Cochlear duct (organ of Corti)** is involved in hearing. This duct has pitch (tonotopic) localization whereby high-frequency sound waves (20,000 Hz) are detected at the base and low-frequency sound waves (20 Hz) are detected at the apex.
 3. **Spiral ganglion of CN VIII** lies in the modiolus of the bony labyrinth.

III. The Membranous and Bony Labyrinth

The membranous labyrinth consists of all the structures derived from the otic vesicle (Table 8-1). The membranous labyrinth is initially surrounded by neural crest cells that form a connective tissue (mesenchyme) covering. This connective tissue becomes cartilaginous, then ossifies to become the **bony labyrinth** of the temporal bone. The connective tissue closest to the membra-

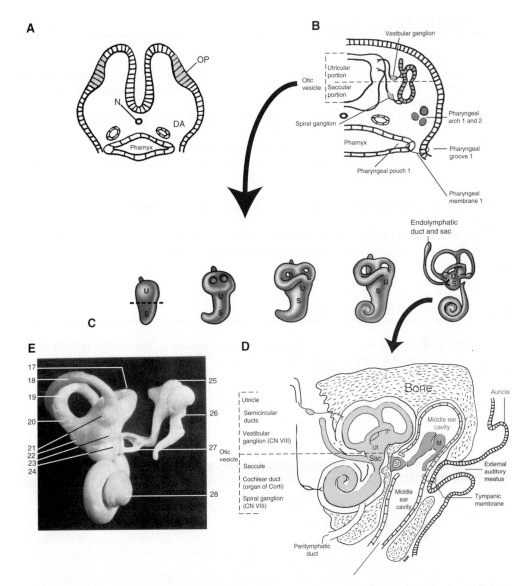

Figure 8-1. Schematic transverse sections showing the formation of the otic placode and otic vesicle from the surface ectoderm. **(A)** The otic placode is distinguished by a thickening of the surface ectoderm. *DA* = dorsal aorta; *N* = notochord; *OP* = otic placode. **(B)** The otic placode invaginates into the underlying connective tissue (mesenchyme) and becomes the otic vesicle. **(C)** The otic vesicle undergoes extensive changes to form the adult membranous labyrinth. *U* = utricle; *S* = saccule. **(D)** The adult ear. *M* = malleus; *I* = incus; *St* = stapes. **(E)** The adult auditory ossicles in connection with the membranous labyrinth (or internal ear). *17* = lateral semicircular canal; *18* = anterior semicircular canal; *19* = posterior semicircular canal; *20* = common crus; *21* = ampulla; *22* = beginning of the endolymphatic duct; *23* = utricle; *24* = saccule; *25* = incus; *26* = malleus; *27* = stapes; *28* = cochlea.

nous labyrinth degenerates, thus forming the **perilymphatic space** containing **perilymph**. This sets up the interesting anatomic relationship whereby the membranous labyrinth is suspended (or floats) within the bony labyrinth by perilymph. Perilymph that is similar in composition to **CSF** communicates with the subarachnoid space via the **perilymphatic duct**.

IV. Middle Ear (see Figure 8-1)

A. **Ossicles of the middle ear**
   1. **Malleus** develops from cartilage of **pharyngeal arch 1** (Meckel's cartilage) and is attached to the tympanic membrane. The malleus is moved by the **tensor tympani muscle**, which is innervated by CN V_3.
   2. **Incus** develops from the cartilage of **pharyngeal arch 1** (Meckel's cartilage). The incus articulates with the malleus and stapes.
   3. **Stapes** develops from the cartilage of **pharyngeal arch 2** (Reichert's cartilage). The stapes is moved by the **stapedius muscle**, which is innervated by CN VII. It is attached to the oval window of the vestibule.

B. **Auditory tube and middle ear cavity** both develop from **pharyngeal pouch 1**.

C. **Tympanic membrane** develops from **pharyngeal membrane 1**. This membrane separates the middle ear from the external auditory meatus of the external ear. It is innervated by CN V_3 and CN IX.

V. External Ear (see Figure 8-1)

A. **External auditory meatus** develops from **pharyngeal groove 1**. The meatus becomes filled with ectodermal cells, forming a temporary **meatal plug** that disappears before birth. The meatus is innervated by **CN V_3 and CN IX.**

B. **Auricle (or pinna)** develops from **six auricular hillocks** that surround pharyngeal groove 1. The auricle is innervated by **CN V_3, CN VII, CN IX, and CN X,** and **cervical nerves C_2 and C_3.**

TABLE 8–1	*Embryonic Ear Structures and Their Adult Derivatives*
Embryonic Structure	**Adult Derivative**
	Internal Ear
Otic vesicle	
Utricular portion	Utricle, semicircular ducts, vestibular ganglion of CN VIII, endolymphatic duct and sac
Saccular portion	Saccule, cochlear duct (organ of Corti) spiral ganglion of CN VIII
	Middle Ear
Pharyngeal arch 1	Malleus, incus, tensor tympani muscle
Pharyngeal arch 2	Stapes, stapedius muscle
Pharyngeal pouch 1	Auditory tube, middle ear cavity
Pharyngeal membrane 1	Tympanic membrane
	External Ear
Pharyngeal groove 1	External auditory meatus
Auricular hillocks	Auricle

CN = cranial nerve.

VI. Congenital Malformations of the Ear (Figure 8-2)

A. Minor auricular malformations are commonly found and raise only cosmetic issues. However, auricular malformations are seen in **Down syndrome (trisomy 21)**, **Patau syndrome (trisomy 13)**, and **Edwards syndrome (trisomy 18)**.

B. Low-set slanted auricles are auricles that are located below a line extended from the corner of the eye to the occiput. This condition may indicate chromosomal abnormalities as indicated above.

C. Preauricular sinus is a narrow tube or shallow pit that has a pinpoint external opening that is most often asymptomatic and of minor cosmetic importance (although infections may occur). The embryologic basis is uncertain but probably involves pharyngeal groove 1.

D. Auricular appendages are skin tags that are commonly found anterior to the auricle (i.e., pre-tragal area) and which raise only cosmetic issues. The embryologic basis is the formation of accessory auricle hillocks.

E. Atresia of the external auditory meatus A **complete atresia** consists of a bony plate in the location of the tympanic membrane. A **partial atresia** consists of a soft tissue plug in the location of the tympanic membrane. This results in conduction deafness and is usually associated with the first arch syndrome. The embryologic basis is the failure of the meatal plug to canalize.

F. Congenital cholesteatoma (epidermoid cyst) is a benign tumor found in the middle ear cavity that results in conduction deafness. The embryologic basis is the proliferation of endodermal cells lining the middle ear cavity.

G. Microtia is a severely disorganized auricle that is associated with other malformations resulting in deafness. The embryologic basis is impaired proliferation or fusion of the auricular hillocks.

H. Congenital deafness The organ of Corti may be damaged by exposure to **rubella virus**, especially during week 7 and week 8 of development.

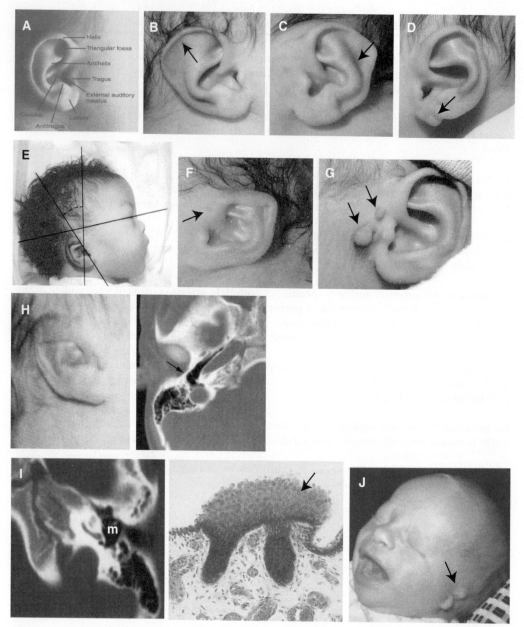

Figure 8-2. (A) Nomenclature of the adult auricle. (B) A minor auricular variation showing minimal folding of the helix (*arrow*), posterior rotation, and mildly low-set auricles. (C) A minor auricular variation showing a partially folded helix with a prominent antihelix (*arrow*). (D) A minor auricular variation showing a cleft lobule (*arrow*). (E) A severely low-set and posteriorly rotated auricle in an infant with Stickler syndrome. (F) Preauricular sinus is shown in the pretragal area (*arrow*). (G) Auricular appendages (i.e., skin tags) are shown in the pretragal area (*arrows*). (H) Atresia of the external auditory meatus. Photograph shows absence of the external auditory meatus in this infant. CT scan shows microtia, absence of aerated external auditory meatus (*), and a bony plate (*arrow*) near the tympanic membrane. (I) Congenital cholesteatoma. CT scan shows a visible mass (*m*) behind the tympanic membrane (*arrow*). Light microscopy shows a large epidermoid formation (*arrow*). (J) Microtia shows a severely disorganized auricle (*arrow*).

STUDY QUESTIONS FOR CHAPTER 8

*Directions: Each of the numbered items or incomplete statements in this section is followed by answers or by completions of the statement. Select the **one** lettered answer or completion that is **best** in each case.*

1. The cochlear duct contains the spiral organ of Corti and is derived from which of the following?

(A) Both ectoderm and mesoderm
(B) Neural crest
(C) Endoderm
(D) Mesoderm
(E) Ectoderm

2. The middle ear cavity

(A) is of mesodermal origin
(B) develops from pharyngeal pouch 1
(C) develops from pharyngeal arch 1
(D) develops from pharyngeal arch 2
(E) develops from the otic vesicle

3. The otic vesicle

(A) gives rise to the bony labyrinth
(B) is found adjacent to the rhomben-cephalon
(C) is derived from neuroectoderm
(D) gives rise to the auricle (pinna)
(E) gives rise to the tympanic membrane

4. The auricle (pinna) of the external ear is innervated by which of the following nerves?

(A) CN V_3
(B) CN V_2
(C) CN XII
(D) CN III
(E) CN VIII

5. The stapedius muscle that moves the stapes ossicle is innervated by

(A) CN V_3
(B) CN XII
(C) CN III
(D) CN VII
(E) cervical nerves C_2 and C_3

6. The utricular portion of the otic vesicle gives rise to the

(A) ductus reuniens
(B) cochlear duct
(C) endolymphatic sac
(D) scala vestibuli
(E) scala tympani

7. The saccular portion of the otic vesicle gives rise to the

(A) organ of Corti
(B) endolymphatic duct
(C) superior semicircular canal
(D) crus commune nonampullare
(E) lateral semicircular canal

8. The tubotympanic recess gives rise to

(A) a conduit that interconnects the middle ear and the nasopharynx
(B) the external auditory meatus
(C) the internal auditory meatus
(D) the facial canal
(E) a conduit that interconnects the perilymphatic space with the subarachnoid space

9. Perilymph enters the subarachnoid space via the

(A) cochlear duct
(B) ductus reuniens
(C) perilymphatic duct
(D) vestibular aqueduct
(E) utriculosaccular duct

10. Pharyngeal groove 1 gives rise to the

(A) internal auditory meatus
(B) external auditory meatus
(C) eustachian tube
(D) cervical sinus
(E) primary tympanic cavity

ANSWERS AND EXPLANATIONS

1. E. The cochlear duct is derived from a thickening of the surface ectoderm called the otic placode.

2. B. The middle ear cavity develops from pharyngeal pouch 1 as it evaginates to form the tubotympanic recess.

3. B. The otic vesicle arises from an invagination of the surface ectoderm called the otic placode. The otic vesicle is found adjacent to the rhombencephalon.

4. A. The auricle (pinna) of the external ear is innervated by cranial nerves V_3 (mandibular division), VII, IX, and X; cervical nerves C_2 and C_3 also innervate the auricle.

5. D. The stapes is innervated by CN VII.

6. C. The utricular region of the otic vesicle gives rise to the endolymphatic sac and duct, and semicircular ducts.

7. A. The saccular region of the otic vesicle gives rise to the cochlear duct, which houses the spiral organ of Corti.

8. A. The tubotympanic recess is derived from pharyngeal pouch 1. It gives rise to the tympanic cavity and the auditory (eustachian) tube; the auditory tube interconnects the tympanic cavity with the nasopharynx.

9. C. The perilymph enters the subarachnoid space of the posterior cranial fossa via the cochlear aqueduct, which contains the perilymphatic duct.

10. B. Pharyngeal groove 1 gives rise to the external auditory meatus.

Eye

I. Development of Optic Vesicle (Figure 9-1)

The development of the optic vesicle begins at day 22 with the formation of **optic sulcus**, which evaginates from the wall of the diencephalon as the **optic vesicle** consisting of **neuroectoderm**. The optic vesicle invaginates and forms a double-layered **optic cup** and **optic stalk**. *PAX6* is the master homeotic gene in eye development. PAX6 is expressed predominately in the optic cup and lens placode. *PAX2* is expressed predominately in the optic stalk.

A. The optic cup and its derivatives   The double-layered optic cup consists of an **outer pigment layer** and **inner neural layer**.
  1. **Retina.**   The outer pigment layer of the optic cup gives rise to the **pigment layer of the retina**. The **intraretinal space** separates the outer pigment layer from the inner neural layer. Although the intraretinal space is obliterated in the adult, it remains a weakened area prone to **retinal detachment**. The inner neural layer of the otic cup gives rise to the **neural layer of the retina** (i.e., the rods and cones, bipolar cells, ganglion cells, etc.).
  2. **Iris** (Figure 9-2).   The epithelium of the iris develops from the anterior portions of both the outer pigment layer and inner neural layer of the optic cup, which explains its histologic appearance of two layers of columnar epithelium. The stroma develops from mesoderm continuous with the choroid. The iris contains the **dilator pupillae muscle** and **sphincter pupillae muscle** that are formed from the epithelium of the outer pigment layer by a transformation of these epithelial cells into contractile cells.
  3. **Ciliary body** (see Figure 9-2).   The epithelium of the ciliary body develops from the anterior portions of both the outer pigment layer and the inner neural layer of the optic cup, which explains its histologic appearance of two layers of columnar epithelium. The stroma develops from mesoderm continuous with the choroid. The ciliary body contains the **ciliary muscle**, which is formed from mesoderm within the choroid. The **ciliary processes** are components of the ciliary body.
     a. The ciliary processes produce **aqueous humor**, which circulates through the posterior and anterior chambers and drains into the venous circulation via the **trabecular meshwork** and the **canal of Schlemm**.
     b. The ciliary processes give rise to the **suspensory fibers** of the lens (ciliary zonule), which attach to and suspend the lens.

B. The optic stalk and its derivatives   The optic stalk contains the **choroid fissure** in which the **hyaloid artery and vein** are found. The hyaloid artery and vein later become the **central artery and vein of the retina**. The optic stalk contains axons from the ganglion cell layer of the retina. The choroid fissure closes during week 7 so that the optic stalk, together with the axons of the ganglion cells, forms the **optic nerve (CN II), optic chiasm, and optic tract**. The optic nerve (CN II) is a tract of the diencephalon and has the following characteristics:

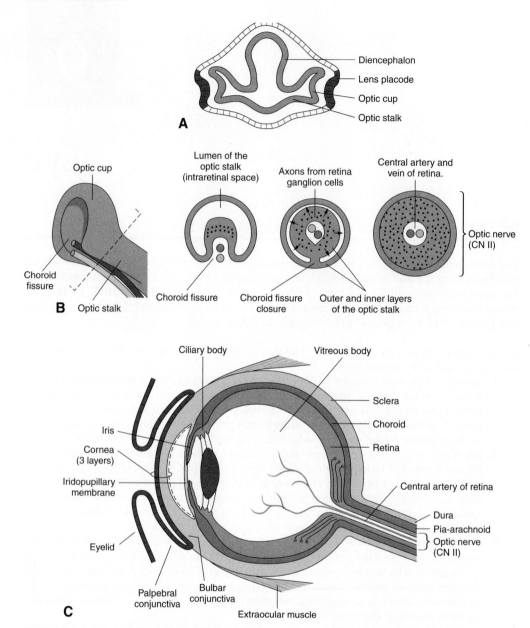

Figure 9-1. (A) The optic cup and optic stalk are evaginations of the diencephalon. The optic cup induces surface ectoderm to differentiate into the lens placode. (B) Formation of the optic nerve (CN II) from the optic stalk. The choroid fissure, which is located on the undersurface of the optic stalk permits access of the hyaloid artery and vein to the inner aspect of the eye. The choroid fissure eventually closes. As ganglion cells form in the retina, axons accumulate in the optic stalk and cause the inner and outer layers of the optic stalk to fuse, obliterating the lumen (or intraretinal space) and forming the optic nerve. (C) The adult eye. Note that the sclera is continuous with the dura mater and the choroid is continuous with the pia-arachnoid. The iridopupillary membrane is normally obliterated.

1. It is not completely myelinated until 3 months after birth; it is myelinated by oligodendrocytes.
2. It is not capable of regeneration after transection.
3. It is invested by the meninges and therefore is surrounded by a subarachnoid space, which plays a role in papilledema.

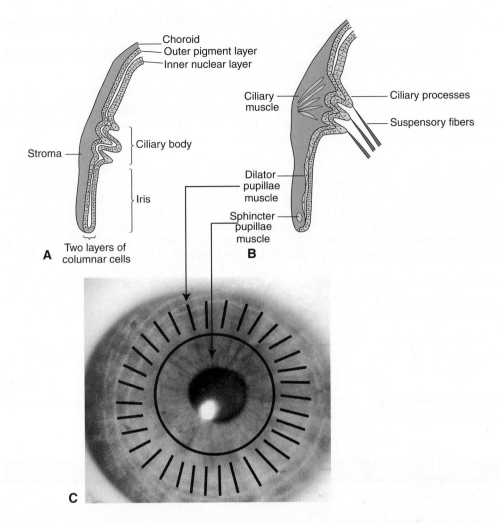

Figure 9-2. (**A** and **B**) Sagittal sections through the developing iris and ciliary body. The iris and ciliary body form from the outer pigment layer and inner neural layer of the optic cup. In the adult, this embryologic origin is reflected histologically by two layers of columnar epithelium that line both the iris and the ciliary body. Note the dilator and sphincter pupillae muscles associated with the iris and the ciliary muscle associated with the ciliary body. (**C**) Photograph of the human eye. Note the radial arrangement (spokelike pattern) of the dilator pupillae muscle around the entire iris as well as the circular arrangement of the sphincter pupillae muscle around the edge of the entire iris.

II. Development of Other Eye Structures

A. Sclera The sclera develops from mesoderm surrounding the optic cup. The sclera forms an outer **fibrous** layer that is continuous with the dura mater posteriorly and the cornea anteriorly.

B. Choroid The choroid develops from mesoderm surrounding the optic cup. The choroid forms a **vascular** layer that is continuous with the pia/arachnoid posteriorly and iris/ciliary body anteriorly.

C. Anterior chamber The anterior chamber develops from mesoderm over the anterior aspect of the eye. It is continuous with the sclera and undergoes vacuolization to form a chamber. The anterior chamber essentially splits the mesoderm into two layers:

1. The mesoderm posterior to the anterior chamber is called the **iridopupillary membrane,** which is normally resorbed before birth.
2. The mesoderm anterior to the anterior chamber develops into the **substantia propria of the cornea** and **corneal endothelium.**

D. Cornea   The cornea develops from both surface ectoderm and mesoderm lying anterior to the anterior chamber. The surface ectoderm forms the **anterior epithelium of the cornea.** The mesoderm forms the **substantia propria of the cornea (i.e., Bowman's layer, stroma, and Descemet's membrane)** and **corneal endothelium.**

E. Lens   The lens develops from surface ectoderm that forms the **lens placode.** The lens placode invaginates to form the **lens vesicle.** The adult lens is completely surrounded by a **lens capsule.** The **lens epithelium** is a simple cuboidal epithelium located beneath the capsule only on the anterior surface. The lens epithelium is mitotically active and migrates to the equatorial region of the lens. The **lens fibers** are prismatic remnants of the lens epithelium that lose their nuclei and organelles. These fibers are filled with cytoskeletal proteins called **filensin** and **α, β, γ-crystallin,** which maintain the conformation and transparency of the lens.

F. Vitreous body   The vitreous body develops from mesoderm that migrates through the choroid fissure and forms a transparent gelatinous substance between the lens and retina. It contains the **hyaloid artery,** which later obliterates to form the **hyaloid canal** of the adult eye.

G. Canal of Schlemm   The canal of Schlemm is found at the sclerocorneal junction called the **limbus** and drains the aqueous humor into the venous circulation. An obstruction of the canal of Schlemm results in increased intraocular pressure (**glaucoma**).

H. Extraocular muscles   The extraocular muscles develop from mesoderm of **somitomeres 1, 2, 3** (also called preotic myotomes) that surround the optic cup.

TABLE 9–1	*Embryonic Eye Structures and Their Adult Derivatives*
Embryonic Structure	**Adult Derivative**
Diencephalon (neuroectoderm) Optic cup	Retina, iris epithelium, dilator and sphincter pupillae muscles of iris, ciliary body epithelium
Optic stalk	Optic nerve (CN II), optic chiasm, optic tract
Surface ectoderm	Lens, anterior epithelium of cornea, bulbar and palpebral conjunctiva
Mesoderm	Sclera, choroid, stroma of iris, stroma of ciliary body, ciliary muscle, substantia propria of cornea, corneal endothelium, vitreous body, central artery and vein of retina, extraocular muscles

III. Congenital Malformations of the Eye (Figure 9-3)

A. Coloboma iridis is a cleft in the iris caused by failure of the choroid fissure to close in week 7 of development and may extend into the ciliary body, retina, choroid, or optic nerve. A **palpebral coloboma**, a notch in the eyelid, results from a defect in the developing eyelid.

B. Congenital cataracts are opacities of the lens and are usually bilateral. They are fairly common and may result from the following: rubella virus infection, toxoplasmosis, congenital syphilis, Down syndrome (trisomy 21), or galactosemia (an inborn error of metabolism).

C. Congenital glaucoma (buphthalmos) is increased intraocular pressure due to abnormal development of the canal of Schlemm or the iridocorneal filtration angle. It is usually genetically determined but may result from maternal rubella infection.

D. Detached retina (see Figure 9-3D) may result from head trauma or may be congenital. The site of detachment is between the outer and inner layers of the optic cup (i.e., between the retinal pigment epithelial layer and outer segment layer of rods and cones of the neural retina).

E. Persistent iridopupillary membrane consists of strands of connective tissue that partially cover the pupil; however, it seldom affects vision.

F. Microphthalmia is a small eye, usually associated with intrauterine infections from the TORCH group of microorganisms (Toxoplasma, other agents, rubella virus, cytomegalovirus, and herpes simplex virus).

G. Anophthalmia is absence of the eye. It is due to failure of the optic vesicle to form.

H. Cyclopia is a single orbit and one eye. It is due to failure of median cerebral structures to develop.

I. Retinocele results from herniation of the retina into the sclera or from failure of the choroid fissure to close.

J. Retrolental fibroplasia (retinopathy of prematurity) is an oxygen-induced retinopathy seen in premature infants.

K. Papilledema is edema of the optic disk (papilla) due to increased intracranial pressure. This pressure is reflected into the subarachnoid space, which surrounds the optic nerve (CN II).

L. Retinitis pigmentosa (RP) is a hereditary degeneration and atrophy of the retina. RP may be transmitted as an autosomal recessive, autosomal dominant, or X-linked trait. It is characterized by a degeneration of the rods, night blindness (nyctalopia), and "gun barrel vision." RP may also be due to abetalipoproteinemia (Bassen-Kornzweig syndrome), which may be arrested with massive doses of vitamin A.

M. Retinoblastoma (RB) is a tumor of the retina that occurs in childhood and develops from precursor cells in the immature retina. The RB gene is located on chromosome 13q and encodes for RB protein that binds to a gene regulatory protein and causes suppression of the cell cycle; that is, the RB gene is a **tumor-suppressor gene** (also called an **anti-oncogene**). A mutation in the RB gene encodes an abnormal RB protein such that there is no suppression of the cell cycle. This leads to the formation of RB. Hereditary RB causes multiple tumors in both eyes. Nonhereditary RB causes one tumor in one eye.

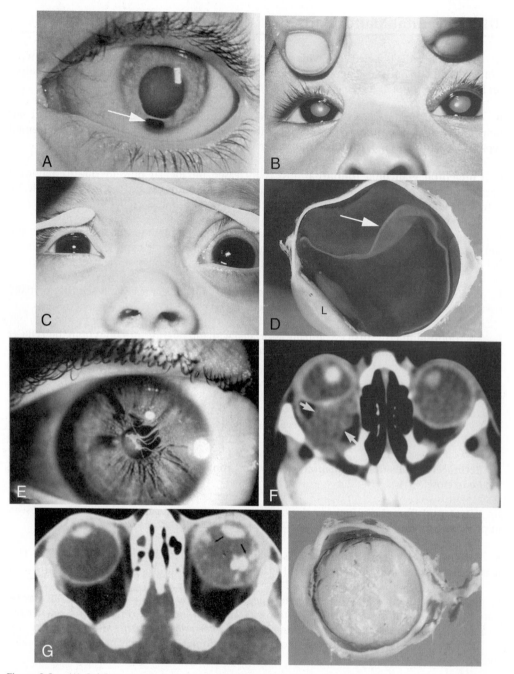

Figure 9-3. **(A)** Coloboma iridis. Note the cleft in the iris (*black spot at arrow*). **(B)** Congenital cataracts. Note the lens opacities in both eyes. **(C)** Congenital glaucoma (buphthalmos). Note the enlarged left eye and normal right eye. **(D)** Detached retina. Note the retina (*arrow*) detached from the choroid and sclera. *L* = lens. **(E)** Persistent iridopupillary membrane. Note the strands of connective tissue that partially cover the pupil. **(F)** Microphthalmia. CT scan shows exophthalmos, small right globe, and a retroocular mass (*arrows*). **(G)** Retinoblastoma. CT scan shows multiple tumor calcifications (*arrows*) within the left intraorbital mass. Photograph shows a large-sized retinoblastoma that fills the entire eye.

Directions: *Each of the numbered items or incomplete statements in this section is followed by answers or by completions of the statement. Select the **one** lettered answer or completion that is **best** in each case.*

1. The surface ectoderm gives rise to which of the following structures?

(A) Dilator pupillae muscle
(B) Retina
(C) Lens
(D) Sclera
(E) Choroid

2. Failure of the choroid fissure to close results in

(A) congenital detached retina
(B) congenital aniridia
(C) congenital aphakia
(D) coloboma iridis
(E) microphthalmos

3. The optic cup is an evagination of which of the following?

(A) Telencephalon
(B) Diencephalon
(C) Mesencephalon
(D) Metencephalon
(E) Myelencephalon

4. The epithelium of the ciliary body is derived from

(A) ectoderm
(B) mesoderm
(C) endoderm
(D) neuroectoderm
(E) neural crest cells

5. Hyperoxygenation of premature infants may result in

(A) congenital glaucoma
(B) microphthalmia
(C) coloboma
(D) retrolental fibroplasia
(E) persistent pupillary membrane

6. The optic nerve is a tract of the diencephalon that is not completely myelinated until

(A) 5 years after birth
(B) 2 years after birth
(C) 1 year after birth
(D) 3 weeks after birth
(E) 3 months after birth

7. The hyaloid canal is found in the

(A) vitreous body
(B) choroid
(C) optic stalk
(D) ciliary body
(E) intraretinal space

8. Aqueous humor is produced by the

(A) choroid plexus
(B) trabecular meshwork
(C) ciliary processes
(D) vitreous body
(E) lens vesicle

9. Aqueous humor enters the venous circulation via

(A) arachnoid villi
(B) scleral canal
(C) hyaloid canal
(D) canal of Schlemm
(E) Cloquet's canal

10. In a detached retina, the site of detachment is found

(A) within the outer plexiform layer
(B) within the inner plexiform layer
(C) between the inner nuclear layer and the outer nuclear layer
(D) between the choriocapillaris and the pigment epithelial layer
(E) between the pigment epithelial layer and the layer of outer segments of rods and cones

ANSWERS AND EXPLANATIONS

1. C. The lens forms from the lens placode that is induced by the optic cup.

2. D. Failure of the choroid (optic) fissure to close results in a cleft of the iris, a coloboma iridis. This defect may extend into the ciliary body, choroid, optic nerve, or retina. Congenital aphakia, absence of the lens, may result from defective development of the lens placode.

3. B. The optic cup and its derivatives, the retina and optic nerve, develop from the diencephalon.

4. D. The ciliary body is derived from the anterior two layers of the optic cup (neuroectoderm), which form the epithelium and form an anterior extension of the choroid (mesoderm).

5. D. Retrolental fibroplasia results from hyperoxygenation of premature infants. In premature infants, high oxygen concentration results in vaso-obliteration of the terminal arterioles, leading to hemorrhage and infarction of the retina. This phenomenon is peculiar to the incompletely vascularized peripheral retina.

6. E. The axons of the optic nerve are not completely myelinated until 3 months after birth. Myelinated axons are normally not found in the retina. The optic nerve is not a true peripheral nerve but a tract of the diencephalon; when severed, the optic nerve does not regenerate. Myelination in the CNS is accomplished by oligodendrocytes; oligodendrocytes are not found in the retina.

7. A. The hyaloid canal (Cloquet's canal) is found in the vitreous body. In early development, a hyaloid artery passes through the vitreous body to perfuse the developing lens; in the late fetal period, this artery obliterates to form the hyaloid canal.

8. C. Aqueous humor is produced by the ciliary processes of the ciliary body. It flows from the posterior chamber, through the pupil, into the anterior chamber, and finally to the canal of Schlemm, which empties into the extraocular veins.

9. D. Aqueous humor enters the venous circulation via the canal of Schlemm. Blockage of this canal results in increased intraocular pressure (glaucoma).

10. E. The site of retinal detachment is between the pigment epithelial layer and the layer of outer segments of rods and cones; this corresponds to the intraretinal space between the inner and outer layers of the optic cup. Retinal detachment occurs when fluid from the vitreous compartment passes through a retinal hole and separates the pigment epithelial layer from the layer of outer segments of rods and cones.

Digestive System

I.   Overview (Figure 10-1)

The **primitive gut tube** is formed from the incorporation of the dorsal part of the yolk sac into the embryo as a result of the craniocaudal folding and lateral folding of the embryo. The primitive gut tube extends from the oropharyngeal membrane to the cloacal membrane and is divided into the **foregut, midgut,** and **hindgut.** Histologically, the general plan of the adult gastrointestinal tract consists of a **mucosa** (epithelial lining and glands, lamina propria, and muscularis mucosae), **submucosa, muscularis externa,** and **adventitia** or **serosa.** Embryologically, the epithelial lining and glands of the mucosa are derived from endoderm, whereas the other components are derived from visceral mesoderm. Early in development, the epithelial lining the gut tube proliferates rapidly and obliterates the lumen. Later, **recanalization** occurs.

II.   Derivatives of the Foregut

Foregut derivatives are supplied by the **celiac trunk.** The exception to this is the esophagus, whereby the intra-abdominal portion of the esophagus is supplied by the celiac trunk, but the intrathoracic portion is supplied by other branches of the aorta.

A. Esophagus
1. **Development.** The foregut is divided into the esophagus dorsally and the trachea ventrally by the **tracheoesophageal folds,** which fuse to form the **tracheoesophageal septum.** The esophagus is initially short but lengthens with descent of the heart and lungs. During development, the endodermal lining of the esophagus proliferates rapidly and obliterates the lumen; later recanalization occurs.
2. **Sources.** The stratified squamous epithelium, mucosal glands, and submucosal glands of the definitive esophagus are derived from endoderm. The lamina propria, muscularis mucosae, submucosa, skeletal muscle and smooth muscle of muscularis externa, and adventitia of the definitive esophagus are derived from visceral mesoderm.
3. **Clinical considerations** (Figure 10-2)
    a. **Esophageal atresia** occurs when the tracheoesophageal septum deviates too far dorsally, causing the esophagus to end as a closed tube. About 33% of patients with esophageal atresia have other congenital defects associated with the VATER (vertebral defects, anal atresia, tracheoesophageal fistula, and renal defects) or VACTERL (similar to VATER but includes cardiovascular defects and upper limb defects) syndromes. It is associated clinically with polyhydramnios (fetus is unable to swallow amniotic fluid) and a tracheoesophageal fistula.

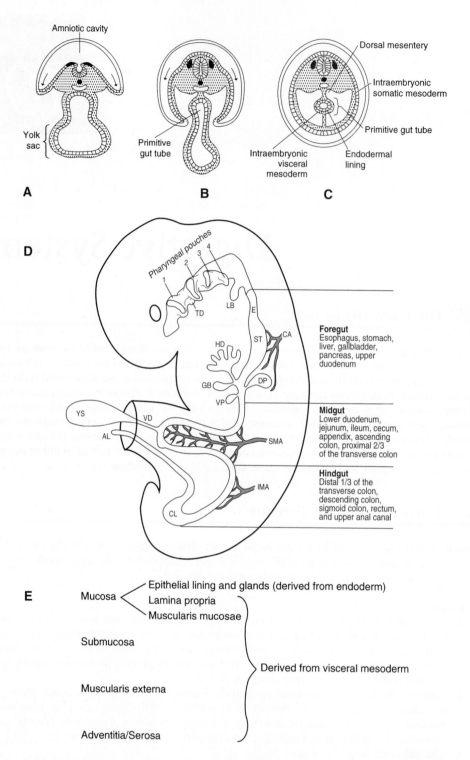

Figure 10-1. (A, B, C) Cross sections of an embryo showing the formation of the primitive gut tube. (D) Development of gastrointestinal tract showing the foregut, midgut, and hindgut along with the adult derivatives. The entire length of the endodermal gut tube is shown from the mouth to the anus. The fates of the lung bud (*LB*), pharyngeal pouches (*1, 2, 3, 4*), and thyroid diverticulum (*TD*) are covered in later chapters. *AL* = allantois; *CA* = celiac artery; *CL* = cloaca; *DP* = dorsal pancreatic bud; *E* = esophagus; *GB* = gallbladder; *HD* = hepatic diverticulum; *IMA* = inferior mesenteric artery; *SMA* = superior mesenteric artery; *ST* = stomach; *VD* = vitelline duct; *VP* = ventral pancreatic bud; *YS* = yolk sac. (E) Diagram showing the general plan of histologic and embryologic organization of the adult gastrointestinal tract.

    b. **Esophageal stenosis** occurs when the lumen of the esophagus is narrowed and usually involves the midesophagus. The stenosis may be caused by submucosal/muscularis externa hypertrophy, remnants of the tracheal cartilaginous ring within the wall of the esophagus, or a membranous diaphragm obstructing the lumen probably due to incomplete recanalization.

    c. **Esophageal duplication** occurs most commonly because of a congenital esophageal cyst that is usually (60% of cases) found in the lower esophagus. Duplication cysts may lie on the posterior aspect of the esophagus where they protrude into the posterior mediastinum or within the wall of the esophagus (i.e., intramural).

    d. **Vascular compression of the esophagus** is caused by the abnormal origin of the **right subclavian artery** due to developmental anomalies of the aortic arches. The anomalous right subclavian artery passes from the aortic arch behind the esophagus and may cause dysphagia (dysphagia lusoria).

    e. **Achalasia** occurs because of the loss of ganglion cells in the myenteric (Auerbach) plexus and is characterized by the failure to relax the lower esophageal sphincter, which causes progressive dysphagia and difficulty in swallowing.

B. Stomach   (Figure 10-3)

    1. **Development.** A fusiform dilatation forms in the foregut in week 4; this gives rise to the **primitive stomach**. The dorsal part of the primitive stomach grows faster than the ventral part, resulting in the greater and lesser curvatures, respectively. The primitive stomach rotates 90° clockwise around its longitudinal axis. The 90° rotation affects all foregut structures and is responsible for the adult anatomic relationship of foregut viscera. As a result of this clockwise rotation, the dorsal mesentery is carried to the left and eventually forms the **greater omentum;** the **left vagus nerve (CN X)** innervates the ventral surface of the stomach; and the **right vagus nerve (CN X)** innervates the dorsal surface of the stomach.

    2. **Sources.** Surface mucous cells lining the stomach, mucous neck cells, parietal cells, chief cells, and enteroendocrine cells comprising the gastric glands of the definitive stomach are derived from endoderm. The lamina propria; muscularis mucosae; submucosa; the outer longitudinal, middle circular, and inner oblique layers of smooth muscle of the muscularis externa; and the serosa of the definitive stomach are derived from visceral mesoderm.

    3. **Clinical considerations. Hypertrophic pyloric stenosis** occurs when the muscularis externa in the pyloric region hypertrophies, causing a narrow pyloric lumen that obstructs food passage. It is associated clinically with projectile, nonbilious vomiting after feeding; a small, palpable mass at the right costal margin; increased incidence has been found in infants treated with the antibiotic erythromycin.

C. Liver   (Figure 10-4)

    1. **Development.** The endodermal lining of the foregut forms an outgrowth **(hepatic diverticulum)** into the surrounding mesoderm of the **septum transversum** through induction by **fibroblast growth factors (FGF-1, FGF-2, and FGF-8)** released by **cardiac mesoderm** (which is in close vicinity). In addition, the differentiation of endoderm into hepatocytes seems to be controlled by the expression of transcription factors: HNF-3β, GATA-4, and **homeobox Hex.** Both HNF-3β and GATA-4 bind to the **albumin gene promoter** (the albumin gene is one of the earliest genes activated in liver development). The mesoderm of the septum transversum is involved in the formation of the **diaphragm**, which explains the intimate gross anatomic relationship between the liver and diaphragm. Cords of hepatoblasts (called **hepatic cords**) from the hepatic diverticulum grow into the mesoderm of the septum transversum where critical hepatoblast/mesoderm interactions occur. Mesodermal factors crucial in this interaction are transcription factor **homeobox Hlx, hepatocyte growth factor (HGF),** and **stress signaling kinase SEK1/MKK4.** The hepatic cords arrange themselves around the **vitelline veins and umbilical veins,** which course through the septum transversum and form the **hepatic sinusoids.** Owing to the

tremendous growth of the liver, the liver bulges into the abdominal cavity, thereby stretching the septum transversum to form the **ventral mesentery**, which consists of the **falciform ligament** and the **lesser omentum**. The falciform ligament contains the **left umbilical vein**, which regresses after birth to form the **ligamentum teres**. The lesser omentum can be divided into the **hepatogastric ligament** and **hepatoduodenal ligament**. The hepatoduodenal ligament contains the **bile duct, portal vein, and hepatic artery** (i.e., **portal triad**).

2. **Sources.** Hepatocytes and the simple columnar or cuboidal epithelium lining the biliary tree of the definitive liver are derived from endoderm. Kupffer cells, hematopoietic cells, endothelium of the sinusoids, and fibroblasts (connective tissue) of the definitive liver are derived from mesoderm.

3. **Clinical considerations.** Congenital malformations of the liver are rare except for minor gross anatomic variations.

D. **Gallbladder and extrahepatic bile ducts**   (Figure 10-4)

1. **Development.** The connection between the hepatic diverticulum and the foregut narrows to form the bile duct. An outgrowth from the bile duct gives rise to the **gallbladder rudiment** and **cystic duct**. The cystic duct divides the bile duct into the common hepatic duct and common bile duct. During development, the endodermal lining of the gallbladder and extrahepatic bile ducts proliferates rapidly and obliterates the lumen; later, recanalization occurs.

2. **Sources.** Simple columnar epithelium lining the definitive gallbladder and simple columnar or cuboidal epithelium lining the definitive extrahepatic bile ducts are derived from endoderm. The lamina propria, muscularis externa, and adventitia of the definitive gallbladder are derived from visceral mesoderm.

3. **Clinical considerations**
   a. **Intrahepatic gallbladder** occurs when the gallbladder rudiment advances beyond the hepatic diverticulum and becomes buried within the substance of the liver.
   b. **Floating gallbladder** occurs when the gallbladder rudiment lags behind the hepatic diverticulum and thereby becomes suspended from the liver by a mesentery. A floating gallbladder is at risk for **torsion**.
   c. **Developmental anomalies of the cystic duct** anatomy are fairly common.
   d. **Developmental anomalies of the gallbladder** anatomy are fairly common whereby two bilobed diverticula and septated gallbladders are found.
   e. **Biliary atresia** is defined as the obliteration of extrahepatic and/or intrahepatic ducts. The ducts are replaced by fibrotic tissue due to acute and chronic inflammation. Biliary atresia is associated clinically with progressive neonatal jaundice with onset soon after birth, white clay-colored stool, and dark-colored urine. The average survival time is 12 to 19 months with a 100% mortality rate.

E. **Pancreas**   (Figure 10-5)

1. **Development.** The **dorsal pancreatic bud** is a direct outgrowth of foregut endoderm whose formation is induced by the notochord. The **ventral pancreatic bud** is a direct outgrowth of foregut endoderm whose formation is induced by hepatic mesoderm. During the earliest stages of pancreatic bud formation, homeobox transcription factors **Pdx-1** and **ISL-1** play an essential role. Within both pancreatic buds, endodermal tubules surrounded by mesoderm branch repeatedly to form acinar cells and ducts (i.e., exocrine pancreas). Isolated clumps of endodermal cells bud from the tubules and accumulate within the mesoderm to form **islet cells** (i.e., endocrine pancreas) in the following sequence (first→last): **alpha cells** (glucagon)→**beta cells** (insulin)→**delta cells** (somatostatin) and **PP cells** (pancreatic polypeptide). Because of the 90° clockwise rotation of the duodenum, the ventral bud rotates dorsally and fuses with the dorsal bud to form the definitive adult pancreas. The ventral bud forms the **uncinate process** and a **portion of the head of the pancreas**. The dorsal bud forms the **remaining portion of the head, body,** and **tail of the**

pancreas. The main pancreatic duct is formed by the anastomosis of the **distal two thirds of the dorsal pancreatic duct** (the proximal third regresses) and the **entire ventral pancreatic duct** (48% incidence). The main pancreatic duct and common bile duct form a single opening (**hepatopancreatic ampulla of Vater**) into the duodenum at the tip of a major papilla (**hepatopancreatic papilla**).

2. **Sources.** Acinar cells, islet cells, and simple columnar or cuboidal epithelium lining the pancreatic ducts of the definitive pancreas are derived from endoderm. Surrounding connective tissue and vascular components of the definitive pancreas are derived from visceral mesoderm.

3. **Clinical considerations**
   a. **Accessory pancreatic duct** develops when the proximal third of the dorsal pancreatic duct persists and opens into the duodenum through a minor papilla at a site proximal to the ampulla of Vater (33% incidence).
   b. **Pancreas divisum** (4% incidence) occurs when the **distal two thirds of the dorsal pancreatic duct** and the **entire ventral pancreatic duct** fail to anastomose and the proximal third of the dorsal pancreatic duct persists, thereby forming two separate duct systems. The dorsal pancreatic duct drains a **portion of the head, body,** and **tail of the pancreas** by opening into the duodenum through a minor papilla. The ventral pancreatic duct drains the **uncinate process** and a **portion of the head of the pancreas** by opening into the duodenum through the major papilla. Patients with pancreas divisum are prone to pancreatitis, especially if the opening of the dorsal pancreatic duct at the minor papilla is small.
   c. **Annular pancreas** occurs when the ventral pancreatic bud fuses with the dorsal bud both dorsally and ventrally, thereby forming a **ring of pancreatic tissue** around the duodenum causing severe **duodenal obstruction.** Newborns and infants are intolerant of oral feeding and often have bilious vomiting. Radiographic evidence of an annular pancreas is indicated by a duodenal obstruction in which a "double bubble" sign is often seen owing to dilation of the stomach and distal duodenum.
   d. **Hyperplasia of pancreatic islets** occurs when fetal islets are exposed to high blood glucose levels, as frequently happens in **infants of diabetic mothers.** Glucose freely crosses the placenta and stimulates fetal islet hyperplasia and insulin secretion, which causes increased fat and glycogen deposition in fetal tissues. This results in increased birth weight of infants at term (i.e., **macrosomia**) and serious episodes of **hypoglycemia** in the postnatal period.

F. **Upper duodenum** develops from the caudal-most part of the foregut.

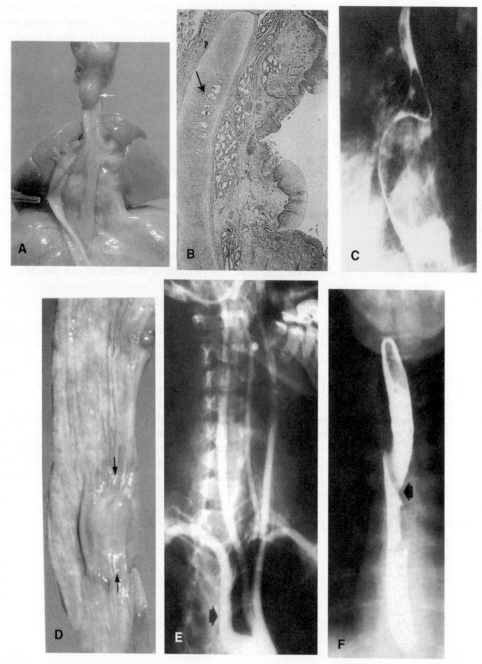

Figure 10-2. **(A)** Esophageal atresia. A posterior view shows that the esophagus terminates blindly in a blunted esophageal pouch (*arrow*). There is a distal esophageal connection with the trachea at the carina (*arrowhead*). **(B)** Esophageal stenosis. This micrograph shows the stratified squamous epithelial lining of the esophagus and submucosal glands. Note that a portion of the muscular wall contains remnants of cartilage (*arrow*), which contributes to a stenosis. **(C and D)** Esophageal duplication cyst. A barium esophagram demonstrates a large intramural duplication cyst in the proximal esophagus. The cyst shows acute angles with the esophageal lumen indicating its intramural location. Gross anatomy photograph of the esophagus shows a large intramural duplication cyst (*arrows*). **(E and F)** Vascular compression of the esophagus. An angiogram reveals an anomalous right subclavian artery (*arrow*) arising from the aortic arch. A barium esophagram in the same patient reveals an oblique compression of the esophagus (*arrow*) due to the anomalous right subclavian artery.

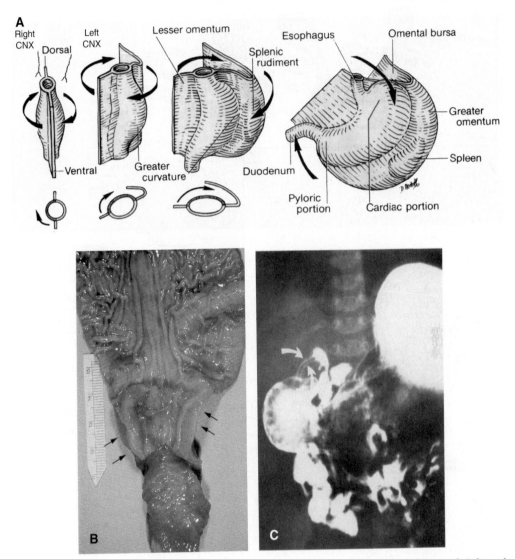

Figure 10-3. **(A)** Diagram depicting the development and 90° rotation of the stomach from week 4 through week 6. **(B and C)** Hypertrophic pyloric stenosis. Gross photograph of the stomach opened along the greater curvature. Note the prominence of the pyloric ring indicated by the *arrows*. Barium contrast radiograph shows the long, narrow double channel of the pylorus (*arrows*) in a patient with hypertrophic pyloric stenosis.

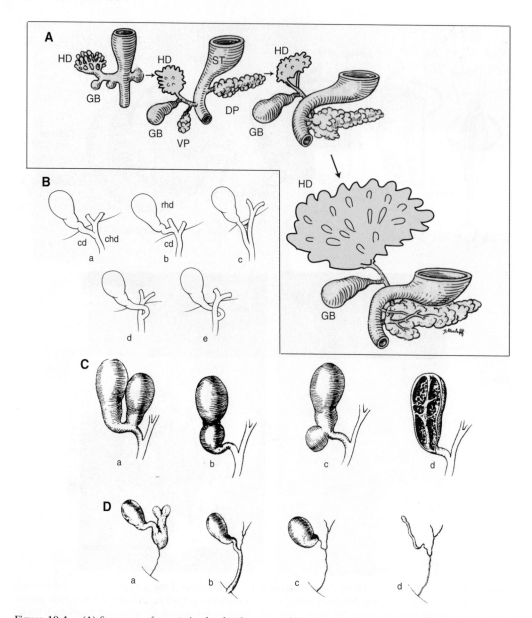

Figure 10-4. **(A)** Sequence of events in the development of the hepatic diverticulum (*HD*) and gallbladder rudiment (*GB*) from week 4 through week 7. *DP* = dorsal pancreatic bud; *ST* = stomach; *VP* = ventral pancreatic bud. **(B)** Developmental anomalies of the cystic duct. (*a*) Cystic duct (*cd*) joins the common hepatic duct (*chd*) directly (most common anatomic arrangement). (*b*) Cystic duct joins the right hepatic duct (*rhd*). (*c*) Low junction of cystic duct with the common hepatic duct. (*d*) Anterior spiral of cystic duct. (*e*) Posterior spiral of cystic duct. **(C)** Developmental anomalies of the gallbladder. (*a*) Two gallbladders. (*b*) Bilobed gallbladder. (*c*) Diverticulum of the gallbladder. (*d*) Septated gallbladder is most likely due to incomplete recanalization of the lumen. **(D)** Different forms of extrahepatic biliary atresia. (*a, b, c*) Partial. (*d*) Complete.

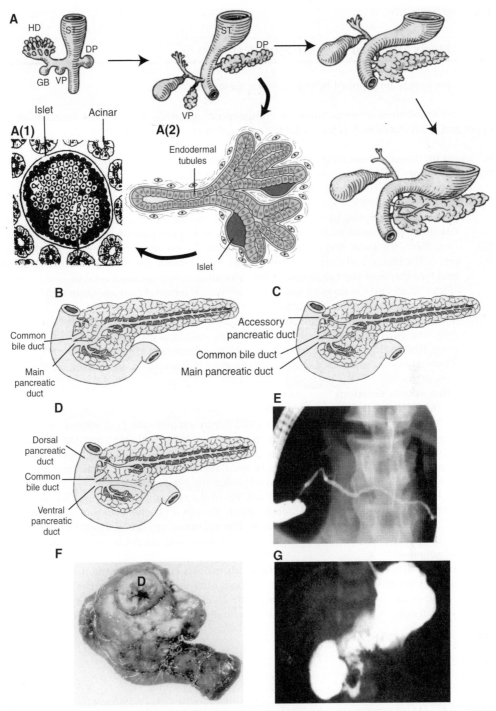

Figure 10-5. (A) Sequence of events in the development of the pancreatic buds from week 4 through week 7. Note that within the pancreatic buds endodermal tubules branch repeatedly to form the exocrine (acinar) pancreas. Islets bud from the endodermal tubules to form the endocrine (islet) pancreas. *DP* = dorsal pancreatic bud; *GB* = gallbladder rudiment; *HD* = hepatic diverticulum; *ST* = stomach; *VP* = ventral pancreatic bud. (B) Normal pattern of the main pancreatic duct (48% incidence in the population). (C) Accessory pancreatic duct (33% incidence in the population). Note that the proximal third of the dorsal pancreatic duct persists. (D and E) Pancreas divisum. Note that distal two thirds of the dorsal pancreatic duct and the ventral pancreatic bud fail to anastomose, thereby forming two separate duct systems. An endoscopic retrograde pancreatogram performed through the accessory minor papilla shows the dorsal pancreatic duct in pancreatic divisum. (F and G) Annular pancreas. Photograph of a pathologic specimen showing a ring of pancreas tissue surrounding the entire duodenum (*D*). Barium contrast radiograph showing partial duodenal obstruction consistent with an annular pancreas.

III.   Derivatives of the Midgut (Figure 10-6)

Midgut derivatives are supplied by the **superior mesenteric artery.**

A. Lower duodenum develops from the cranial-most part of the midgut. The junction of the upper and lower duodenum is just distal to the opening of the common bile duct.

B. Jejunum, ileum, cecum, appendix, ascending colon, and the proximal two thirds of the transverse colon   (see Figure 10-6)
  1. **Development.** The midgut forms a U-shaped loop (**midgut loop)** that herniates through the primitive umbilical ring into the extraembryonic coelom (i.e., **physiologic umbilical herniation**) beginning at week 6. The midgut loop consists of a **cranial limb** and a **caudal limb.** The cranial limb forms the **jejunum** and **upper part of the ileum.** The caudal limb forms the **cecal diverticulum,** from which the **cecum** and **appendix** develop; the rest of the caudal limb forms the **lower part of the ileum, ascending colon,** and **proximal two thirds of the transverse colon.** The midgut loop rotates a total of 270° counterclockwise around the superior mesenteric artery as it returns to the abdominal cavity, thus reducing the physiologic herniation, around week 11.
  2. **Sources.** Simple columnar absorptive cells lining midgut derivatives, goblet cells, Paneth cells, and enteroendocrine cells comprising the intestinal glands are derived from endoderm. The lamina propria, muscularis mucosae, submucosa, inner circular and outer longitudinal smooth muscle of the muscularis externa, and serosa are derived from visceral mesoderm.
  3. **Clinical considerations**
     a. **Omphalocele** occurs when abdominal contents herniate through the umbilical ring and persist outside the body covered variably by a translucent peritoneal membrane sac (a light-gray, shiny sac) protruding from the base of the umbilical cord. Large omphaloceles may contain stomach, liver, and intestines. Small omphaloceles contain only intestines. Omphaloceles are usually associated with other congenital anomalies (e.g., trisomy 13, trisomy 18, or Beckwith-Wiedemann syndrome).
     b. **Gastroschisis** occurs when there is a defect in the ventral abdominal wall usually to the right of the umbilical ring through which there is a massive evisceration of intestines (other organs may also be involved). The intestines are not covered by a peritoneal membrane, are directly exposed to amniotic fluid, and are thickened and covered with adhesions.
     c. **Ileal diverticulum (Meckel's diverticulum)** occurs when a remnant of the vitelline duct persists, thereby forming an outpouching located on the **antimesenteric border** of the ileum. The outpouching may connect to the umbilicus via a fibrous cord or fistula. A Meckel's diverticulum is usually located about 30 cm proximal to the

Figure 10-6.   (A) Diagram depicting the 270° counterclockwise rotation of the midgut loop. *Striped area* indicates the caudal limb. Note that after the 270° rotation, the cecum and appendix are located in the upper abdominal cavity. Later in development, there is growth in the direction indicated by the *bold arrow* so that the cecum and appendix end up in the lower right quadrant. *SMA* = superior mesenteric artery. **(B)** Omphalocele. **(C)** Gastroschisis. **(D)** Meckel's diverticulum *(arrow).* *IL* = ileum. **(E)** Nonrotation of midgut loop. Note small intestines *(SI)* on the right side and large intestines *(LI)* on left side. **(F)** Volvulus. Note the twisting *(arrow)* of the small intestines around the axis of the mesentery. **(G)** Type II atresia. Note the fibrous cord *(arrow).* **(H)** Type IIIa atresia. Note the gap in the mesentery (*). **(I)** Duplication. Note the larger diameter of normal bowel segment *(N)* and the smaller diameter of the duplicated segment *(D).* Atretic areas *(arrows)* are indicated in the duplicated segment.

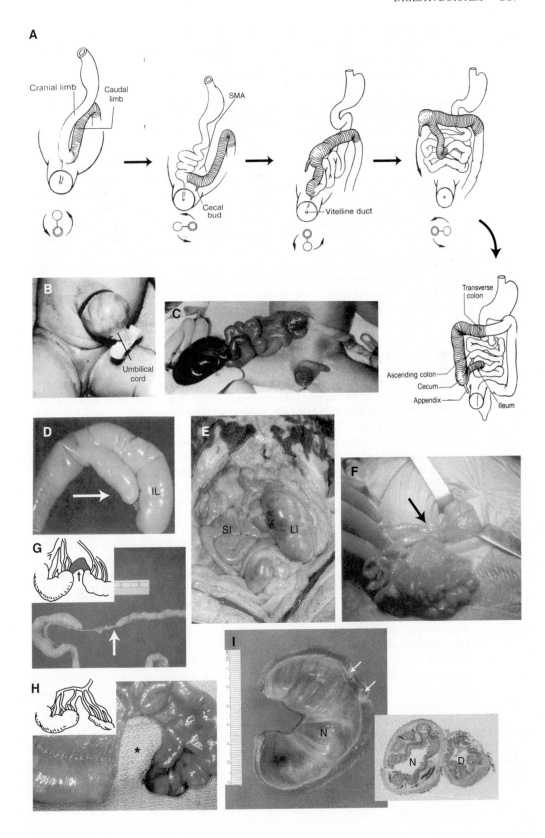

ileocecal valve in infants and varies in length from 2 to 15 cm. **Heterotopic gastric mucosa** may be present, which leads to ulceration, perforation, or gastrointestinal bleeding, especially if a large number of parietal cells are present. It is associated clinically with symptoms resembling appendicitis and bright-red or dark-red stools (i.e., bloody).

d. **Nonrotation of the midgut loop** occurs when the midgut loop rotates only 90° counterclockwise, thereby positioning the small intestine entirely on the right side and the large intestine entirely on the left side with the cecum located either in the left upper quadrant or the left iliac fossa.

e. **Malrotation of the midgut loop** occurs when the midgut loop undergoes only partial counterclockwise rotation. This results in the cecum and appendix lying in a subpyloric or subhepatic location and the small intestine suspended by only a vascular pedicle (i.e., not a broad mesentery). A major clinical complication of malrotation is **volvulus** (twisting of the small intestines around the vascular pedicle), which may cause necrosis due to compromised blood supply. (Note: The abnormal position of the appendix due to malrotation of the midgut should be considered when diagnosing appendicitis.)

f. **Reversed rotation of the midgut loop** occurs when the midgut loop rotates clockwise instead of counterclockwise, causing the large intestine to enter the abdominal cavity first. This results in the large intestine anatomically located posterior to the duodenum and superior mesenteric artery.

g. **Intestinal atresia and stenosis** Atresia occurs when the lumen of the intestines is completely occluded, whereas stenosis occurs when the lumen of the intestines is narrowed. The causes of these conditions seem to be failed recanalization and/or an ischemic intrauterine event ("vascular accident"). **Type I atresia** is characterized by a membranous septum or diaphragm of mucosa and submucosa that obstructs the lumen. **Type II atresia** is characterized by two blind bowel ends connected by a fibrous cord with an intact mesentery. **Type IIIa atresia** is characterized by two blind bowel ends separated by a gap in the mesentery. **Type IIIb atresia** ("apple peel" atresia) is characterized by a bowel segment (distal to the atresia) that is shortened, coiled around a mesentery remnant, and lacking a blood supply from the superior mesentery artery (blood supply to this bowel segment is via collateral circulation). **Type IV atresia** is characterized by multiple atresias throughout the bowel having the appearance of a "string of sausages." Proximal atresias are associated clinically with polyhydramnios and bilious vomiting early after birth. Distal atresias are associated clinically with normal amniotic fluid, abdominal distention, later vomiting, and failure to pass meconium.

h. **Duplication of the intestines** occurs when a segment of the intestines is duplicated as a result of abnormal recanalization (most commonly near the ileocecal valve). The duplication is found on the mesenteric border, its lumen generally communicates with the normal bowel, shares the same blood supply as the normal bowel, is lined by normal intestinal epithelium but heterotopic gastric and pancreatic tissue has been identified. It is associated clinically with an abdominal mass, bouts of abdominal pain, vomiting, chronic rectal bleeding, intussusception, and perforation.

i. **Intussusception** occurs when a segment of bowel invaginates or telescopes into an adjacent bowel segment leading to obstruction or ischemia. This is one of the most common causes of obstruction in children under 2 years of age, is most often idiopathic, and most commonly involves the ileum and colon (i.e., ileocolic). It is associated clinically with acute onset of intermittent abdominal pain, vomiting, bloody stools, diarrhea, and somnolence.

j. **Retrocecal and retrocolic appendix** occurs when the appendix is located on the posterior side of the cecum or colon, respectively. These anomalies are very common and important to remember during appendectomies. Note: The appendix is normally found on the medial side of the cecum.

IV.   Derivatives of the Hindgut (Figure 10-7)

Hindgut derivatives are supplied by the **inferior mesenteric artery**.

A. **Distal third of the transverse colon, descending colon, sigmoid colon**
   1. **Development.** The cranial end of the hindgut develops into the distal third of the transverse colon, descending colon, and sigmoid colon. The terminal end of the hindgut is an endoderm-lined pouch called the **cloaca**, which contacts the surface ectoderm of the **proctodeum** to form the **cloacal membrane**.
   2. **Sources.** Simple columnar absorptive cells lining hindgut derivatives, goblet cells, and enteroendocrine cells comprising the intestinal glands are derived from endoderm. The lamina propria, muscularis mucosae, submucosa, inner circular and outer longitudinal (taeniae coli) smooth muscle of the muscularis externa, and serosa are derived from visceral mesoderm.

B. **Rectum and upper anal canal**
   1. **Development.** The cloaca is partitioned by the **urorectal septum** into the **rectum and upper anal canal** and the **urogenital sinus**. The cloacal membrane is partitioned by the urorectal septum into the **anal membrane** and **urogenital membrane**. Note: The urorectal septum fuses with the cloacal membrane at the future site of the gross anatomic **perineal body**.
   2. **Sources.** As mentioned above, IV.A.2.
   3. **Clinical considerations**
      a. **Colonic aganglionosis (Hirschsprung disease)** is caused by the arrest of the caudal migration of neural crest cells. The hallmark is the absence of ganglionic cells in the myenteric and submucosal plexuses most commonly in the sigmoid colon and rectum resulting in a narrow segment of colon (i.e., the colon fails to relax). Although the ganglionic cells are absent, there is a proliferation of hypertrophied nerve fiber bundles. The most characteristic functional finding is the failure of internal anal sphincter to relax after rectal distention (i.e., abnormal rectoanal reflex). Mutations of the **RET proto-oncogene** (chromosome 10q11.2) have been associated with Hirschsprung disease. It is associated clinically with a distended abdomen, inability to pass meconium, gushing of fecal material upon rectal digital examination, and a loss of peristalsis in the colon segment distal to the normal innervated colon.
      b. **Rectovesical, rectourethral, and rectovaginal fistulas** are abnormal communications between the rectum and urinary bladder (rectovesical), rectum and urethra (rectourethral), and rectum and vagina (rectovaginal) due to abnormal formation of the urorectal septum. These fistulas are associated clinically with the presence of meconium in the urine or vagina.

V.   Anal Canal (see Figure 10-7)

A. **Development**   The **upper anal canal** develops from the **hindgut**. The **lower anal** canal develops from the **proctodeum**, which is an invagination of surface ectoderm caused by a proliferation of mesoderm surrounding the anal membrane. The dual components (hindgut and proctodeum) involved in the embryologic formation of the entire anal canal determine the gross anatomy of this area, which becomes important when considering the characteristics and metastasis of anorectal tumors. The junction between the upper and lower anal canals is indicated by the **pectinate line,** which also marks the site of the former **anal membrane.** In the adult, the pectinate line is located at the lower border of the anal columns.

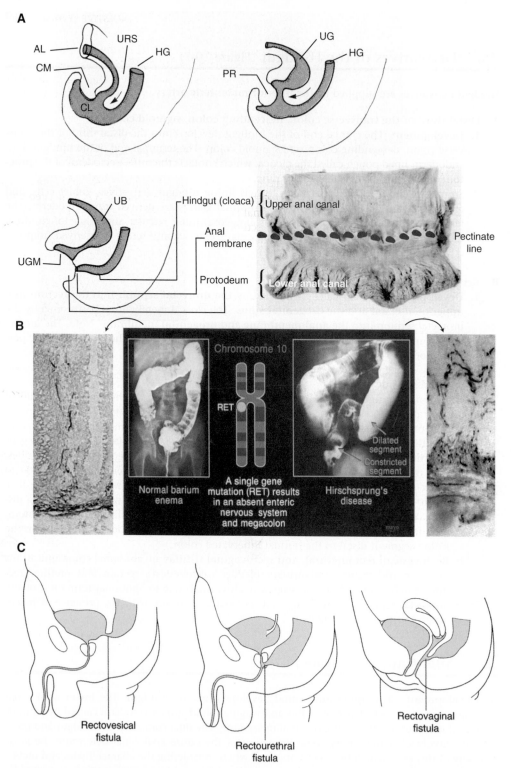

Figure 10-7. **(A)** Diagram depicting the partitioning of the cloaca (*CL*) by urorectal septum (URS). *AL* = allantois; *CM* = cloacal membrane; *HG* = hindgut; *PR* = proctodeum; *UB* = urinary bladder; *UG* = urogenital sinus; *UGM* = urogenital membrane. The *bold arrow* shows the direction of growth of the urorectal septum. **(B)** Hirschsprung disease. Micrographs show nerve fibers stained for acetylcholinesterase. Note the proliferation of hypertrophied nerve fiber bundles in Hirschsprung disease. **(C)** Rectovesical fistula, rectourethral fistula, and rectovaginal fistula. A rectourethral fistula that generally occurs in males is associated with the prostatic urethra and is therefore sometimes called a rectoprostatic fistula.

120

B. Sources   The simple columnar epithelium lining the upper anal canal is derived from endoderm, whereas the simple columnar and stratified columnar epithelia lining the lower anal canal are derived from ectoderm. The lamina propria, muscularis mucosae, submucosa, muscularis externa consisting of the internal and external anal sphincters, and adventitia are derived from mesoderm.

C. Clinical considerations
   1. **Imperforate anus** occurs when the anal membrane fails to perforate; a layer of tissue separates the anal canal from the exterior.
   2. **Anal agenesis** occurs when the anal canal ends as a blind sac **below the puborectalis muscle** due to abnormal formation of the urorectal septum. It is usually associated with rectovesical, rectourethral, or rectovaginal fistula.
   3. **Anorectal agenesis** occurs when the rectum ends as a blind sac **above the puborectalis muscle** due to abnormal formation of the urorectal septum. It is the most common type of anorectal malformation and is usually associated with a rectovesical, rectourethral, or rectovaginal fistula.
   4. **Rectal atresia** occurs when both the rectum and the anal canal are present but remain unconnected either because of abnormal recanalization or a compromised blood supply causing focal atresia.

VI. Mesenteries

The primitive gut tube is suspended within the peritoneal cavity of the embryo by the **ventral mesentery** and **dorsal mesentery**, from which all adult mesenteries are derived (Table 10-1).

TABLE 10-1	*Derivation of Adult Mesenteries*
Embryonic Mesentery	**Adult Mesentery**
Ventral	Lesser omentum (hepatoduodenal and hepatogastric ligaments), falciform ligament of liver, coronary ligament of liver, triangular ligament of liver
Dorsal	Greater omentum (gastrorenal, gastrosplenic, gastrocolic, and splenorenal ligaments), mesentery of small intestine, mesoappendix, transverse mesocolon, sigmoid mesocolon

*Directions: Each of the numbered items or incomplete statements in this section is followed by answers or by completions of the statement. Select the **one** lettered answer or completion that is **best** in each case.*

1. Pancreatic islets consist of alpha, beta, and delta cells, which secrete glucagon, insulin, and somatostatin, respectively. These cells are derived from

(A) mesoderm
(B) endoderm
(C) ectoderm
(D) neuroectoderm
(E) neural crest cells

2. A 2-month-old baby with severe jaundice also has dark-colored urine (deep yellow) and white clay-colored stool. Which of the following disorders might be suspected?

(A) Esophageal stenosis
(B) Annular pancreas
(C) Hypertrophic pyloric stenosis
(D) Extrahepatic biliary atresia
(E) Duodenal atresia

3. A 28-day-old baby is brought to the physician because of projectile vomiting after feeding. Until this time, the baby has had no problems in feeding. On examination, a small knot is palpated at the right costal margin. Which of the following disorders might be suspected?

(A) Esophageal stenosis
(B) Annular pancreas
(C) Hypertrophic pyloric stenosis
(D) Extrahepatic biliary atresia
(E) Duodenal atresia

4. Which of the following arteries supplies foregut derivatives of the digestive system?

(A) Celiac trunk
(B) Superior mesenteric artery
(C) Inferior mesenteric artery
(D) Right umbilical artery
(E) Intercostal artery

5. The most common type of anorectal malformation is

(A) imperforate anus
(B) anal agenesis
(C) anorectal agenesis
(D) rectal atresia
(E) colonic aganglionosis

6. The simple columnar or cuboidal epithelium lining the extrahepatic biliary ducts is derived from

(A) mesoderm
(B) endoderm
(C) ectoderm
(D) neuroectoderm
(E) neural crest cells

7. A 4-day-old baby boy has not defecated since coming home from the hospital even though feeding has been normal without any excessive vomiting. Rectal examination reveals a normal anus, anal canal, and rectum. However, a large fecal mass is found in the colon, and a large release of flatus and feces follows the rectal examination. Which of the following conditions would be suspected?

(A) Imperforate anus
(B) Anal agenesis
(C) Anorectal agenesis
(D) Rectal atresia
(E) Colonic aganglionosis

8. Which one of the following structures is derived from the midgut?

(A) Appendix
(B) Stomach
(C) Liver
(D) Pancreas
(E) Sigmoid colon

9. A 3-month-old baby girl presents with a swollen umbilicus that has failed to heal normally. The umbilicus drains secretions, and there is passage of fecal material through the umbilicus at times. What is the most likely diagnosis?

(A) Omphalocele
(B) Gastroschisis
(C) Anal agenesis
(D) Ileal diverticulum
(E) Intestinal stenosis

10. The midgut loop normally herniates through the primitive umbilical ring into the extraembryonic coelom during week 6 of development. Failure of the intestinal loops to return to the abdominal cavity by week 11 results in the formation of

(A) omphalocele
(B) gastroschisis
(C) anal agenesis
(D) ileal diverticulum
(E) intestinal stenosis

11. Kupffer cells present in the adult liver are derived from

(A) mesoderm
(B) endoderm
(C) ectoderm
(D) neuroectoderm
(E) neural crest cells

12. The simple columnar and stratified columnar epithelia lining the lower part of the anal canal is derived from

(A) mesoderm
(B) endoderm
(C) ectoderm
(D) neuroectoderm
(E) neural crest cells

13. A baby born to a young woman whose pregnancy was complicated by polyhydramnios was placed in the intensive care unit because of repeated vomiting containing bile. The stomach was markedly distended, and only small amounts of meconium had passed through the anus. What is the most likely diagnosis?

(A) Esophageal stenosis
(B) Annular pancreas
(C) Hypertrophic pyloric stenosis
(D) Extrahepatic biliary atresia
(E) Duodenal atresia

ANSWERS AND EXPLANATIONS

1. B. Pancreatic islets form as isolated clumps of cells that bud from endodermal tubules.

2. D. The baby is suffering from extrahepatic biliary atresia, which results from failure of the bile ducts to recanalize during development. This prevents bile from entering the duodenum.

3. C. The baby is suffering from hypertrophic pyloric stenosis. This occurs when the smooth muscle in the pyloric region of the stomach hypertrophies and obstructs passage of food. The hypertrophied muscle can be palpated at the right costal margin. The exact cause of this condition is not known.

4. A. The artery that supplies foregut derivatives of the digestive system is the celiac trunk. The celiac trunk consists of the left gastric artery, splenic artery, and common hepatic artery. The superior mesenteric artery supplies the midgut, and the inferior mesenteric artery supplies the hindgut.

5. C. The most common type of malformation involving the anal canal and rectum is anorectal agenesis, in which the rectum ends as a blind sac above the puborectalis muscle. The anal canal may form normally but does not connect with the rectum. This malformation is accompanied by various fistulas.

6. B. The epithelium lining the extrahepatic biliary ducts is derived from endoderm. The intrahepatic biliary ducts are also derived from endoderm.

7. E. This baby boy suffers from colonic aganglionosis, or Hirschsprung disease, which results in the retention of fecal material, causing the normal colon to enlarge. The retention of fecal material results from a lack of peristalsis in the narrow segment of colon distal to the enlarged colon. A biopsy of the narrow segment of colon would reveal the absence of parasympathetic ganglion cells in the myenteric plexus caused by failure of neural crest migration.

8. A. The appendix is derived from the midgut. The midgut normally undergoes a 270° counterclockwise rotation during development; malrotation of the midgut may result in the appendix lying in the upper part of the abdominal cavity, which may affect a diagnosis of appendicitis.

9. D. This baby girl has an ileal diverticulum (Meckel's diverticulum), which occurs when a remnant of the vitelline duct persists. In this case, a fistula is present whereby contents of the ileum can be discharged onto the surface of the skin.

10. A. An omphalocele results when intestinal loops fail to return to the abdominal cavity. Instead, the intestinal loops remain in the umbilical cord covered by amnion.

11. A. Kupffer cells are actually macrophages and are derived from mesoderm. Hepatocytes and the epithelial lining of the intrahepatic biliary tree are derived from endoderm.

12. C. The anal canal is formed from two components, the hindgut and proctodeum. The epithelium lining the lower anal canal is derived from ectoderm lining the proctodeum.

13. E. This baby is suffering from duodenal atresia at a level distal to the opening of the common bile duct. This causes a reflux of bile and its presence in the vomitus. The pregnancy was complicated by polyhydramnios because the duodenal atresia prevented passage of amniotic fluid into the intestines for absorption.

Respiratory System

I. Upper Respiratory System

The upper respiratory system consists of the **nose, nasopharynx,** and **oropharynx.**

II. Lower Respiratory System (Figure 11-1)

The lower respiratory system consists of the **larynx, trachea, bronchi,** and **lungs.** The first sign of development is the formation of the **respiratory diverticulum** in the ventral wall of the primitive foregut during week 4. The distal end of the respiratory diverticulum enlarges to form the **lung bud.** The lung bud divides into two **bronchial buds** that branch into the **main (primary), lobar (secondary), segmental (tertiary),** and **subsegmental bronchi.** The respiratory diverticulum initially is in open communication with the foregut, but eventually they become separated by indentations of mesoderm, the **tracheoesophageal folds.** When the tracheoesophageal folds fuse in the midline to form the **tracheoesophageal septum,** the foregut is divided into the trachea ventrally and esophagus dorsally. The **Hox-complex, FGF-10** (fibroblast growth factor), **BMP-4** (bone morphogenetic protein), **N-*myc*** (a proto-oncogene), **syndecan** (a proteoglycan), **tenascin** (an extracellular matrix protein), and **epimorphin** (a protein) appear to play a role in development of the respiratory system.

A. Development of the larynx The opening of the respiratory diverticulum into the foregut becomes the **laryngeal orifice.** The **laryngeal epithelium** and **glands** are derived from endoderm. The **laryngeal muscles** are derived from somitomeric mesoderm of pharyngeal arches 4 and 6 and therefore are innervated by branches of the vagus nerve (CN X), that is, the superior laryngeal nerve and recurrent laryngeal nerve, respectively. The **laryngeal cartilages (thyroid, cricoid, arytenoid, corniculate,** and **cuneiform)** are derived from somitomeric mesoderm of pharyngeal arches 4 and 6.

B. Development of the trachea
1. **Sources.** The tracheal epithelium and glands are derived from endoderm. The tracheal smooth muscle, connective tissue, and C-shaped cartilage rings are derived from visceral mesoderm.
2. **Clinical considerations. Tracheoesophageal fistula** is an abnormal communication between the trachea and esophagus that results from improper division of foregut by the tracheoesophageal septum. It is generally associated with **esophageal atresia** and **polyhydramnios.** Clinical features include excessive accumulation of saliva or mucus in the nose and mouth; episodes of gagging and cyanosis after swallowing milk; abdominal distention after crying; and reflux of gastric contents into lungs, causing pneumonitis. Diagnostic features include inability to pass a catheter into the infant's stomach and radiographs demonstrating air in the stomach.

C. Development of the bronchi

1. **Stages of development.** The lung bud divides into two bronchial buds. In week 5 of development, bronchial buds enlarge to form **main (primary) bronchi.** The right main bronchus is larger and more vertical than the left main bronchus; this relationship persists throughout adult life and accounts for the greater likelihood of foreign bodies lodging on the right side than on the left. The main bronchi further subdivide into **lobar (secondary) bronchi** (three on the right side and two on the left side, corresponding to the lobes of the adult lung). The lobar bronchi further subdivide into **segmental (tertiary) bronchi** (10 on the right side and 9 on the left side), which further subdivide into **subsegmental bronchi.** The segmental bronchi are the primordia of the **bronchopulmonary segments,** which are morphologically and functionally separate respiratory units of the lung. As the bronchi develop, they expand laterally and caudally into a space known as the primitive pleural cavity. The visceral mesoderm covering the outside of the bronchi develops into **visceral pleura,** and somatic mesoderm covering the inside of the body wall develops into **parietal pleura.** The space between the visceral and parietal pleura is called the **pleural cavity.**

2. **Sources.** The bronchial epithelium and glands are derived from endoderm. The bronchial smooth muscle, connective tissue, and cartilage are derived from visceral mesoderm.

3. **Clinical considerations** (Figure 11-2)

   a. **Bronchopulmonary segment** is a segment of lung tissue supplied by a segmental (tertiary) bronchus. Surgeons can resect diseased lung tissue along bronchopulmonary segments rather than removing the entire lobe.

   b. **Congenital lobar emphysema (CLE)** is characterized by progressive overdistention of one of the upper lobes or the right middle lobe with **air.** The term emphysema is a misnomer because there is no destruction of the alveolar walls. Although the exact etiology remains unknown, many cases involve **collapsed bronchi** due to **failure of bronchial cartilage formation.** In this situation, air can be inspired through collapsed bronchi, but cannot be expired. During the first few days of life, fluid may be trapped in the involved lobe, producing an opaque, enlarged hemithorax. Later, the fluid is resorbed, and the classic radiologic appearance of an emphysematous lobe with generalized radiolucency (hyperlucent) is apparent.

   c. **Congenital bronchogenic cysts** represent an abnormality in bronchial branching and may be found within the mediastinum (most commonly) or intrapulmonary. Intrapulmonary cysts are round, solitary, sharply marginated, and **fluid-filled,** and they do not initially communicate with the tracheobronchial tree. Since intrapulmonary bronchogenic cysts contain fluid, they appear as water-density masses on chest radiographs. These cysts may become air-filled as a result of infection or instrumentation.

D. Development of the lungs

1. **Periods of development** (Figure 11-3). The lung matures in a proximal-distal direction, beginning with the largest bronchi and proceeding outward. As a result, lung development

Figure 11-1. Development of respiratory system at 4 weeks (**A**), 5 weeks (**B**), and 6 weeks (**C**). Both lateral ▶ views and cross-sectional views are shown. Note the relationship of the respiratory diverticulum (*RD*) and foregut (*F*). *Curved arrows* indicate the movement of the tracheoesophageal folds (*TEF*) as the tracheoesophageal septum (*TES*) forms between the trachea (*T*) and esophagus (*E*). B = bronchial buds; LL = left lung; RL = right lung; VM = visceral mesoderm. (**D to H**) Five different anatomic types of esophagus and trachea malformations. (**D**) Esophageal atresia with a tracheoesophageal fistula at distal third end of the trachea. This is the most common type, occurring in 82% of cases. The AP radiograph of this malformation shows an enteric tube (*arrow*) coiled in the upper esophageal pouch. The air in the bowel indicates a distal tracheoesophageal fistula. (**E**) Esophageal atresia only, occurring in 9% of the cases. (**F**) H-type tracheoesophageal fistula only, occurring in 6% of the cases. The barium swallow radiograph shows a normal esophagus (*E*), but dye has spilled into the trachea (*T*) through the fistula and outlines the upper trachea and larynx. (**G**) Esophageal atresia with a tracheoesophageal fistula at both proximal and distal ends, occurring in 2% of the cases. (**H**) Esophageal atresia with a tracheoesophageal fistula at the proximal end, occurring in 1% of the cases.

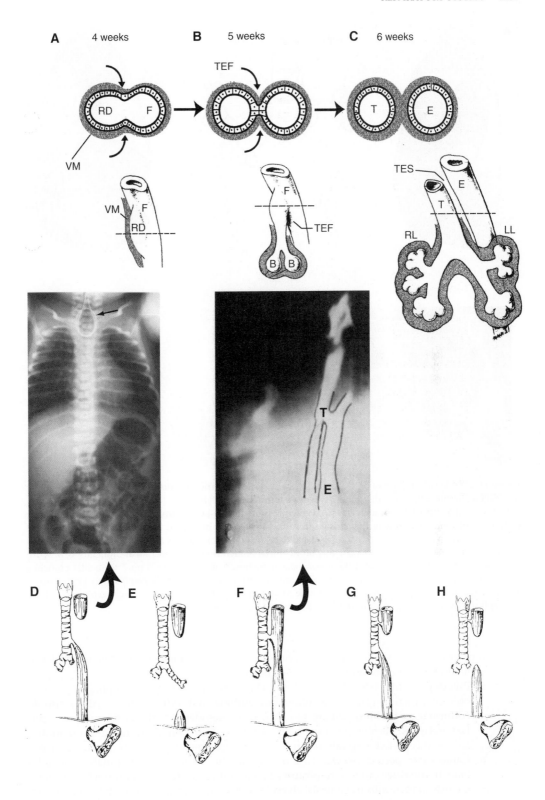

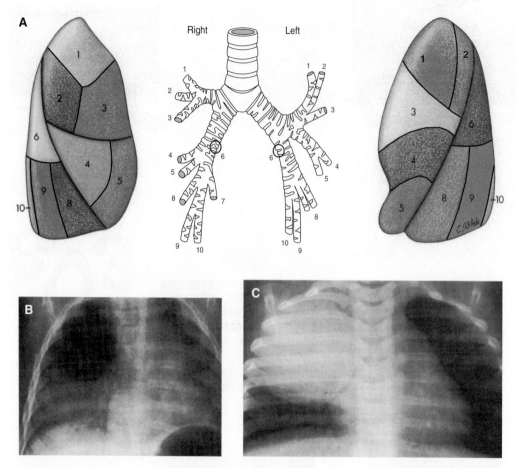

Figure 11-2. **(A)** Distribution of bronchopulmonary segments and their relationship to the tracheobronchial tree. Segmental bronchi of the right and left lungs are numbered. Right lung: 1, 2, 3: segmental bronchi that branch from the upper lobar bronchus; 4, 5: segmental bronchi that branch from the middle lobar bronchus; 6, 7, 8, 9, 10: segmental bronchi that branch from the lower lobar bronchus. Note that bronchopulmonary segment 7 is not represented on the outer costal surface of the right lung (7 is located on the inner mediastinal surface). Left lung: 1, 2, 3, 4, 5: segmental bronchi that branch from the upper lobar bronchus; 6, 8, 9, 10: segmental bronchi that branch from the lower lobar bronchus. Note that there is no 7 segmental bronchus associated with the left lung. **(B)** Congenital lobar emphysema. Expiratory AP radiograph shows a hyperlucent area in the emphysematous right upper lobe due to air-trapping. **(C)** Congenital bronchogenic cyst. AP radiograph shows large opaque area in the right upper lobe due to a fluid-filled cyst.

is heterogeneous; proximal pulmonary tissue will be in a more advanced period of development than distal pulmonary tissue (see Box on page 131).

a. **Pseudoglandular period (weeks 7–16).** During this period, the developing lung resembles an exocrine gland. The numerous **endodermal tubules** are lined by **simple columnar epithelium** and are surrounded by mesoderm containing a **modest capillary network**. Each endodermal tubule branches into 15 to 25 **terminal bronchioles**. During this period, respiration is not possible and premature infants cannot survive.

b. **Canalicular period (weeks 16–24).** During this period, the terminal bronchioles branch into three or more **respiratory bronchioles**. The respiratory bronchioles subsequently branch into three to six **alveolar ducts**. The terminal bronchioles, respiratory bronchioles, and alveolar ducts are now lined by a **simple cuboidal epithelium** and are surrounded by mesoderm containing a **prominent capillary network**. Premature infants born before week 20 rarely survive.

c. **Terminal sac period (week 24–birth).** During this period, **terminal sacs** bud off the alveolar ducts and then dilate and expand into the surrounding mesoderm. The terminal sacs are separated from each other by **primary septa**. The simple cuboidal epithelium within the terminal sacs differentiates into **Type I pneumocytes** (thin, flat cells that make up part of the blood–air barrier) and **Type II pneumocytes** (which produce surfactant). The terminal sacs are surrounded by mesoderm containing a **rapidly proliferating capillary network**. The capillaries make intimate contact with the terminal sacs and thereby establish a **blood–air barrier** with the Type I pneumocytes. **Premature infants born between week 25 and week 28 can survive with intensive care**. Adequate vascularization and surfactant levels are the most important factors for the survival of premature infants.

d. **Alveolar period (week 32–age 8 years).** During this period, terminal sacs are partitioned by **secondary septa** to form adult **alveoli**. About 20 to 70 million alveoli are present at birth. About 300 to 400 million alveoli are present by 8 years of age. The major mechanism for the increase in the number of alveoli is formation of secondary septa that partition existing alveoli. After birth, the increase in the size of the lung is due to an **increase in the number of respiratory bronchioles**. On chest radiographs, lungs of a newborn infant are denser than an adult lung because of the fewer number of mature alveoli.

2. **Clinical considerations**

a. **Aeration at birth** is the replacement of lung liquid with air in the newborn's lungs. In the fetal state, the functional residual capacity (FRC) of the lung is filled with liquid secreted by fetal lung epithelium via Cl^- transport using CFTR (cystic fibrosis transmembrane protein). At birth, lung liquid is eliminated by a reduction in lung liquid secretion via Na^+ transport by Type II pneumocytes and resorption into pulmonary capillaries (major route) and lymphatics (minor route). Lungs of a stillborn baby would sink when placed in water because they contain fluid rather than air.

b. **Respiratory distress syndrome (RDS)** (Figure 11-4) is caused by a deficiency or absence of **surfactant**. This surface active agent is composed of **cholesterol** (50%), **dipalmitoylphosphatidylcholine** (DPPC; 40%), and **surfactant proteins A, B, and C** (10%), and it coats the inside of alveoli to maintain alveolar patency. RDS is prevalent in premature infants (accounts for 50%–70% of deaths in premature infants), infants of diabetic mothers, infants who experienced fetal asphyxia or maternofetal hemorrhage (damages Type II pneumocytes), and multiple birth infants. Clinical signs include dyspnea, tachypnea, inspiratory retractions of chest wall, expiratory grunting, cyanosis, and nasal flaring. Treatments include administration of betamethasone (a corticosteroid) to the mother for several days before delivery (i.e., antenatal) to increase surfactant production, postnatal administration of an artificial surfactant solution, and postnatal high-frequency ventilation. RDS in premature infants cannot be discussed without mentioning **germinal matrix hemorrhage** (GMH). The germinal matrix is the site of proliferation of neuronal and glial precursors in the developing brain, which is located above the caudate nucleus, in the floor of the lateral ventricles, and the caudothalamic groove. The germinal matrix also contains a rich network of fragile, thin-walled blood vessels. The brain of the premature infant lacks the ability to autoregulate the cerebral blood pressure. Consequently, increased arterial blood pressure in these blood vessels leads to rupture and hemorrhage into the germinal matrix. This leads to significant neurologic sequelae, including cerebral palsy, mental retardation, and seizures. Antenatal corticosteroid administration has a clear role in reducing the incidence of GMH in premature infants.

c. **Pulmonary agenesis** is the complete absence of a lung or a lobe and its bronchi. This is a rare condition caused by failure of bronchial buds to develop. Unilateral pulmonary agenesis is compatible with life.

d. **Pulmonary aplasia** is the absence of lung tissue but the presence of a rudimentary bronchus.

e. **Pulmonary hypoplasia (PH)** is a poorly developed bronchial tree with abnormal histology. PH classically involves the right lung in association with right-sided obstructive

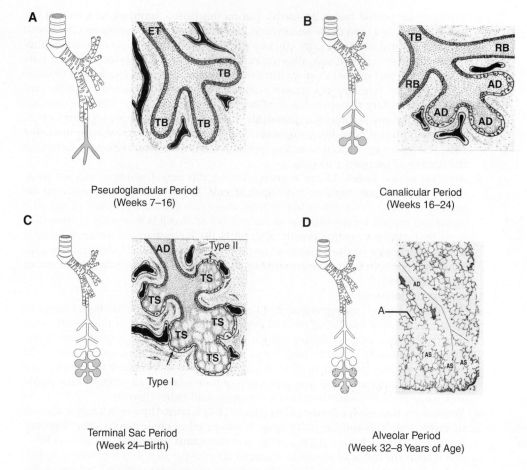

congenital heart defects. PH can also be found in association with **congenital diaphragmatic hernia** (i.e., herniation of abdominal contents into the thorax), which compresses the developing lung. In addition, PH can be found in association with **bilateral renal agenesis**, which causes an insufficient amount of amniotic fluid (oligohydramnios) to be produced, which in turn increases pressure on the fetal thorax.

Pseudoglandular Period (Weeks 7–16)

- The developing lung resembles an exocrine gland whereby numerous **endodermal tubules** are lined by **simple columnar epithelium** and are surrounded by mesoderm containing a **modest capillary network**.
- Each endodermal tubule branches into 15–25 **terminal bronchioles.**
- **Respiration is not possible and premature infants cannot survive.**

Canalicular Period (Weeks 16–24)

- The terminal bronchioles branch into 3 or more **respiratory bronchioles.**
- The respiratory bronchioles subsequently branch into 3–6 **alveolar ducts.**
- The terminal bronchioles, respiratory bronchioles, and alveolar ducts are now lined by a **simple cuboidal epithelium** and are surrounded by mesoderm containing a **prominent capillary network.**
- **Premature infants born before week 20 rarely survive.**

Terminal Sac Period (Week 24–Birth)

- The alveolar ducts bud off **terminal sacs,** which dilate and expand into the surrounding mesoderm.
- The terminal sacs are separated from each other by **primary septa**.
- The simple cuboidal epithelium within the terminal sacs differentiates into **Type I pneumocytes** (thin, flat cells that make up part of the blood–air barrier) and **Type II pneumocytes** (which secrete surfactant).
- The terminal sacs are surrounded by mesoderm containing a **rapidly proliferating capillary network**. The capillaries make intimate contact with the terminal sacs and thereby establish a **blood–air barrier** with the Type I pneumocytes.
- **Premature infants born between week 25 and week 28 can survive with intensive care.** Adequate vascularization and surfactant levels are the most important factors for the survival of premature infants.

Alveolar Period (Week 32–8 Years of Age)

- The terminal sacs are partitioned by **secondary septa** to form adult **alveoli**. About 20–70 million alveoli are present at birth. About 300–400 million alveoli are present by 8 years of age.
- The major mechanism for the increase in the number of alveoli is formation of secondary septa that partition existing alveoli.
- After birth, the increase in the size of the lung is due to an **increase in the number of respiratory bronchioles**.
- On chest radiographs, lungs of a newborn infant are denser than an adult lung because of the fewer number of mature alveoli.

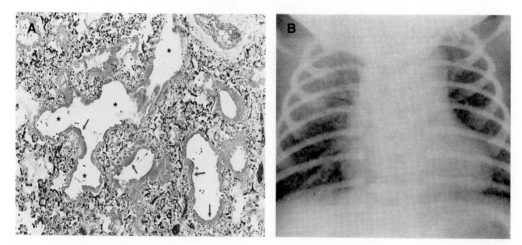

Figure 11-4.   Respiratory distress syndrome (RDS). **(A)** Light micrograph. The pathologic hallmarks are acinar atelectasis (i.e., collapse of the respiratory acinus, which includes the respiratory bronchioles, alveolar ducts, and alveoli), dilation of terminal bronchioles (*), and deposition of an eosinophilic hyaline membrane material (*arrows*), which consists of fibrin and necrotic cells. **(B)** AP radiograph. The radiologic hallmarks consist of a bell-shaped thorax due to underaeration and reticulogranularity of the lungs caused by acinar atelectasis.

STUDY QUESTIONS FOR CHAPTER 11

*Directions: Each of the numbered items or incomplete statements in this section is followed by answers or by completions of the statement. Select the **one** lettered answer or completion that is **best** in each case.*

1. A young mother brings her recently born infant into your office and complains that the infant gags and chokes after swallowing milk. A physical examination indicates excessive saliva and mucus around the mouth and nose, abdominal distention, pneumonitis, and radiographs indicate air in the infant's stomach. What is the most likely cause?

(A) Hypertrophic pyloric stenosis
(B) Tracheoesophageal fistula
(C) Congenital lobar emphysema
(D) Respiratory distress syndrome
(E) Pulmonary hypoplasia

2. Within hours after birth, a baby, whose mother is diabetic, had a rising respiratory rate and labored breathing. The baby became cyanotic and died. Postmortem histologic examination revealed collapsed alveoli lined with eosinophilic material. What is the diagnosis?

(A) Congenital emphysema
(B) Respiratory distress syndrome
(C) Cystic fibrosis
(D) Tracheoesophageal fistula
(E) Pulmonary carcinoma

3. The trachea is lined with pseudostratified ciliated columnar epithelium with goblet cells. This epithelium is derived from

(A) neuroectoderm
(B) endoderm
(C) ectoderm
(D) visceral mesoderm
(E) mesoderm of fourth and sixth pharyngeal arches

4. Smooth muscle, connective tissue, and cartilage of primary bronchi are derived from which one of the following sources?

(A) Neuroectoderm
(B) Endoderm
(C) Ectoderm
(D) Visceral mesoderm
(E) Mesoderm of pharyngeal arches 4 and 6

5. Components of the blood–air barrier in the lung are derived from which of the following sources?

(A) Ectoderm only
(B) Visceral mesoderm only

(C) Visceral mesoderm and ectoderm
(D) Endoderm and ectoderm
(E) Visceral mesoderm and endoderm

6. The respiratory diverticulum initially is in open communication with the primitive foregut. Which of the following embryonic structures is responsible for separating these two structures?

(A) Laryngotracheal groove
(B) Posterior esophageal folds
(C) Laryngotracheal diverticulum
(D) Tracheoesophageal septum
(E) Bronchopulmonary segment

7. Collapsed bronchi caused by failure of bronchial cartilage development is indicative of which one of the following congenital malformations?

(A) Congenital bronchial cysts
(B) Congenital neonatal emphysema
(C) Tracheoesophageal fistula
(D) Hyaline membrane disease
(E) Pulmonary hypoplasia

8. Pulmonary hypoplasia is commonly associated with which condition?

(A) Hyaline membrane disease
(B) Diaphragmatic hernia
(C) Tracheoesophageal fistula
(D) Congenital bronchial cysts
(E) Congenital neonatal emphysema

9. Development of which one of the following is the first sign of respiratory system development?

(A) Tracheoesophageal septum
(B) Hypobranchial eminence
(C) Primitive foregut
(D) Tracheoesophageal fistula
(E) Respiratory diverticulum

10. In which stage of lung maturation is the blood–air barrier established?

(A) Embryonic period
(B) Pseudoglandular period
(C) Canalicular period
(D) Terminal sac period
(E) Alveolar period

ANSWERS AND EXPLANATIONS

1. B. Tracheoesophageal fistula is an abnormal communication between the trachea and esophagus that results from an improper division of the foregut by the tracheoesophageal septum. It is generally associated with esophageal atresia and polyhydramnios.

2. B. Respiratory distress syndrome is common in premature infants and infants of diabetic mothers. It is caused by a deficiency or absence of surfactant. Collapsed alveoli and eosinophilic material consisting of fibrin (hyaline membrane) can be observed histologically, indicating associated hyaline membrane disease.

3. B. The epithelial lining of the entire respiratory system (from tracheal epithelium to Type I pneumocytes lining alveoli) is derived from endoderm.

4. D. The epithelium of primary bronchi is derived from endoderm; the other components are derived from visceral mesoderm.

5. E. The blood–air barrier comprises the structures through which gaseous exchange occurs between air in alveoli and blood in pulmonary capillaries. The attenuated pulmonary epithelium (Type I pneumocytes) is derived from endoderm. The simple, squamous epithelium (endothelium) lining pulmonary capillaries is derived from visceral mesoderm.

6. D. When the tracheoesophageal folds fuse in the midline, they form the tracheoesophageal septum. This septum is responsible for separating the adult trachea ventrally from the esophagus dorsally.

7. B. Congenital neonatal emphysema is a malformation involving the bronchi. One or more lobes of the lungs are overdistended with air because air can be inspired through collapsed bronchi, but cannot be expired.

8. B. During normal development, a space is provided for the prolific growth of the bronchial buds in a lateral and caudal direction. This space, which is part of the intraembryonic coelom, is called the primitive pleural cavity. If this space is reduced by herniation of abdominal viscera, lung development will be severely compromised.

9. E. Development of the respiratory system begins in week 4; the first sign of development is formation of the respiratory diverticulum in the ventral wall of the primitive foregut.

10. D. The simple cuboidal epithelium within the terminal sacs differentiate into pneumocytes within the terminal sac period. The rapidly proliferating capillary network makes intimate contact with the terminal sacs, and the blood–air barrier is established with Type I pneumocytes. These events take place in the terminal sac period, which runs from embryonic week 24 until birth.

Head and Neck

I. Pharyngeal Apparatus (Figure 12-1; Table 12-1)

Consists of the **pharyngeal arches, pharyngeal pouches, pharyngeal grooves,** and **pharyngeal membranes** all of which contribute greatly to the formation of the head and neck. The pharyngeal apparatus is first observed in week 4 of development and gives the embryo its distinctive appearance. There are five pharyngeal arches (1, 2, 3, 4, and 6), four pharyngeal pouches (1, 2, 3, and 4), four pharyngeal grooves (1, 2, 3, and 4), and four pharyngeal membranes (1, 2, 3, and 4). Pharyngeal arch 5 and pharyngeal pouch 5 completely regress in the human. Aortic arch 5 also completely regresses (see Chapter 5). The **Hox complex** and **retinoic acid** appear to be important factors in early head and neck formation. A lack or excess of retinoic acid causes striking facial anomalies.

A. Pharyngeal arches (1, 2, 3, 4, and 6) contain **somitomeric mesoderm** and **neural crest cells**. In general, the mesoderm differentiates into **muscles** and **arteries** (i.e., aortic arches 1–6), whereas neural crest cells differentiate into **bone** and **connective tissue**. In addition, each pharyngeal arch has a **cranial nerve** associated with it.

B. Pharyngeal pouches (1, 2, 3, and 4) are evaginations of endoderm lining the foregut.

C. Pharyngeal grooves (1, 2, 3, and 4) are invaginations of ectoderm located between each pharyngeal arch.

D. Pharyngeal membranes (1, 2, 3, and 4) are structures consisting of ectoderm, intervening mesoderm and neural crest, and endoderm located between each pharyngeal arch.

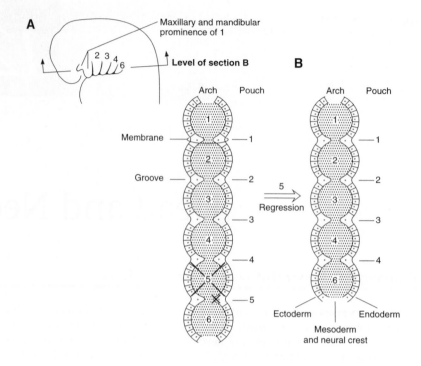

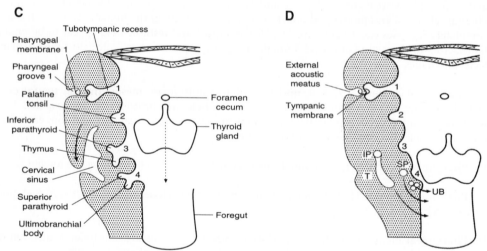

Figure 12-1. **(A)** Drawing of lateral view of an embryo in week 4 of development, showing the pharyngeal arches. Note that pharyngeal arch 1 consists of a maxillary prominence and a mandibular prominence, which can cause some confusion in numbering of the arches. **(B)** A schematic diagram indicating a convenient way to understand the numbering of the arches and pouches. The *X*s indicate regression of pharyngeal arch 5 and pouch 5. **(C and D)** Schematic diagrams of the fate of the pharyngeal pouches, grooves, and membranes. **(C)** *Solid arrow* indicates the downward growth of pharyngeal arch 2, thereby forming a smooth contour at the neck region. *Dotted arrow* indicates downward migration of the thyroid gland. **(D)** *Curved arrows* indicate direction of migration of the inferior parathyroid (*IP*), thymus (*T*), superior parathyroid (*SP*), and ultimobranchial bodies (*UB*). Note that the parathyroid tissue derived from pharyngeal pouch 3 is carried farther caudally by the descent of the thymus than parathyroid tissue from pharyngeal pouch 4.

TABLE 12–1	*Adult Derivatives of Pharyngeal Arches, Pouches, Grooves, and Membranes*

Arch	Nerve	Adult Derivatives
1	CN V	**Mesoderm:** Muscles of mastication, mylohyoid, anterior belly of digastric, tensor veli palatini, tensor tympani **Neural Crest:** Maxilla, mandible, incus, malleus, zygomatic bone, squamous temporal bone, palatine bone, vomer, sphenomandibular ligament
2	CN VII	**Mesoderm:** Muscles of facial expression, posterior belly of digastric, stylohyoid, stapedius **Neural Crest:** Stapes, styloid process, stylohyoid ligament, lesser horn and upper body of hyoid bone
3	CN IX	**Mesoderm:** Stylopharyngeus, common carotid arteries, internal carotid arteries **Neural Crest:** Greater horn and lower body of hyoid bone
4	CN X (superior laryngeal nerve)	**Mesoderm:** Muscles of soft palate (except tensor veli palatini), muscles of the pharynx (except stylopharyngeus) cricothyroid, cricopharyngeus, laryngeal cartilages, right subclavian artery, arch of aorta **Neural Crest:** none
6	CN X (recurrent laryngeal nerve)	**Mesoderm:** Intrinsic muscles of larynx (except cricothyroid), upper muscles of the esophagus, laryngeal cartilages, pulmonary arteries, ductus arteriosus **Neural Crest:** none
Pouch		
1		Epithelial lining of auditory tube and middle ear cavity
2		Epithelial lining of palatine tonsil crypts
3		Inferior parathyroid gland Thymus
4		Superior parathyroid gland Ultimobranchial body[a]
Groove		
1		Epithelial lining of the external auditory meatus
2,3,4		Obliterated
Membrane		
1		Tympanic membrane
2,3,4		Obliterated

[a]Neural crest cells migrate into the ultimobranchial body to form parafollicular cells (C cells) of the thyroid which secrete calcitonin.

II.   Development of the Thyroid Gland

In the midline of the floor of the pharynx, the endodermal lining of the foregut forms the **thyroid diverticulum.** The thyroid diverticulum migrates caudally, passing ventral to the hyoid bone and laryngeal cartilages. During this migration, the thyroid remains connected to the tongue by the **thyroglossal duct,** which later is obliterated. The site of the thyroglossal duct is indicated in the adult by the **foramen cecum.**

III.   Development of the Tongue (Figure 12-2A)

A. The **oral part (anterior two thirds) of the tongue** forms from the **median tongue bud** and **two distal tongue buds** that develop in the floor of the pharynx associated with **pharyngeal arch 1.** The distal tongue buds overgrow the median tongue bud and fuse in the midline, forming the **median sulcus.** The oral part is characterized by **filiform papillae** (no taste buds), **fungiform papillae** (taste buds present), **foliate papillae** (taste buds present; poorly developed in humans), and **circumvallate papillae** (taste buds present). General sensation from the mucosa is carried by the **lingual branch of the trigeminal nerve (CN V).** Taste sensation from the mucosa is carried by the **chorda tympani branch of the facial nerve (CN VII).**

B. The **pharyngeal part (posterior third) of the tongue** forms from the **copula** and **hypobranchial eminence** that develop in the floor of the pharynx associated with **pharyngeal arches 2, 3, and 4.** The hypobranchial eminence overgrows the copula, thereby eliminating any contribution of pharyngeal arch 2 in the formation of the definitive adult tongue. The line of fusion between the oral and pharyngeal parts of the tongue is indicated by the **terminal sulcus.** The pharyngeal part is characterized by the **lingual tonsil,** which, along with the palatine tonsil and pharyngeal tonsil (adenoids), forms **Waldeyer's ring.** General sensation from the mucosa is carried primarily by the **glossopharyngeal nerve (CN IX).** Taste sensation from the mucosa is carried predominantly by the **glossopharyngeal nerve (CN IX).**

C. **Muscles of the tongue**   The intrinsic muscles and extrinsic muscles (styloglossus, hyoglossus, genioglossus, and palatoglossus) are derived from myoblasts that migrate into the tongue region from **occipital somites.** Motor innervation is supplied by the **hypoglossal nerve (CN XII),** except for palatoglossus muscle, which is innervated by CN X.

IV.   Development of the Face (see Figure 12-2B)

The face is formed by three swellings: the **frontonasal prominence, maxillary prominence** (pharyngeal arch 1), and **mandibular prominence** (pharyngeal arch 1). Bilateral ectodermal thickenings called **nasal placodes** develop on the ventrolateral aspects of the frontonasal prominence. The nasal placodes invaginate into the underlying mesoderm to form the **nasal pits,** thereby producing a ridge of tissue that forms the **medial nasal prominence** and **lateral nasal prominence.** A deep groove called the **nasolacrimal groove** forms between the maxillary prominence and the lateral nasal prominence and eventually forms the **nasolacrimal duct** and **lacrimal sac.**

Figure 12-2.   (A) Development of the tongue at week 5 and in the newborn. **(B)** Development of the face at ▶ week 6 and week 10. **(C)** Development of the palate from week 5 through week 10. (*1*) Horizontal section as indicated shows the intermaxillary segment and maxillary prominence with palatine shelves growing toward the midline (*arrows*). (*2,3*) Coronal sections showing movements of the palatine shelves (*single arrows*) and fusion with the nasal septum (*double arrows*). (*4*) A horizontal section as indicated of the adult palate. *Insets for 1–4* show the roof of the mouth. *Arrows* indicate open communication between the nasal cavities and mouth. Level of sections in *1* and *4* is noted in top drawing.

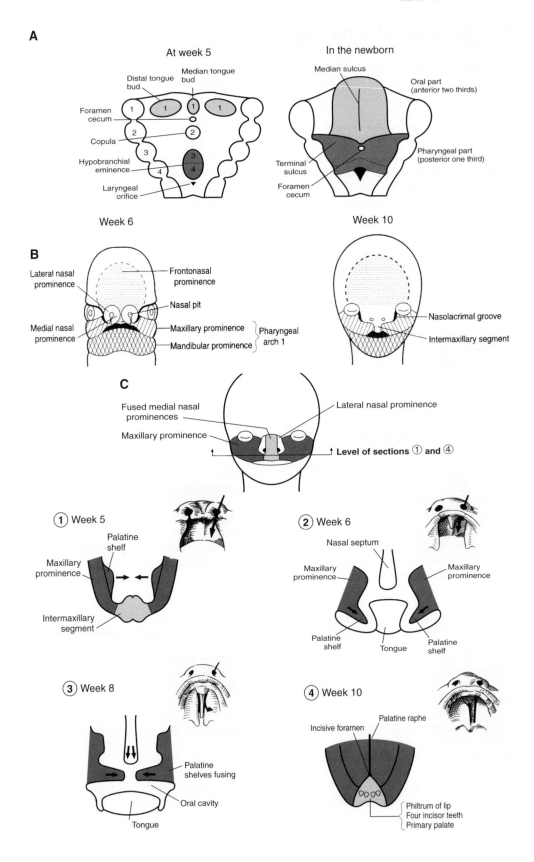

A

At week 5

Distal tongue bud
Median tongue bud

Foramen cecum

Copula

Hypobranchial eminence

Laryngeal orifice

In the newborn

Median sulcus

Oral part (anterior two thirds)

Terminal sulcus

Foramen cecum

Pharyngeal part (posterior one third)

Week 6

B

Lateral nasal prominence

Frontonasal prominence

Medial nasal prominence

Nasal pit

Maxillary prominence

Mandibular prominence

Pharyngeal arch 1

Week 10

Nasolacrimal groove

Intermaxillary segment

C

Fused medial nasal prominences

Maxillary prominence

Lateral nasal prominence

Level of sections ① and ④

① Week 5

Palatine shelf

Maxillary prominence

Intermaxillary segment

② Week 6

Nasal septum

Maxillary prominence

Maxillary prominence

Palatine shelf

Tongue

Palatine shelf

③ Week 8

Palatine shelves fusing

Oral cavity

Tongue

④ Week 10

Incisive foramen

Palatine raphe

Philtrum of lip
Four incisor teeth
Primary palate

V. Development of the Palate (see Figure 12-2C)

A. The **intermaxillary segment** forms when the medial growth of the maxillary prominences causes the two medial nasal prominences to fuse together at the midline. The intermaxillary segment forms the **philtrum of the lip, four incisor teeth,** and the **primary palate.**

B. The **secondary palate** forms from outgrowths of the maxillary prominences called the **palatine shelves.** Initially, the palatine shelves project downward on either side of the tongue but later attain a horizontal position and fuse along the **palatine raphe** to form the **secondary palate.** The primary and secondary palates fuse at the **incisive foramen** to form the **definitive palate.** Bone develops in both the primary palate and the anterior part of the secondary palate. Bone does not develop in the posterior part of the secondary palate, which eventually forms the **soft palate** and **uvula.** The **nasal septum** develops from the medial nasal prominences and fuses with the definitive palate.

VI. Development of the Mouth

The mouth is formed from a surface depression called the **stomodeum,** which is lined by ectoderm, and the **cephalic end of the foregut,** which is lined by endoderm. The stomodeum and foregut meet at the **oropharyngeal membrane.** The epithelium of the **oral part of the tongue, hard palate, sides of the mouth, lips, parotid gland and ducts, Rathke's pouch,** and **enamel of the teeth** are derived from ectoderm. The epithelium of the **pharyngeal part of the tongue, floor of the mouth, palatoglossal fold, palatopharyngeal fold, soft palate, sublingual gland and ducts,** and **submandibular gland and ducts** are derived from endoderm.

VII. Development of the Nasal Cavities

The nasal placodes deepen considerably to form the nasal pits and finally the **nasal sacs.** The nasal sacs remain separated from the oral cavity by the **oronasal membrane,** but it soon ruptures; the nasal cavities and oral cavity are then continuous via the **primitive choanae.** Swellings in the lateral wall of each nasal cavity form the **superior, middle, and inferior conchae.** In the roof of each nasal cavity, the ectoderm of the nasal placode forms a thickened patch, the **olfactory epithelium.** Olfactory epithelium contains **sustentacular cells, basal cells,** and **ciliated cells.** These ciliated cells are bipolar neurons that give rise to the **olfactory nerve (CN I),** have a lifespan of 1–2 months, and are continuously regenerated.

VIII. Clinical Considerations (Figure 12-3)

A. First arch syndrome results from abnormal development of **pharyngeal arch 1** and produces various facial anomalies. It is caused by a lack of migration of neural crest cells into pharyngeal arch 1. Two well-described first arch syndromes are **Treacher Collins syndrome** and **Pierre Robin syndrome.**

B. A **pharyngeal fistula** occurs when **pharyngeal pouch 2** and **pharyngeal groove 2** persist, thereby forming a patent opening from the internal tonsillar area to the external neck. It is generally found along the **anterior border of the sternocleidomastoid muscle.**

C. A **pharyngeal cyst** occurs when parts of the **pharyngeal grooves 2, 3, and 4,** which are normally obliterated, persist, thereby forming a cyst. A pharyngeal cyst is generally found near the **angle of the mandible.**

D. Ectopic thymus, parathyroid, or **thyroid tissue** results from the abnormal migration of these glands from their embryonic position to their definitive adult location. Glandular tissue may be found anywhere along their migratory path.

E. A **thyroglossal duct cyst** occurs when parts of the thyroglossal duct persist and thereby form a cyst. It is most commonly located in the midline near the hyoid bone, but may also be located at the base of the tongue; it is then called a **lingual cyst.**

F. Congenital hypothyroidism (cretinism) occurs when a thyroid deficiency exists during the early fetal period owing to a severe lack of dietary iodine, thyroid agenesis, or mutations involving the biosynthesis of thyroid hormone. This condition causes impaired skeletal growth and mental retardation. Congenital hypothyroidism is characterized by dry, rough skin, wide-set eyes, periorbital puffiness, a flat, broad nose, and a large protuberant tongue.

G. Cleft palate has multifactorial causes. It is classified as anterior or posterior. The anatomic landmark that separates anterior from posterior cleft palate defects is the incisive foramen.
1. **Anterior cleft palate** occurs when the palatine shelves fail to fuse with the primary palate.
2. **Posterior cleft palate** occurs when the palatine shelves fail to fuse with each other and with the nasal septum.
3. **Anteroposterior cleft palate** occurs when there is a combination of both defects.

H. Cleft lip has multifactorial causes. Cleft lip and cleft palate are distinct malformations based on their embryologic formation, even though they often occur together. They may occur unilaterally or bilaterally. Unilateral cleft lip is the most common congenital malformation of the head and neck. It results from the following:
1. The maxillary prominence fails to fuse with the medial nasal prominence.
2. The underlying somitomeric mesoderm and neural crest fail to expand, resulting in a **persistent labial groove.**

I. DiGeorge syndrome occurs when **pharyngeal pouches 3 and 4** fail to differentiate into the thymus and parathyroid glands. It is usually accompanied by facial anomalies resembling first arch syndrome, cardiovascular anomalies due to abnormal neural crest cell migration during formation of the aorticopulmonary septum, immunodeficiency due to absence of thymus gland, and hypocalcemia due to absence of parathyroid glands.

J. Ankyloglossia (tongue-tie) occurs when the frenulum of the tongue extends to the tip of the tongue, preventing protrusion.

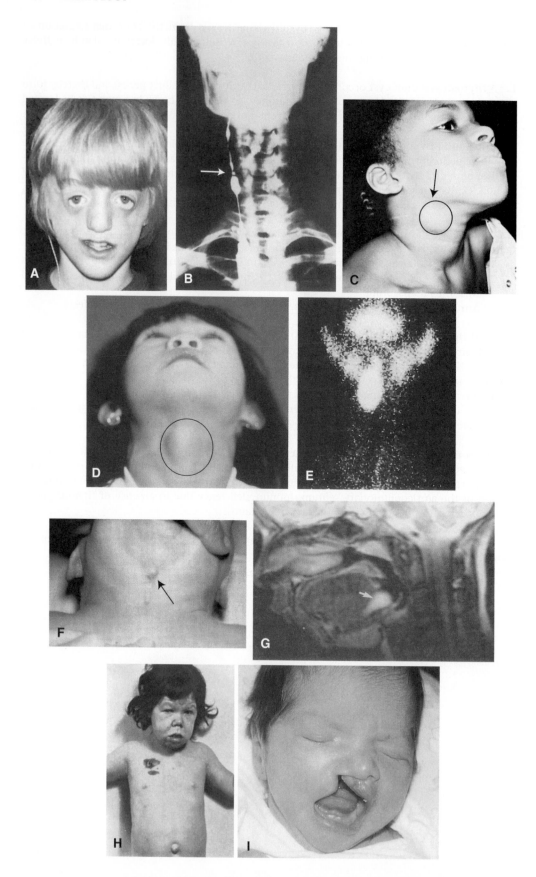

◀ **Figure 12-3.** **(A)** Treacher Collins syndrome (mandibulofacial dysostosis) is characterized by underdevelopment of the zygomatic bones, mandibular hypoplasia, lower eyelid colobomas, downward-slanting palpebral fissures, and malformed external ears (note the hearing aid cord). This is an autosomal-dominant genetic disorder involving a gene locus on chromosome 5q31.3-q33.3. **A.** From McMillan JA, DeAngelis CD, Feigin RD, et al. eds. *Oski''s Pediatrics: Principles and Practice,* 3rd ed. Philadelphia: Lippincott Williams & Wilkins, 1999:394. **(B)** Pharyngeal fistula. A radiograph after injection of a contrast medium demonstrates the course of the fistula through the neck (*arrow*). The fistula may begin inside the throat near the tonsils, travel through the neck, and open to the outside near the anterior border of the sternocleidomastoid muscle. **(C)** Pharyngeal cyst. A fluid-filled cyst (*circle*) near the angle of the mandible (*arrow*). **(D and E)** Ectopic thyroid tissue. A sublingual thyroid mass (*circle*) is seen in a 5-year-old euthyroid girl. A technetium pertechnetate (Tc 99m) scan localizes the position and the extent of the sublingual thyroid gland. There is no evidence of functioning thyroid tissue in the lower neck (i.e., normal anatomic position). **(F)** Thyroglossal duct cyst. A thyroglossal duct cyst (*arrow*) is one of the most common congenital anomalies in the neck and is found along the midline most frequently below the hyoid bone. **(G)** Lingual cyst. MRI shows a mass of thyroid tissue (*arrow*) at the base of the tongue. **(H)** Congenital hypothyroidism (cretinism). This child shows impaired skeletal growth and mental retardation. Note the dry, rough skin (myxedema) and protuberant tongue. **(I)** Unilateral cleft lip and cleft palate.

STUDY QUESTIONS FOR CHAPTER 12

1. The most common site of a thyroglossal cyst is the

(A) dorsal aspect of neck
(B) anterior border of sternocleidomastoid muscle
(C) superior mediastinum
(D) midline close to the hyoid bone
(E) base of the tongue

2. Taste sensation from the oral part (anterior two thirds) of the tongue is predominantly carried by the

(A) trigeminal nerve (CN V)
(B) chorda tympani branch of the facial nerve (CN VII)
(C) glossopharyngeal nerve (CN IX)
(D) superior laryngeal branch of the vagus nerve (CN X)
(E) recurrent laryngeal branch of the vagus nerve (CN X)

3. The intermaxillary segment forms via the fusion of the

(A) maxillary prominences
(B) mandibular prominences
(C) palatine shelves
(D) lateral nasal prominences
(E) medial nasal prominences

4. The most common site of a pharyngeal fistula is the

(A) dorsal aspect of neck
(B) anterior border of sternocleidomastoid muscle
(C) superior mediastinum
(D) midline close to the hyoid bone
(E) base of the tongue

5. What is the most common congenital malformation of the head and neck region?

(A) Anterior cleft palate
(B) Posterior cleft palate
(C) Thyroglossal duct cyst
(D) Unilateral cleft lip
(E) Ankyloglossia

6. Which pharyngeal arch is associated with Treacher Collins syndrome?

(A) Pharyngeal arch 1
(B) Pharyngeal arch 2
(C) Pharyngeal arch 3
(D) Pharyngeal arch 4
(E) Pharyngeal arch 6

7. During surgery for removal of a thyroid tumor, a number of small masses of glandular tissue are noted just lateral to the thyroid gland. Metastasis from the thyroid tumor is suspected, but histologic analysis of a biopsy reveals parathyroid tissue and remnants of thymus. How can this finding be explained?

(A) Tumor tissue has differentiated into normal tissue
(B) A parathyroid gland tumor is also present
(C) Ectopic glandular tissue is commonly found in this region
(D) Patient has DiGeorge syndrome
(E) The glandular tissue is a result of a thyroglossal duct cyst

8. A newborn presents with midfacial and mandibular hypoplasia, defects of the first pharyngeal arch consistent with the diagnosis of Treacher Collins syndrome. What structure would most likely be involved with this syndrome?

(A) Hyoid bone
(B) Stapes
(C) Malleus
(D) Thyroid gland
(E) Inferior parathyroid gland

ANSWERS AND EXPLANATIONS

1. D. The thyroid gland forms from a diverticulum in the midline of the floor of the pharynx. The thyroid migrates caudally and passes ventral to the hyoid bone. During this migration, the thyroid remains connected to the tongue by the thyroglossal duct. If a part of the thyroglossal duct persists, a cyst develops, usually near the hyoid bone.

2. B. Taste sensation from the mucosa for the oral part of the tongue is carried by the chorda tympani branch of the facial nerve (CN VII). This part of the tongue forms from pharyngeal arch 1, so the trigeminal nerve (CN V) will carry sensory innervation from the mucosa.

3. E. The intermaxillary segment, which plays a critical role in the formation of the definitive adult palate, forms when the two medial nasal prominences fuse in the midline.

4. B. A pharyngeal fistula forms when pharyngeal pouch 2 and pharyngeal groove 2 persist. Therefore, these fistulas are found on the lateral aspect of the neck, usually along the anterior border of the sternocleidomastoid muscle.

5. D. Unilateral cleft lip is the most common congenital malformation of the head and neck. Cleft lip occurs when the maxillary prominences fail to fuse with the medial nasal prominences and when the underlying somitomeric mesoderm and neural crest fail to proliferate, resulting in a persistent labial groove. Cleft lip occurs in 1 of 900 births and may be unilateral or bilateral.

6. A. First arch syndrome results from abnormal development of pharyngeal arch 1 due to a lack of migration of neural crest cells. Treacher Collins syndrome is associated with underdevelopment of the zygomatic bone, down-slanting palpebral fissures, and deformed lower eyelids and external ears.

7. C. The parathyroid and thymus migrate in a caudal and medial direction during development; therefore, ectopic glandular tissue may be found anywhere along the migratory path.

8. C. The malleus is the only structure on this list derived from the neural crest of the first pharyngeal arch.

CHAPTER

13

Urinary System

I.   Overview (Figure 13-1)

The **intermediate mesoderm** forms a longitudinal elevation along the dorsal body wall called the **urogenital ridge**. A portion of the urogenital ridge forms the **nephrogenic cord**, which gives rise to the urinary system. The nephrogenic cord develops into three sets of nephric structures: the **pronephros, mesonephros,** and **metanephros.** The homeobox genes, *Lim-1* and *Pax-2*, are important in the early stages of kidney development.

A. The **pronephros** develops by the differentiation of mesoderm within the nephrogenic cord to form **pronephric tubules** and the **pronephric duct**. The pronephros is the cranialmost nephric structure and is a transitory structure that regresses completely by week 5. The pronephros is not functional in humans.

B. The **mesonephros** develops by the differentiation of mesoderm within the nephrogenic cord to form **mesonephric tubules** and the **mesonephric duct (wolffian duct).** The mesonephros is the middle nephric structure and is a partially transitory structure. Most of the mesonephric tubules regress, but the mesonephric duct persists and opens into the urogenital sinus. The mesonephros is functional for a short period.

C. The **metanephros** develops from an outgrowth of the mesonephric duct (called the **ureteric bud**) and from a condensation of mesoderm within the nephrogenic cord called the **metanephric mesoderm.** It is the caudalmost nephric structure. The metanephros begins to form at week 5 and is functional in the fetus at about week 10. It develops into the **definitive adult kidney.** The fetal kidney is divided into lobes in contrast to the definitive adult kidney, which has a smooth contour.

II.   Development of the Metanephros

A. Development of the collecting system   The ureteric bud is an outgrowth of the mesonephric duct. This outgrowth is regulated by **WT-1** (an anti-oncogene), **GDNF** (glial cell line-derived neurotrophic factor), and **c-Ret** (a tyrosine kinase receptor). The ureteric bud initially penetrates the metanephric mesoderm, and then undergoes repeated branching to form the **ureters, renal pelvis, major calyces, minor calyces,** and **collecting ducts.**

B. Development of the nephron   The inductive influence of the collecting ducts causes the metanephric mesoderm to differentiate into **metanephric vesicles** which later give rise to primitive **S-shaped renal tubules,** which are critical to nephron formation. The S-shaped renal tubules differentiate into the **connecting tubule, distal convoluted tubule, loop of Henle, proximal convoluted tubule,** and **Bowman's capsule.** Tufts of capillaries called **glomeruli** protrude into

Bowman's capsule. Nephron formation is complete at birth, but functional maturation of nephrons continues throughout infancy.

C. **Tissue sources**
  1. The transitional epithelium lining the ureter, pelvis, major calyx, and minor calyx and the simple cuboidal epithelium lining the collecting tubules are derived from mesoderm of the ureteric bud.
  2. The simple cuboidal epithelium lining the connecting tubule and distal convoluted tubule, the simple squamous epithelium lining the loop of Henle, the simple columnar epithelium lining the proximal convoluted tubule, and the podocytes and simple squamous epithelium lining Bowman's capsule are derived from metanephric mesoderm.

III.   Relative Ascent of the Kidneys

The fetal metanephros is located at vertebral level **S1-S2**, whereas the definitive adult kidney is located at vertebral level **T12-L3**. The change in location results from a disproportionate growth of the embryo caudal to the metanephros. During the relative ascent, the kidneys **rotate 90°** causing the hilum, which initially faces ventrally, to finally face medially.

IV.   Blood Supply of the Kidneys

During the relative ascent of the kidneys, the kidneys receive their blood supply from arteries at progressively higher levels until the definitive renal arteries develop at **L2**. Arteries formed during the ascent may persist and are called **supernumerary arteries**. Supernumerary arteries are **end arteries**. Therefore, any damage to them results in necrosis of kidney parenchyma.

V.   Development of the Urinary Bladder (Figure 13-2)

The urinary bladder is formed from the upper portion of the **urogenital sinus**, which is continuous with the **allantois**. The allantois becomes a fibrous cord called the **urachus** (or **median umbilical ligament** in the adult). The lower ends of the mesonephric ducts become incorporated into the posterior wall of the bladder to form the **trigone of the bladder**. The mesonephric ducts eventually open into the urogenital sinus below the bladder. The **transitional epithelium** lining the urinary bladder is derived from endoderm because of its etiology from the urogenital sinus and gut tube.

VI.   Development of the Female Urethra (see Figure 13-2)

The female urethra is formed from the lower portion of the urogenital sinus. The female urethra develops endodermal outgrowths into the surrounding mesoderm to form the **urethral glands** and **paraurethral glands of Skene** (which are homologous to the prostate gland in the male). The paraurethral glands of Skene open on each side of the external urethral orifice. The female urethra ends at **navicular fossa**, which empties into the **vestibule of the vagina**, which also forms from the urogenital sinus. The vestibule of the vagina develops endodermal outgrowths into the surrounding mesoderm to form the **lesser vestibular glands** and **greater vestibular glands of Bartholin** (which are homologous to the bulbourethral glands of Cowper in the male). The greater vestibular glands of Bartholin open on each side of the vaginal orifice. The transitional epithelium and stratified squamous epithelium lining the female urethra are derived from endoderm.

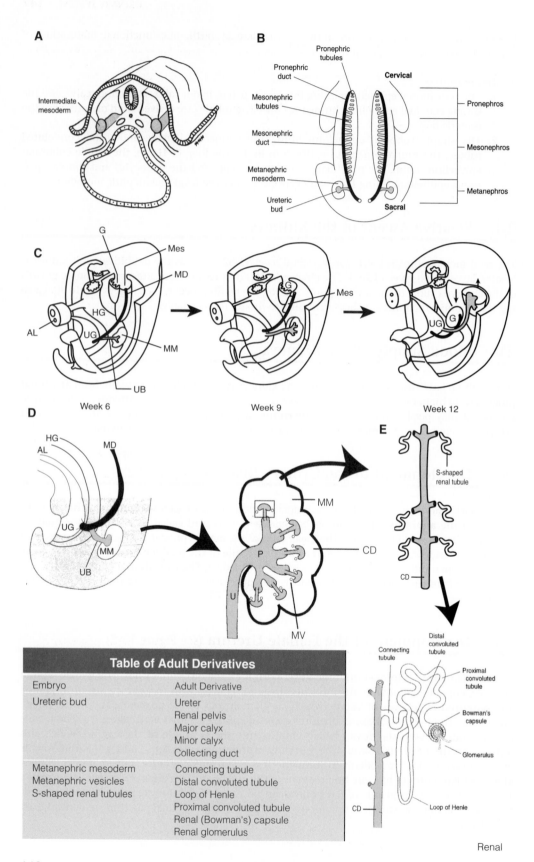

A

Intermediate mesoderm

B

Pronephric tubules
Pronephric duct
Mesonephric tubules
Mesonephric duct
Metanephric mesoderm
Ureteric bud

Cervical

Sacral

Pronephros
Mesonephros
Metanephros

C

G
Mes
MD
HG
AL
UG
MM
UB

Week 6

Mes
G

Week 9

UG
G

Week 12

D

HG
AL
MD
UG
MM
UB

MM
P
CD
U
MV

E

S-shaped renal tubule

CD

Connecting tubule
Distal convoluted tubule
Proximal convoluted tubule
Bowman's capsule
Glomerulus
Loop of Henle
CD

Table of Adult Derivatives	
Embryo	Adult Derivative
Ureteric bud	Ureter
	Renal pelvis
	Major calyx
	Minor calyx
	Collecting duct
Metanephric mesoderm	Connecting tubule
Metanephric vesicles	Distal convoluted tubule
S-shaped renal tubules	Loop of Henle
	Proximal convoluted tubule
	Renal (Bowman's) capsule
	Renal glomerulus

Renal

VII. Development of the Male Urethra (see Figure 13-2)

A. Prostatic urethra, membranous urethra, bulbous urethra, and proximal part of penile urethra These parts of the urethra are formed from the lower portion of the urogenital sinus. The transitional epithelium and stratified columnar epithelium lining these parts of the urethra are derived from endoderm.

   1. **The prostatic urethra** develops endodermal outgrowths into the surrounding mesoderm to form the **prostate gland**. The posterior wall of the prostatic urethra has an elevation called the **urethral crest**. The **prostatic sinus** is a groove on either side of the urethral crest that receives most of the prostatic ducts from the prostate gland. At a specific site along the urethral crest, there is an ovoid enlargement called the **seminal colliculus** (also called the **verumontanum**), which contains the **openings of the ejaculatory ducts** and the **prostatic utricle** (a vestigial remnant of the paramesonephric ducts in the male that is involved in the development of the vagina and uterus).
   2. **The membranous urethra** develops endodermal outgrowths into the surrounding mesoderm to form the **bulbourethral glands of Cowper**.
   3. **The bulbous urethra** contains the openings of the bulbourethral glands of Cowper.
   4. **The proximal part of the penile urethra** develops endodermal outgrowths into the surrounding mesoderm to form **urethral glands of Littré**.

B. The **distal part of the penile urethra** is formed from an ingrowth of surface ectoderm called the **glandular plate**. The glandular plate joins the proximal penile urethra and becomes canalized to form the **navicular fossa**. **Ectodermal septa** appear lateral to the navicular fossa and become canalized to form the **foreskin**. The stratified squamous epithelium lining of the distal penile urethra is derived from ectoderm.

VIII. Clinical Considerations (Figure 13-3)

A. Renal agenesis occurs when the ureteric bud fails to develop, thereby eliminating the induction of metanephric vesicles and nephron formation.

   1. **Unilateral renal agenesis** is relatively common (more common in males). Therefore, a physician should never assume a patient has two kidneys. This situation is asymptomatic and compatible with life because the remaining kidney hypertrophies.

Figure 13-1. (A) Cross-sectional view of an embryo at week 4, illustrating the intermediate mesoderm as a cord of mesoderm that extends from the cervical to sacral levels that forms the urogenital ridge and nephrogenic cord. (B) Frontal view of an embryo, depicting the pronephros, mesonephros, and metanephros. Note that nephric structures develop from cervical through sacral levels. (C) Diagrams show the relationship between the gonad, mesonephros, and metanephros during development at week 6, week 9, and week 12. Note that the gonad descends (*arrow*) while the metanephros ascends (*arrow*). AL = allantois; C = cloaca; G = gonad; HG = hindgut; MD = mesonephric duct; Mes = mesonephros; MM = metanephric mesoderm; UB = ureteric bud; UG = urogenital sinus. (D) Lateral view of the embryo showing the relationship between the ureteric bud (UB; *shaded*), metanephric mesoderm (MM), and mesonephric duct (MD; *black*). In addition, note the urogenital sinus (UG), hindgut (HD), and allantois (AL). Lateral view of a fetal kidney. *Shaded area* indicates structures formed from the ureteric bud. Note the repeated branching of the ureteric bud into the metanephric mesoderm (MM). At the tip of the each collecting duct (CD), the formation of metanephric vesicles (MV) is induced. Note the lobulated appearance of a fetal kidney. P = pelvis; U = ureter. (E) Enlarged view of the rectangle, illustrating the further branching of a collecting duct (CD; *shaded*) and the formation of primitive S-shaped renal tubules. (F) Diagram shows a collecting duct (CD) and the components of a mature adult nephron. A summary table of derivatives is shown.

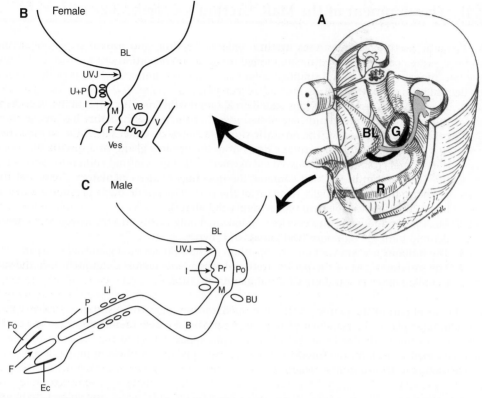

Figure 13-2. **(A)** Diagram of an embryo showing the development of the upper portion of the urogenital sinus into the urinary bladder (*BL*) and the lower portion into the female and male urethra. *G* = gonad; *R* = rectum. **(B)** Female urethra. The bladder (*BL*), membranous portion of the female urethra (*M*), and navicular fossa (*F*) are shown emptying into the vestibule of the vagina (*Ves*). In addition, the urethrovesical junction (*UVJ*) and intermuscular incisura (*I*) are shown. *U+P* = urethral and paraurethral glands of Skene; *VB* = lesser and greater vestibular glands of Bartholin; *V* = vagina. **(C)** Male urethra. The bladder (*BL*), prostatic urethra (*Pr*), membranous urethra (*M*), bulbous urethra (*B*), proximal part of the penile urethra (*P*), and navicular fossa (*F*) are shown. In addition, the urethrovesical junction (*UVJ*) and intermuscular incisura (*I*) are shown. *Bu* = bulbourethral glands of Cowper; *Ec* = ectodermal septa; *Fo* = foreskin; *Li* = urethral glands of Littré; *Pr* = prostate gland.

    2. Bilateral renal agenesis is relatively uncommon. It causes oligohydramnios, which causes compression of the fetus, resulting in **Potter syndrome** (deformed limbs, wrinkly skin, and abnormal facial appearance). Infants with bilateral renal agenesis are usually stillborn or die shortly after birth.

B. Renal hypoplasia occurs when there is a congenitally small kidney with no pathologic evidence of dysplasia.

C. Renal dysplasia occurs when there is a disorganization of renal parenchyma with abnormally developed and immature nephrons.

D. Renal ectopia occurs when one or both kidneys fail to ascend and therefore remain in the pelvis or lower lumbar area (i.e., **pelvic kidney**). In some cases, two pelvic kidneys fuse to form a solid mass, commonly called a **pancake kidney**.

E. Renal fusion The most common type of renal fusion is the **horseshoe kidney.** A horseshoe kidney occurs when the inferior poles of the kidneys fuse across the midline. Normal ascent of the kidneys is arrested because the fused portion gets trapped behind the **inferior mesenteric artery**. Kidney rotation is also arrested so that the hilum faces ventrally.

F. **Renal artery stenosis** is the most common cause of renovascular hypertension in children. The stenosis may occur in the main renal artery of segmental renal arteries.

G. **Ureteropelvic junction obstruction (UPJ)** occurs when there is an obstruction to the urine flow from the renal pelvis to the proximal ureter. UPJ is the most common congenital obstruction of the urinary tract. If there is severe uteropelvic atresia, a **multicystic dysplastic kidney** is found in which the cysts are actually dilated calyces. In this case, the kidney consists of grapelike, smooth-walled cysts of variable size. Between the cysts are found dysplastic glomeruli and atrophic tubules.

H. **Childhood polycystic kidney disease (PCKD)** is an autosomal recessive disease that has been mapped to the short arm of chromosome 6 (p6). In childhood PCKD, the kidneys are huge and spongy and contain numerous cysts caused by the dilatation of collecting ducts and tubules that severely compromise kidney function. Childhood PCKD is associated clinically with cysts of the liver, pancreas, and lungs. Treatment includes dialysis and kidney transplant.

I. **Wilms' tumor (WT)** is the **most common renal malignancy of childhood**. Patients with WT present with a large, solitary, well-circumscribed mass that, on cut section, is soft, homogeneous, and tan-gray in color. WT is interesting histologically in that this tumor tends to recapitulate different stages of embryologic formation of the kidney so that three classic histologic areas are described: a stromal area; a blastemal area of tightly packed embryonic cells; and a tubular area.

J. **Ureteropelvic duplications** occur when the ureteric bud prematurely divides before penetrating the metanephric blastema. This results in either a double kidney or duplicated ureter and renal pelvis. The term **duplex kidney** refers to a configuration in which two ureters drain one kidney.

K. **Exstrophy of the bladder** occurs when the posterior wall of the urinary bladder is exposed to the exterior. It is caused by a failure of the anterior abdominal wall and anterior wall of the bladder to develop properly. It is associated clinically with urine drainage to the exterior and epispadias. Surgical reconstruction is difficult and prolonged.

L. **Urachal fistula or cyst** occurs when a remnant of the allantois persists, thereby forming a fistula or cyst. It is found along the midline on a path from the umbilicus to the apex of the urinary bladder. A urachal fistula forms a direct connection between the urinary bladder and the outside of the body at the umbilicus causing **urine drainage** from the umbilicus.

M. An **ectopic opening of the ureter** occurs when the ureteric bud fails to separate from the mesonephric duct, which results in the opening of the ureter to be carried to a point distal to its normal position. The most common ectopic opening is a **lateral ureteral ectopia** in which the opening is lateral to its normal position.
    1. **In males**, the ectopic openings are most commonly located in the prostatic urethra, ejaculatory ducts, ductus deferens, or rectum. Because the ectopic openings all are located above the external urethral sphincter, boys with an ectopic opening of the ureter do not present with urine incontinence.
    2. **In females**, the ectopic openings are most commonly located in the urethra, vestibule, or vagina. Because the ectopic openings all are located below the external urethral sphincter, girls with an ectopic opening of the ureter generally present with urine incontinence.

N. Ureterocele
    1. A **simple ureterocele** occurs when the distal end of the ureter has a cystlike protrusion into the submucosal layer of the urinary bladder.
    2. An **ectopic ureterocele** occurs when the distal end of the ureter has a cystlike protrusion into the submucosal layer of the urinary bladder that is almost invariably associated with

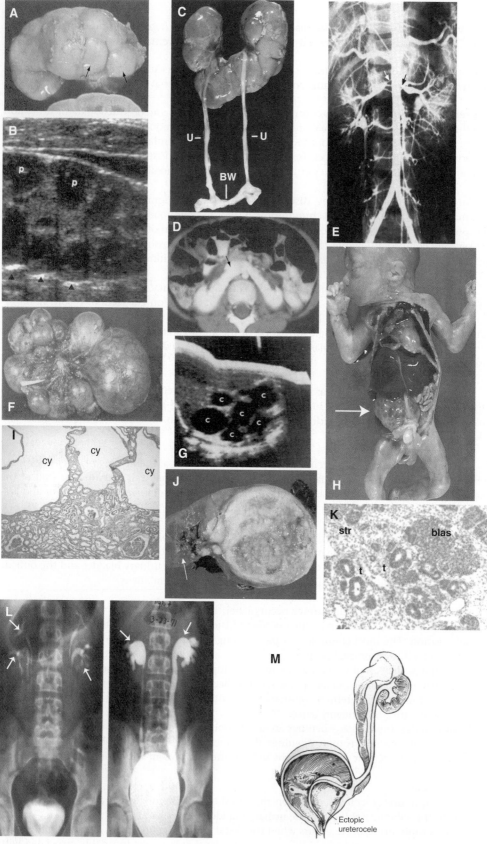

152

an ectopic ureter and duplication. In this situation, the ureterocele is at the end of the ureter from the upper renal segment and is located inferior to the other ureter opening.

IX. Development of the Suprarenal Gland (Figure 13-4)

A. Cortex The cortex forms from two episodes of mesoderm proliferation that occurs between the root of the dorsal mesentery and the gonad. The first episode forms the inner **fetal cortex.** The second episode forms the outer **adult cortex,** whereby mesoderm proliferation occurs at the periphery of the fetal cortex. During the fetal period and at birth, the suprarenal glands are very large because of the size of the fetal cortex. The suprarenal glands become smaller as the fetal cortex involutes rapidly during the first 2 weeks after birth and continues to involute during the first year of life. The zona glomerulosa and zona fasciculata of the adult cortex are present at birth, but the zona reticularis is not formed until age 3 years.

B. Medulla The medulla forms when neural crest cells aggregate at the medial aspect of the fetal cortex and eventually become surrounded by the fetal and adult cortex. The neural crest cells differentiate into **chromaffin cells,** which stain yellow-brown with chromium salts. Chromaffin cells can be found in extrasuprarenal sites at birth, but these sites normally regress completely by puberty. In a normal adult, chromaffin cells are found only in the suprarenal medulla.

C. Clinical considerations
1. **Neuroblastoma (NB).** NB is a common extracranial neoplasm containing **primitive neuroblasts** (small cells arranged in **Homer-Wright pseudorosettes**) of **neural crest origin.** NB occurs mainly in children and is found in extra-adrenal sites usually along the sympathetic chain ganglia (60%) or within the adrenal medulla (40%). NB metastasizes widely to the bone marrow, bone, and lymph nodes. A common laboratory finding is increased urine vanillylmandelic acid (VMA) and metanephrine levels.
2. **Pheochromocytoma (PH).** PH is a relatively rare neoplasm that contains both epinephrine and norepinephrine. PH occurs mainly in adults 40–60 years old and is generally found in the region of the adrenal gland; however, it may be found in extrasuprarenal sites. PH is associated with persistent or paroxysmal hypertension, anxiety, tremor, profuse sweating, pallor, chest pain, and abdominal pain. Laboratory findings include increased urine VMA and metanephrine levels, inability to suppress catecholamines with clonidine, and hyperglycemia. PH is treated by surgery or phenoxybenzamine (an α-adrenergic antagonist).

◄ **Figure 13-3.** (**A and B**) Normal newborn kidney. Photograph shows the normal lobation pattern (*arrows*). Sonogram shows mounds (*arrowheads*) that indicate the fetal lobes. The renal pyramids (*p*) are less echoic than the surrounding renal cortex. (**C and D**) Horseshoe kidney. Photograph of a horseshoe kidney. *BW* = bladder wall; *U* = ureter. CT shows the isthmus of renal tissue (*arrow*) that extends across the midline. (**E**) Renal artery stenosis. Angiogram shows bilateral renal artery stenosis (*arrows*). (**F and G**) Multidysplastic kidney. Photograph shows numerous cysts. Sonogram shows many anechoic cysts (*C*) separated by renal septa. (**H and I**) Childhood polycystic kidney disease. Photograph of an infant with polycystic kidney (*arrow*). Light micrograph shows large, fluid-filled cysts (*CY*) throughout the substance of the kidney. Between the cysts, some functioning nephrons can be observed. (**J and K**) Wilms' tumor. Photograph shows Wilms' tumor extending from normal kidney tissue (*arrow*). Light micrograph shows that tumor is characterized histologically by recognizable attempts to recapitulate embryonic development of the kidney. In this regard, the following three components are seen: (a) metanephric blastema elements (*blas*) consisting of clumps of small, tightly packed embryonic cells; (b) stromal elements (*str*); and (c) epithelial elements generally in the form of abortive attempts at forming tubules (*t*) or glomeruli. (**L**) Ureteropelvic duplication. The intravenous urogram shows bilateral duplication of the collecting system (*arrows*). The cystogram shows reflux into both of the lower collecting systems (*arrows*) only. (**M**) Ectopic ureterocele. The ectopic ureterocele is shown at the end of an enlarged ureter from the upper renal segment. The opening of the enlarged ureter is located inferior to the normal-sized ureter from the lower renal segment.

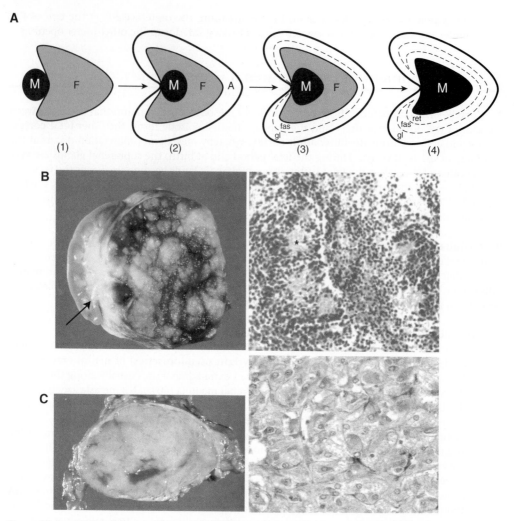

Figure 13-4. **(A)** Development of the suprarenal gland. (*1*) At week 6, the fetal cortex (*F*) and medulla (*M*) at the medial aspect of the adrenal gland are apparent. (*2*) At week 9, the adult cortex (*A*) has formed at the periphery of the fetal cortex. Note that the medulla is completely surrounded by the adult and fetal cortex. (*3*) At birth, the fetal cortex is still present, and the adult cortex has differentiated into the zona glomerulosa (*gl*) and zone fasciculate (*fas*). (*4*) At 3 years of age, the fetal cortex has completely involuted, thus reducing the size of the suprarenal gland. The adult cortex has further differentiated to form the zona reticularis (*ret*). **(B)** Neuroblastoma. Neuroblastomas vary in size from 1 cm to filling the entire abdomen. They are generally soft and white to gray-pink. As the size increases, the tumors become hemorrhagic and undergo calcification and cyst formation. Note the nodular appearance of this tumor with the kidney apparent on the its left border (*arrow*). Light micrograph shows that the neoplastic cells are small, primitive-looking cells with dark nuclei and scant cytoplasm. The cells are generally arranged as solid sheets, and some cells arrange around a central fibrillar area forming Homer-Wright pseudorosettes (*). **(C)** Pheochromocytoma. Pheochromocytomas vary in size from 3 to 5 cm in diameter. They are gray-white to pink-tan. Exposure of the cut surface often results in darkening of the surface due to formation of yellow-brown adrenochrome pigment. Light micrograph shows neoplastic cells that have abundant cytoplasm with small centrally located nuclei. The cells are generally separated into clusters that are also separated by a slender stroma and numerous capillaries. Numerous cytoplasmic hyaline eosinophilic globules are sometimes present; these are derived from membranes of secretory granules.

3. **Congenital adrenal hyperplasia (CAH).** CAH is caused most commonly by mutations in genes for enzymes involved in adrenocortical steroid biosynthesis (e.g., **21-hydroxylase deficiency, 11β-hydroxylase deficiency**). In 21-hydroxylase deficiency (90% of all cases), there is virtually no synthesis of the cortisol or aldosterone so that intermediates are funneled into androgen biosynthesis thereby elevating androgen levels. The elevated levels of androgens lead to **masculinization of a female fetus** (i.e., **female pseudointersexuality**). Female pseudointersexuality produces the following clinical findings: mild clitoral enlargement, complete labioscrotal fusion with a phalloid organ, or macrogenitosomia (in the male fetus). Since cortisol cannot be synthesized, negative feedback to the adenohypophysis does not occur, so ACTH continues to stimulate the adrenal cortex resulting in adrenal hyperplasia. Since aldosterone cannot be synthesized, the patient presents with **hyponatremia ("salt-wasting")** with adjoining **dehydration** and **hyperkalemia**. Treatment includes immediate infusion of intravenous saline and long-term steroid hormone replacement, both cortisol and mineralocorticoids (9α-fludrocortisone).

STUDY QUESTIONS FOR CHAPTER 13

Directions: Each of the numbered items or incomplete statements in this section is followed by answers or by completions of the statement. Select the **one** lettered answer or completion that is **best** in each case.

1. When does the metanephros become functional?

(A) At week 3 of development
(B) At week 4 of development
(C) At week 10 of development
(D) Just before birth
(E) Just after birth

2. A urachal cyst is a remnant of the

(A) urogenital sinus
(B) urogenital ridge
(C) cloaca
(D) allantois
(E) mesonephric duct

3. During surgery for a benign cyst on the kidney, the surgeon notes that the patient's right kidney has two ureters and two renal pelves. This malformation is

(A) an abnormal division of the pronephros
(B) an abnormal division of the mesonephros
(C) formation of an extra mass of intermediate mesoderm
(D) a premature division of the metanephric blastema
(E) a premature division of the ureteric bud

4. The transitional epithelium lining the urinary bladder is derived from

(A) ectoderm
(B) endoderm
(C) mesoderm
(D) endoderm and mesoderm
(E) neural crest cells

5. The transitional epithelium lining the ureter is derived from

(A) ectoderm
(B) endoderm
(C) mesoderm
(D) endoderm and mesoderm
(E) neural crest cells

6. The podocytes of Bowman's capsule are derived from

(A) ectoderm
(B) endoderm

(C) mesoderm
(D) endoderm and mesoderm
(E) neural crest cells

7. The proximal convoluted tubules of the definitive adult kidney are derived from the

(A) ureteric bud
(B) metanephric vesicle
(C) mesonephric duct
(D) mesonephric tubules
(E) pronephric tubules

8. The trigone on the posterior wall of the urinary bladder is formed by the

(A) incorporation of the lower end of the mesonephric ducts
(B) incorporation of the lower end of the pronephric ducts
(C) incorporation of the metanephric blastema
(D) incorporation of the mesonephric tubules
(E) incorporation of the pronephric tubules

9. A 6-year-old girl presents with a large abdominal mass just superior to the pubic symphysis. The mass is tender when palpated and fixed in location. During surgery, a fluid-filled mass is noted, which is connected to the umbilicus superiorly and to the urinary bladder inferiorly. What is the diagnosis?

(A) Pelvic kidney
(B) Horseshoe kidney
(C) Polycystic disease of the kidney
(D) Urachal cyst
(E) Exstrophy of the bladder

10. Immediately after birth of a boy, a moist, red protrusion of tissue is noted just superior to his pubic symphysis. After observation, urine drainage is noted from the upper lateral corners of this tissue mass. What is the diagnosis?

(A) Pelvic kidney
(B) Horseshoe kidney
(C) Polycystic disease of the kidney
(D) Urachal cyst
(E) Exstrophy of the bladder

ANSWERS AND EXPLANATIONS

1. C. The metanephros begins to form at week 5 and starts to function in the fetus at about week 10. The pronephros is not functional in humans; it is the interim kidney, which functions until the metanephros is ready.

2. D. The upper end of the urogenital sinus is in patent communication with the allantois, which lies in the umbilical cord. The allantois normally regresses and forms a fibrous cord. If a remnant persists, it forms a urachal cyst or sinus.

3. E. The ureteric bud seems to be preprogrammed to undergo repeated divisions. These divisions normally begin on contact with the metanephric blastema. If the ureteric bud undergoes division prematurely, duplication of the ureter and renal pelvis occurs. In some circumstances, two separate kidneys form.

4. B. The transitional epithelium lining the urinary bladder is derived from endoderm because the urinary bladder develops from the upper end of the urogenital sinus. The origin of the urogenital sinus can be traced back to the gut tube, which is lined by endoderm.

5. C. The transitional epithelium lining the ureter is derived from mesoderm because the ureter develops from the ureteric bud. The ureteric bud is a diverticulum from the mesonephric duct whose origin can be traced back to the intermediate mesoderm.

6. C. The podocytes of Bowman's capsule develop from the metanephric vesicles, which are of mesodermal origin.

7. B. The distal convoluted tubule, loop of Henle, proximal convoluted tubule, and Bowman's capsule all are derived from the metanephric vesicle.

8. A. The lower end of the mesonephric ducts is incorporated into the posterior wall of the urinary bladder. The mesonephric ducts contribute to the connective tissue component of the posterior wall at the trigone. It is generally believed that the transitional epithelium lining the entire bladder (even the trigone) is of endodermal origin.

9. D. A urachal cyst or sinus forms from a remnant of the allantois and is found along the midline on a path from the umbilicus to the apex of the urinary bladder. The epithelium lining the cyst produces secretions that gradually fill the remnant with fluid. Very rarely, the entire allantois persists, forming a fistula that is patent from the urinary bladder to the exterior at the umbilicus.

10. E. The moist, red tissue mass that is exposed to the exterior is actually the posterior wall of the urinary bladder. This is called exstrophy of the bladder and is caused when the anterior abdominal wall and anterior wall of the bladder fail to form. The ureters open onto the posterior wall; therefore, urine drainage is apparent.

Female Reproductive System

I.   The Indifferent Embryo

The genotype of the embryo (46,XX or 46,XY) is established at fertilization. **During weeks 1–6**, the embryo remains in a sexually indifferent or undifferentiated stage. This means that genetically female embryos and genetically male embryos are phenotypically indistinguishable. **During week 7**, the indifferent embryo begins phenotypic sexual differentiation. **By week 12**, female or male characteristics of the external genitalia can be recognized. **By week 20**, phenotypic differentiation is complete.

A.   Phenotypic sexual differentiation is determined by the *Sry* **gene** located on the short arm of the Y chromosome and may result in individuals with a **female phenotype**, an **intersex phenotype**, or a **male phenotype**. The *Sry* gene encodes for a protein called **testes-determining factor (TDF)**. TDF is a 220-amino acid nonhistone protein that contains a highly conserved DNA-binding region called a **high-mobility group box**. As the indifferent gonad develops into the testes, Leydig cells and Sertoli cells differentiate to produce **testosterone** and **müllerian inhibiting factor (MIF)**, respectively. In the presence of TDF, testosterone, and MIF, the indifferent embryo is directed to the male phenotype. In the absence of TDF, testosterone, and MIF, the indifferent embryo is directed to the female phenotype.

B.   The components of the indifferent embryo that are remodeled to form the adult female reproductive system include the **gonads, genital ducts**, and **primordia of external genitalia**. Phenotypic sexual differentiation occurs in a sequence beginning with the gonads, then the genital ducts, and finally the primordia of external genitalia.

II.   Development of the Gonads (Figure 14-1)

A.   The Ovary   The **intermediate mesoderm** forms a longitudinal elevation along the dorsal body wall, the **urogenital ridge**. The coelomic epithelium and underlying mesoderm of the urogenital ridge proliferate to form the **gonadal ridge**. **Primary sex cords** develop from the gonadal ridge and incorporate primordial germ cells (XX genotype), which migrate into the gonad from the wall of the yolk sac. Primary sex cords extend into the medulla and develop into the **rete ovarii**, which eventually degenerates. Later, **secondary sex cords** develop and incorporate primordial germ cells as a thin **tunica albuginea** forms. The secondary sex cords break apart and form isolated cell clusters called **primordial follicles**, which contain **primary oocytes** surrounded by a layer of **simple squamous cells**. Primary oocytes, simple squamous cells, and connective tissue stroma of the ovary are derived from mesoderm.

B.   Relative descent of the ovaries   The ovaries originally develop within the abdomen but later undergo a relative descent into the pelvis as a result of disproportionate growth of the upper abdominal region away from the pelvic region. Other factors in this movement are uncertain but probably include the **gubernaculum**. The gubernaculum is a band of fibrous tissue along the posterior wall that extends from the medial pole of the ovary to the uterus at the junction of the uterine tubes, forming the **ovarian ligament**. The gubernaculum then continues into the labia majora, forming the **round ligament of the uterus**. The peritoneum evaginates alongside the gubernaculum to form the **processus vaginalis**, which is obliterated in the female later in development.

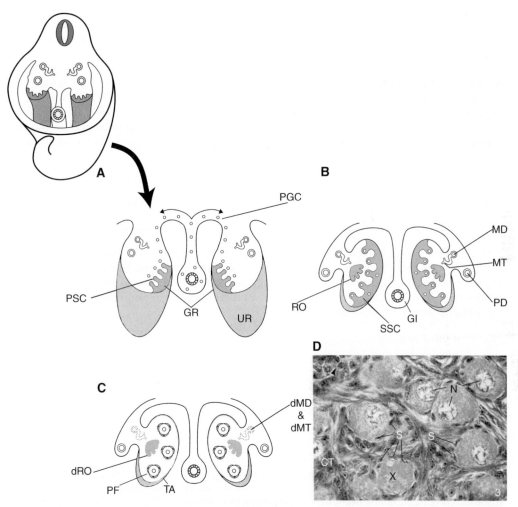

Figure 14-1.   Diagram indicating the differentiation of the gonad in the female. (**A**) Gonad in the indifferent embryo. (**B**) Ovary at week 12. (**C**) Ovary at week 20. *dMD* = degenerating mesonephric duct; *dMT* = degenerating mesonephric tubules; *dRO* = degenerating rete ovarii; *GI* = gut tube; *GR* = gonadal ridge; *MD* = mesonephric duct; *MT* = mesonephric tubules; *PD* = paramesonephric duct; *PF* = primordial follicles; *PGC* = primordial germ cells; *PSC* = primary sex cords; *RO* = rete ovarii; *SSC* = secondary sex cords; *TA* = tunica albuginea; *UR* = urogenital ridge. (**D**) Light micrograph of the definitive adult ovary showing several primordial follicles. Each primordial follicle consists of a primary oocyte surrounded by a single layer of simple squamous cells (*S*). The nucleus (*N*) of the primary oocyte is typically large, but many times the nucleus is not in the plane of section so that only cytoplasm of the primary oocyte is observed (*X*). *CT* = connective tissue.

III. Development of the Genital Ducts (Figure 14-2)

A. Paramesonephric (müllerian) ducts develop as invaginations of the lateral surface of the urogenital ridge. The cranial portions develop into the **uterine tubes**. The caudal portions fuse in the midline to form the **uterovaginal primordium** and thereby bring together two peritoneal folds called the **broad ligament**. The uterovaginal primordium develops into the **uterus, cervix, and superior third of the vagina**. The paramesonephric ducts project into the dorsal wall of the cloaca and induce the formation of the **sinovaginal bulbs**. The sinovaginal bulbs fuse to form the solid **vaginal plate**, which canalizes and develops into the **inferior two thirds of the vagina**. Although the vagina has a dual origin, most authorities agree that the epithelial lining of the entire vagina is of endodermal origin. Vestigial remnants of the paramesonephric duct may be found in the adult female and are called the **hydatid of Morgagni**.

B. Mesonephric (wolffian) ducts and tubules develop in the female as part of the urinary system, since these ducts are critical in the formation of the definitive metanephric kidney. However, they degenerate in the female after formation of the metanephric kidney. Vestigial remnants of the mesonephric ducts may be found in the adult female called the **appendix vesiculosa** and **Gartner's duct**. Vestigial remnants of the mesonephric tubules may be found in the adult female called the **epoöphoron** and **paroöphoron**.

IV. Development of the Primordia of the External Genitalia (Figure 14-3)

A proliferation of mesoderm around the cloacal membrane causes the overlying ectoderm to rise up so that three structures are visible externally: **phallus, urogenital folds,** and **labioscrotal swellings**. The phallus forms the **clitoris (glans clitoris, corpora cavernosa clitoris,** and **vestibular bulbs)**. The urogenital folds form the **labia minora**. The labioscrotal swellings form the **labia majora** and **mons pubis**.

Figure 14-2. **(A–C)** Lateral view of the embryo. **(A)** At week 5, paired paramesonephric ducts (*PD*) begin to ▶ form along the lateral surface of the urogenital ridge at the mesonephros (*Mes*) and grow in close association to the mesonephric duct (*MD*). **(B)** At week 6, the paramesonephric ducts (*PD*) grow caudally and project into the dorsal wall of the cloaca (*C*) and induce the formation of the sinovaginal bulbs (not shown). The mesonephric ducts (*MD*) continue to prosper. **(C)** At week 9, the caudal portions of the paramesonephric ducts (*PD*) fuse in the midline to form the uterovaginal primordium (*UVP*), and the sinovaginal bulbs fuse to form the vaginal plate (*VP*) at the urogenital sinus (*UG*). During this time period, the mesonephric duct and mesonephric tubules both degenerate in the female (*dMD* [degenerating mesonephric duct] and *dMT* [degenerating mesonephric tubules]). *R* = rectum. **(D)** Genital ducts in the indifferent embryo. **(E)** Lateral view showing the dual origin of the vagina. **(F)** Female components and vestigial remnants (*dotted lines*) at birth. **(G)** Location of various cysts within the female reproductive tract that are encountered clinically. The formation of cysts is related to vestigial remnants of the genital ducts. *1,* Hydatid cyst of Morgagni arises from hydatid of Morgagni, which is a remnant of the paramesonephric duct. *2,* Kobelt's cyst arises from the appendix vesiculosa, which is a remnant of the mesonephric duct. *3,* Cyst of the epoöphoron (Type II) arises from the epoöphoron, which is a remnant of the mesonephric tubules. *4,* Cyst of the paroöphoron arises from the paroöphoron, which is a remnant of the mesonephric tubules. *5,* Gartner's duct cyst arises from the duct of Gartner, which is a remnant of the mesonephric duct.

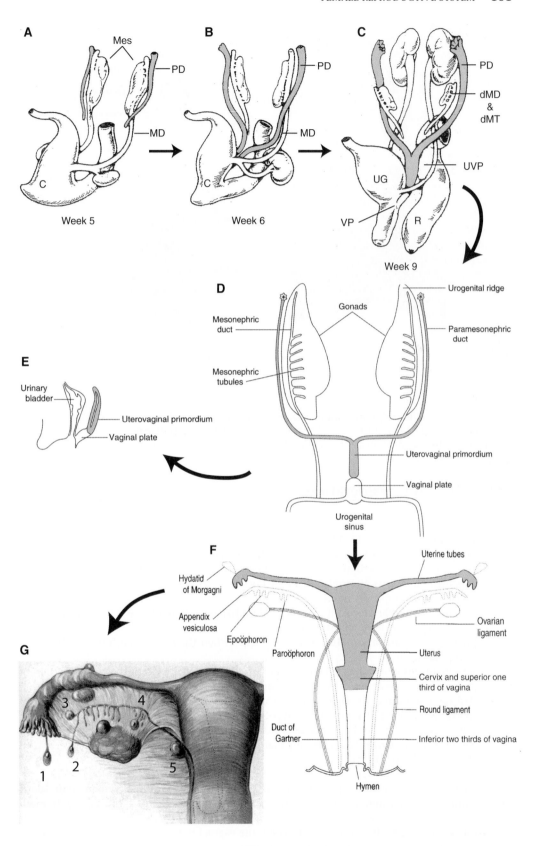

A

Mes

PD

MD

C

Week 5

B

PD

MD

C

Week 6

C

PD

dMD
&
dMT

UVP

UG

VP

R

Week 9

D

Urogenital ridge

Mesonephric
duct

Gonads

Paramesonephric
duct

Mesonephric
tubules

Uterovaginal primordium

Vaginal plate

Urogenital
sinus

E

Urinary
bladder

Uterovaginal primordium

Vaginal plate

F

Hydatid
of Morgagni

Uterine tubes

Appendix
vesiculosa

Ovarian
ligament

Epoöphoron

Uterus

Paroöphoron

Cervix and superior one
third of vagina

Round ligament

Duct of
Gartner

Inferior two thirds of vagina

Hymen

G

3   4

1   2   5

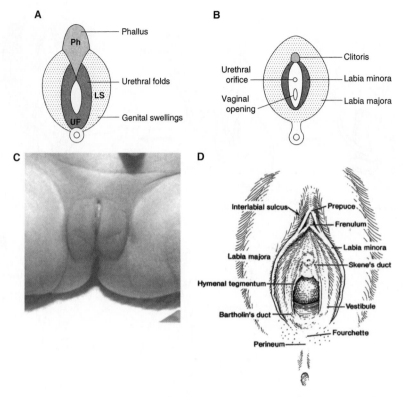

Figure 14-3. (**A** and **B**) Diagrams indicating the differentiation of the phallus (*Ph*), urogenital folds (*UF*), and labioscrotal swellings (*LS*) in the female. (**A**) At week 5. (**B**) At birth. (**C**) Appearance of normal female genitalia at birth. (**D**) Diagram of the gross anatomy of the vulvar region in the adult female.

V.   Clinical Considerations

A. **Uterine anomalies**   (Figure 14-4)
   1. **Müllerian hypoplasia or agenesis anomalies (Class I)** involving the paramesonephric ducts can result in vaginal, cervical, uterine, uterine tube, or combined anomalies.
   2. **Unicornuate uterus anomalies (Class II)** occur when one paramesonephric duct fails to develop or incompletely develops.
   3. **Didelphys (double uterus) anomalies (Class III)** occur when there is a complete lack of fusion of the paramesonephric ducts.
   4. **Bicornuate uterus anomalies (Class IV)** occur when there is partial fusion of the paramesonephric ducts.
   5. **Septate uterus anomalies (Class V)** occur when the medial walls of the caudal portion of the paramesonephric ducts partially or completely fail to resorb.
   6. **DES-related anomalies.** Diethylstilbestrol (DES) was used until 1970 in the treatment of abortions, preeclampsia, diabetes, and preterm labor. For female offspring (i.e., daughters) exposed to DES in utero, an increased incidence of vaginal and cervical adenocarcinoma has been documented. In addition, many uterine anomalies, which include T-shaped uterus have been observed.

B. **Hymen variations** (Figure 14-5) include **crescentic hymen, annular hymen, redundant hymen, imperforate hymen, cribriform hymen, microperforate hymen, and septate hymen**.

C. **Atresia of the vagina is** a condition in which the vaginal lumen is blocked because of a failure of the vaginal plate to canalize and form a lumen.

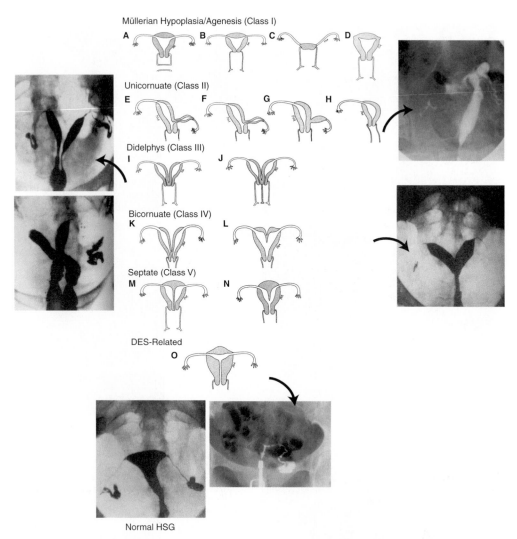

Müllerian Hypoplasia/Agenesis (Class I)

Unicornuate (Class II)

Didelphys (Class III)

Bicornuate (Class IV)

Septate (Class V)

DES-Related

Normal HSG

Figure 14-4. Diagram depicting various congenital anomalies of the uterus and vagina. (**A–D**) Müllerian hypoplasia and agenesis anomalies Class I. (**A**) Lower vagina agenesis. (**B**) Cervix agenesis. (**C**) Uterus and cervix hypoplasia. (**D**) Uterine tube agenesis. (**E–H**) Unicornuate anomalies Class II. (**E**) Unicornuate uterus with a communicating rudimentary horn. (**F**) Unicornuate uterus with a noncommunicating rudimentary horn. (**G**) Unicornuate uterus with a rudimentary horn containing no uterine cavity. (**H**) Unicornuate uterus. A hysterosalpingography (HSG) shows a single lenticular-shaped uterine canal with no evidence of a rudimentary right horn. There is filling of the left uterine tube. (**I** and **J**) Didelphys (double uterus) anomalies Class III. (**I**) Didelphys with normal vagina. HSG shows a double uterus with a single normal vagina (*top panel*). (**J**) Didelphys with complete vaginal septum. HSG shows a double uterus with a double vagina due to vaginal septum (*bottom panel*). This 17-year-old girl uses two tampons during menses. (**K** and **L**) Bicornuate anomalies Class IV. (**K**) Bicornuate uterus with complete division down to the internal os. (**L**) Bicornuate uterus with partial division. HSG shows the uterine cavity partitioned into two channels. (**M** and **N**) Septate uterus anomalies Class V. (**M**) Septate uterus with complete septum down to the external os. (**N**) Septate uterus with partial septum. (**O**) DES-related uterus anomalies. These anomalies typically result in a T-shaped uterus. HSG shows a T-shaped uterus. HSG of normal female reproductive tract is shown for comparison.

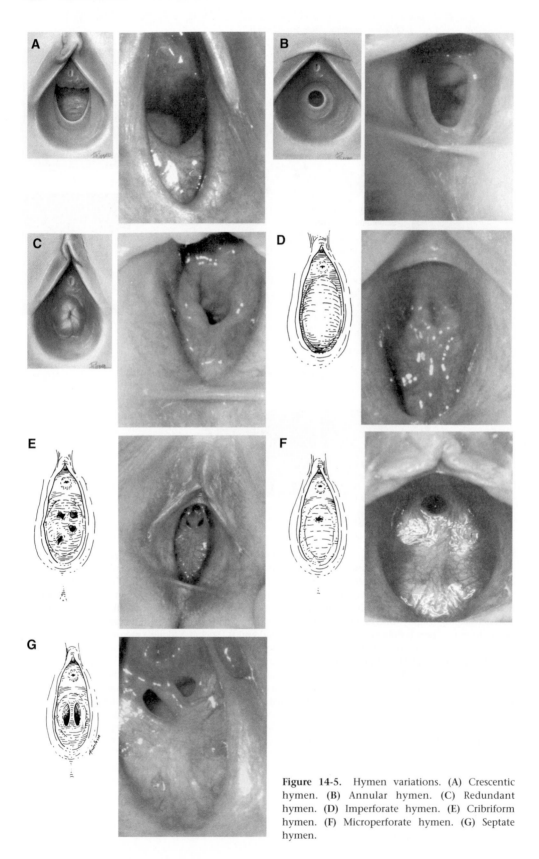

Figure 14-5. Hymen variations. **(A)** Crescentic hymen. **(B)** Annular hymen. **(C)** Redundant hymen. **(D)** Imperforate hymen. **(E)** Cribriform hymen. **(F)** Microperforate hymen. **(G)** Septate hymen.

STUDY QUESTIONS FOR CHAPTER 14

Directions: Each of the numbered items or incomplete statements in this section is followed by answers or by completions of the statement. Select the **one** lettered answer or completion that is **best** in each case.

1. The indifferent embryo begins phenotypic sexual differentiation during

(A) week 3 of development
(B) week 5 of development
(C) week 7 of development
(D) week 12 of development
(E) week 20 of development

2. The indifferent embryo completes phenotypic sexual differentiation during

(A) week 3 of development
(B) week 5 of development
(C) week 7 of development
(D) week 12 of development
(E) week 20 of development

3. After the sinovaginal bulbs have proliferated and fused, they form a solid core of endodermal cells called the

(A) vestibule of the vagina
(B) uterovaginal primordium
(C) urogenital sinus
(D) vaginal plate
(E) clitoris

4. A structure found within the adult female pelvis formed from the gubernaculum is the

(A) broad ligament
(B) suspensory ligament of the ovary
(C) round ligament of the uterus
(D) medial umbilical ligament
(E) median umbilical ligament

5. The labia minora arise embryologically from which of the following structures?

(A) Phallus
(B) Labioscrotal swellings
(C) Sinovaginal bulbs
(D) Urogenital folds
(E) Paramesonephric duct

6. The uterine tubes of the adult female are derived embryologically from which of the following?

(A) Mesonephric duct
(B) Mesonephric tubules
(C) Paramesonephric duct
(D) Paramesonephric tubules
(E) Uterovaginal primordium

ANSWERS AND EXPLANATIONS

1. C. The embryo during weeks 1–6 remains in an indifferent or undifferentiated stage. The embryo begins phenotypic sexual differentiation during week 7.

2. E. By week 12, female and male characteristics can be recognized. By week 20, phenotypic sexual differentiation is complete.

3. D. The sinovaginal bulbs proliferate, fuse, and form the vaginal plate under the inductive influence of the paramesonephric ducts. The vaginal plate then canalizes to form the inferior two thirds of the vagina.

4. C. The round ligament of the uterus and the ovarian ligament both form from the gubernaculum.

5. D. In the female, the urogenital folds remain unfused and form the labia minora.

6. C. The cranial portion of the paramesonephric ducts form the uterine tubes.

Male Reproductive System

I. The Indifferent Embryo

The genotype of the embryo (46,XX or 46,XY) is established at fertilization. **During weeks 1–6,** the embryo remains in a sexually indifferent or undifferentiated stage. This means that genetically female embryos and genetically male embryos are phenotypically indistinguishable. **During week 7**, the indifferent embryo begins phenotypic sexual differentiation. **By week 12**, female or male characteristics of the external genitalia can be recognized. **By week 20**, phenotypic differentiation is complete.

A. Phenotypic sexual differentiation is determined by the *Sry* gene located on the short arm of the Y chromosome and may result in individuals with a **female phenotype**, an **intersex phenotype**, or a **male phenotype**. The *Sry* gene encodes for a protein called **testes-determining factor (TDF)**. TDF is a 220-amino acid nonhistone protein that contains a highly conserved DNA-binding region called a **high-mobility group box**. As the indifferent gonad develops into the testes, Leydig cells and Sertoli cells differentiate to produce **testosterone** and **müllerian inhibiting factor (MIF)**, respectively. In the presence of TDF, testosterone, and MIF, the indifferent embryo is directed to the male phenotype. In the absence of TDF, testosterone, and MIF, the indifferent embryo is directed to the female phenotype.

B. The components of the indifferent embryo that are remodeled to form the adult female reproductive system include the **gonads, genital ducts**, and **primordia of external genitalia**. Phenotypic sexual differentiation occurs in a sequence beginning with the gonads, then the genital ducts, and finally the primordia of external genitalia.

II. Development of the Gonads (Figure 15-1)

A. The testes   The **intermediate mesoderm** forms a longitudinal elevation along the dorsal body wall, the **urogenital ridge**. The coelomic epithelium and underlying mesoderm of the urogenital ridge proliferate to form the **gonadal ridge**. **Primary sex cords** develop from the gonadal ridge and incorporate primordial germ cells (XY genotype), which migrate into the gonad from the wall of the yolk sac. The Y chromosome carries a gene on its short arm that codes for **testes-determining factor (TDF)**, which is crucial to testes differentiation. The primary sex cords extend into the medulla of the gonad and lose their connection with the surface epithelium as the thick **tunica albuginea** forms. The primary sex cords form the **seminiferous cords, tubuli recti**, and **rete testis**. Seminiferous cords consist of **primordial germ cells** and **sustentacular (Sertoli) cells**, which secrete **MIF**. The mesoderm between the seminiferous cords gives rise to the **interstitial (Leydig) cells**, which secrete **testosterone**. The primordial germ cells, sustentacular (Sertoli) cells, interstitial (Leydig) cells, and connective tissue stroma of the testes are derived from mesoderm. The seminiferous cords remain as solid cords until puberty when they acquire a lumen and are then called **seminiferous tubules**.

B. Relative descent of the testes   The testes originally develop within the abdomen but later undergo a relative descent into the scrotum as a result of disproportionate growth of the upper abdominal region away from the pelvic region. Other factors involved in this movement are uncertain but probably include the **gubernaculum**. The gubernaculum is a band of fibrous tissue along the posterior wall that extends from the caudal pole of the testes to the scrotum. Remnants of the gubernaculum in the adult male serve to anchor the testes within the scrotum. The peritoneum evaginates alongside the gubernaculum to form the **processus vaginalis.** Later in development, most of the processus vaginalis is obliterated except at its distal end, which remains as a peritoneal sac called the **tunica vaginalis** of the testes.

III.   Development of the Genital Ducts (Figure 15-2)

A. Paramesonephric (müllerian) ducts develop as invaginations of the lateral surface of the urogenital ridge. The cranial portions run parallel with the mesonephric ducts. The caudal portions fuse in the midline to form the uterovaginal primordium. Under the influence of MIF, the

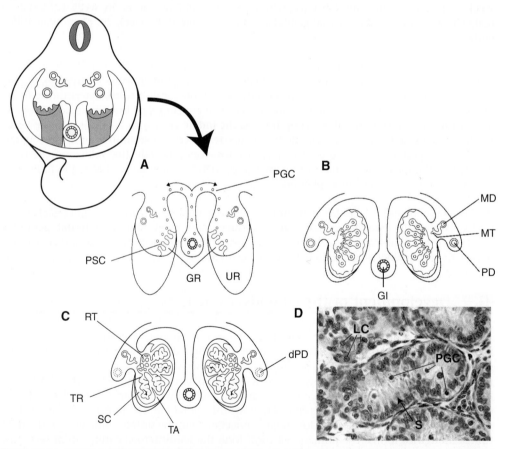

Figure 15-1.   Diagram indicating the differentiation of the gonad in the male. **(A)** Gonad in the indifferent embryo. **(B)** Testes at week 7. **(C)** Testes at week 20. *dPD* = degenerating paramesonephric duct; *GI* = gut tube; *GR* = gonadal ridge; *MD* = mesonephric duct; *MT* = mesonephric tubules; *PD* = paramesonephric duct; *PGC* = primordial germ cells; *PSC* = primary sex cords; *RT* = rete testis; *SC* = seminiferous cords; *TA* = tunica albuginea; *TR* = tubuli recti; *UR* = urogenital ridge. **(D)** Light micrograph of a prepubertal testis showing seminiferous cords composed of primordial germ cells *(PGC)* and Sertoli cells *(S)*. Leydig cells *(LC)* are found surrounding the seminiferous cords in the interstitial space.

cranial portions of the paramesonephric ducts and the uterovaginal primordium regress. Vestigial remnants of the paramesonephric duct (called the **appendix testis**) may be found in the adult male.

B. Mesonephric (wolffian) ducts and tubules develop in the male as part of the urinary system, since these ducts are critical in the formation of the definitive metanephric kidney. The mesonephric ducts then proceed to additionally form the **epididymis, ductus deferens, seminal vesicle,** and **ejaculatory duct.** A few mesonephric tubules in the region of the testes form the **efferent ductules** of the testes. Vestigial remnants of the mesonephric duct (called the **appendix epididymis**) may be found in the adult male. Vestigial remnants of mesonephric tubules (called the **paradidymis**) also may be found in the adult male.

IV. Development of the Primordia of the External Genitalia
(Figure 15-3)

A proliferation of mesoderm around the cloacal membrane causes the overlying ectoderm to rise up so that three structures are visible externally: **phallus, urogenital folds,** and **labioscrotal swellings.** The phallus forms the **penis (glans penis, corpora cavernosa penis,** and **corpus spongiosum penis).** The urogenital folds form the **ventral aspect of the penis (i.e., penile raphe).** The labioscrotal swellings form the **scrotum.**

V. Clinical Considerations

A. **Male anomalies**   (Figure 15-4)
  1. **Hypospadias** occurs when the urethral folds fail to fuse completely, resulting in the external urethral orifice opening onto the ventral surface of the penis. It is generally associated with a poorly developed penis that curves ventrally, known as **chordee.**
  2. **Epispadias** occurs when the external urethral orifice opens onto the dorsal surface of the penis. It is generally associated with **exstrophy of the bladder.**
  3. **Undescended testes (cryptorchidism)** occurs when the testes fail to descend into the scrotum. Descent of the testes is evident within 3 months after birth. Bilateral cryptorchidism results in **sterility.** The undescended testes may be found in the abdominal cavity or in the inguinal canal.
  4. **Hydrocele of the testes** occurs when a small patency of the processus vaginalis remains so that peritoneal fluid can flow into the processus vaginalis, which results in a fluid-filled cyst near the testes.
  5. **Congenital inguinal hernia** occurs when a large patency of the processus vaginalis remains so that a loop of intestine herniates into the scrotum or labia majora. It is most common in males and is generally associated with cryptorchidism.

B. **Other anomalies of the reproductive system**   (Figure 15-5)
  1. **Intersexuality.** Because the early embryo goes through an indifferent stage, events may occur whereby a fetus does not progress toward either of the two usual phenotypes but gets caught in an intermediate stage known as intersexuality. Intersexuality is classified according to the histologic appearance of the **gonad** and **ambiguous genitalia. True intersexuality** occurs when an individual has both ovarian and testicular tissue (ovotestes) histologically, ambiguous genitalia, and a 46,XX genotype. True intersexuality is a rare condition whose cause is poorly understood.
  2. **Female pseudointersexuality (FP)** occurs when an individual has only ovarian tissue histologically and has masculinization of the female external genitalia. These individuals have a **46,XX genotype.** FP is most often observed clinically in association with a condition in which the fetus produces an **excess of androgens (e.g., congenital adrenal hyperplasia [CAH]).** CAH is caused most commonly by mutations in genes for enzymes

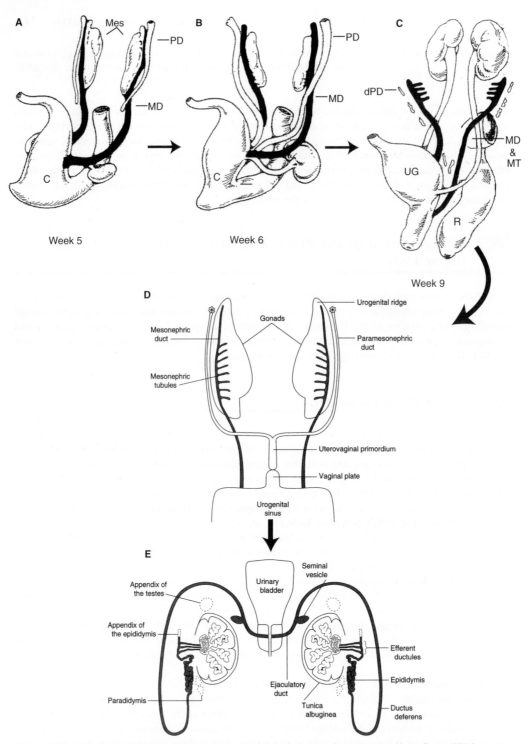

Figure 15-2. (A–C) Lateral view of the embryo. **(A)** At week 5, paired paramesonephric ducts (*PD*) begin to form along the lateral surface of the urogenital ridge at the mesonephros (*Mes*) and grow in close association to the mesonephric duct (*MD*). *C* = cloaca. **(B)** At week 6, the paramesonephric ducts (*PD*) grow caudally and project into the dorsal wall of the cloaca (*C*) and induce the formation of the sinovaginal bulbs (not shown). The mesonephric ducts (*MD*) continue to prosper. **(C)** At week 9, the mesonephric ducts (*MD*) and mesonephric tubules establish contact with the testes and develop into definitive adult structures. During this time period, the paramesonephric ducts degenerate in the male (*dPD*). *MT* = mesonephric tubules; *R* = rectum; *UG* = urogenital sinus. **(D)** Genital ducts in the indifferent embryo. **(E)** Male components and vestigial remnants (*dotted lines*). The mesonephric ducts/tubules and their derivatives are shaded.

A

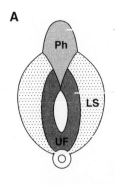

B

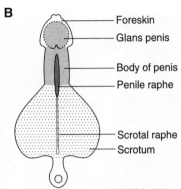

Foreskin

Glans penis

Body of penis

Penile raphe

Scrotal raphe

Scrotum

Figure 15-3. **(A and B)** Diagrams indicating the differentiation of the phallus (*Ph*), urogenital folds (*UF*), and labioscrotal swellings (*LS*) in the male. **(A)** At week 5. **(B)** At birth.

involved in adrenocortical steroid biosynthesis (e.g., **21-hydroxylase deficiency, 11β-hydroxylase deficiency**). **In 21-hydroxylase deficiency (90% of all cases)**, there is virtually no synthesis of the cortisol or aldosterone so that intermediates are funneled into androgen biosynthesis, thereby elevating androgen levels. The elevated levels of androgens lead to **masculinization of a female fetus**. FP produces the following clinical findings: mild clitoral enlargement, complete labioscrotal fusion with a phalloid organ, and macrogenitosomia (in the male fetus). Because cortisol cannot be synthesized, negative feedback to the adenohypophysis does not occur. Therefore, adrenocorticotropic hormone continues to stimulate the adrenal cortex, resulting in adrenal hyperplasia. Because aldosterone cannot be synthesized, the patient presents with **hyponatremia ("salt-wasting")** with **dehydration** and **hyperkalemia**. Treatment includes immediate infusion of intravenous saline and long-term steroid hormone replacement, both cortisol and mineralocorticoids (9α-fludrocortisone).

3. **Male pseudointersexuality (MP)** occurs when an individual has only testicular tissue histologically and has various stages of stunted development of the male external genitalia. These individuals have a **46,XY genotype**. MP is most often observed clinically in association with a condition in which the fetus produces a **lack of androgens (and MIF)**. This is caused most frequently by mutations in genes for androgen steroid biosynthesis (e.g., **5α-reductase 2 deficiency** or **17β-hydroxysteroid dehydrogenase**). Normally, 5α-reductase 2 catalyzes the conversion of testosterone→dihydrotestosterone, and 17β HSD 3 catalyzes the conversion of androstenedione→testosterone. An increased **T:DHT (testosterone:dihydrotestosterone) ratio** is diagnostic (normal = 5; 5α-reductase 2 deficiency = 20–60). The reduced levels of androgens lead to the **feminization of a male fetus**. MP produces the following clinical findings: underdevelopment of the penis and scrotum (microphallus, hypospadias, and bifid scrotum) and of the prostate gland. The epididymis, ductus deferens, seminal vesicle, and ejaculatory duct are normal. These clinical findings have led to inference that DHT is essential in the development of the penis and scrotum (external genitalia) and prostate gland in genotypic XY fetus. At puberty, these individuals demonstrate a striking virilization.

4. **Complete androgen insensitivity (CAIS or testicular feminization syndrome)** occurs when a fetus with a 46,XY genotype develops testes and female external genitalia with a rudimentary vagina; uterus and uterine tubes are generally absent. The testes may be found in the labia majora and are surgically removed to circumvent malignant tumor formation. These individuals present as normal-appearing females, and their psychosocial orientation is female despite their genotype. The most common cause is a mutation in the gene for the **androgen receptor**. Even though the developing male fetus is exposed to normal levels of androgens, the lack of androgen receptors renders the phallus, urogenital folds, and labioscrotal swellings unresponsive to androgens.

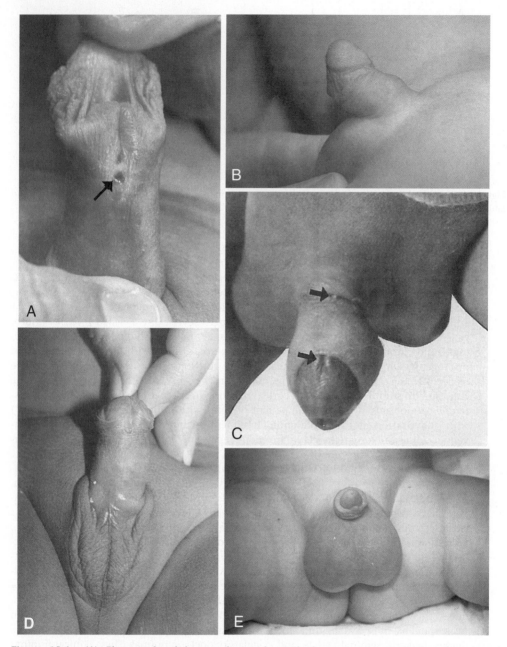

Figure 15-4. (A) Photograph of hypospadias with urethral opening on ventral surface (*arrow*). (B) Photograph of chordee. Note that the penis is poorly developed and bowed dorsally. (C) Photograph of epispadias with two urethral openings on the dorsal surface of the penis (*arrows*). (D) Photograph of cryptorchidism. Note that both testes have not descended into the scrotal sac. (E) Photograph of bilateral hydrocele.

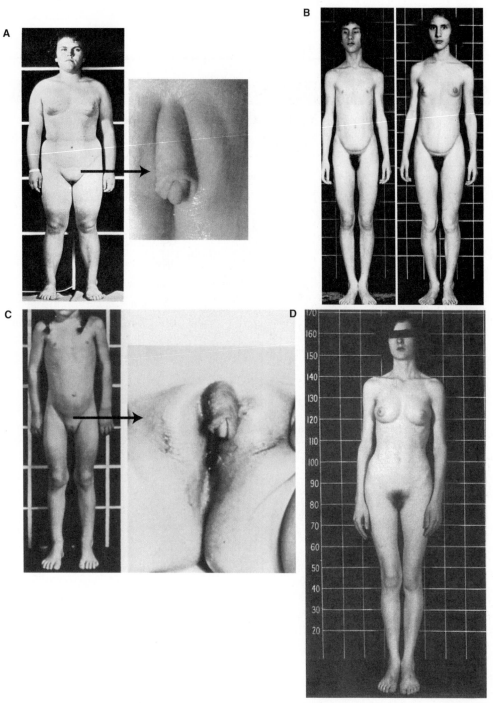

Figure 15-5. **(A)** A patient (XX genotype) with female pseudointersexuality due to congenital adrenal hyperplasia. Masculinization of female external genitalia is apparent with fusion of the labia majora and enlarged clitoris (see *arrow* to *inset*). **(B)** A patient (XX genotype) with female pseudointersexuality due to congenital adrenal hyperplasia (i.e., 21-hydroxylase deficiency). This 10-year-old girl is clearly masculinized (*left panel*). After 9 months of cortisone therapy, there is marked improvement (*right panel*). **(C)** A patient (XY genotype) with male pseudointersexuality. Stunted development of male external genitalia is apparent. The stunted external genitalia fooled parents and physician into thinking that this XY infant was a girl. In fact, this child was raised as a girl (note pigtails). As this child neared puberty, testosterone levels increased and clitoral enlargement ensued. This alarmed the parents and the child was brought in for clinical evaluation. **(D)** A patient (XY genotype) with complete androgen insensitivity (CAIS or testicular feminization). Complete feminization of male external genitalia is apparent.

173

VI.   Summary (Table 15-1)

TABLE 15-1	Female and Male Reproductive Systems Development	
Adult Female	**Indifferent Embryo**	**Adult Male**
Ovary, ovarian follicles, rete ovarii	Gonads	Testes, seminiferous tubules, tubuli recti, rete testis, Leydig cells, Sertoli cells
Uterine tubes, uterus, cervix, superior third of vagina	Paramesonephric duct	—
Hydatid of Morgagni[a]		*Appendix testis*[a]
—	Mesonephric duct	Epididymis, ductus deferens, seminal vesicle, ejaculatory duct
Appendix vesiculosa, Gartner's duct[a]		*Appendix epididymis*[a]
—	Mesonephric tubules	Efferent ductules
Epoöphoron, paroöphoron[a]		*Paradidymis*[a]
Glans clitoris, corpora cavernosa clitoris, vestibular bulbs	Phallus	Glans penis, corpora cavernosa penis, corpus spongiosum
Labia minora	Urogenital folds	Ventral aspect of penis
Labia majora, mons pubis	Labioscrotal swellings	Scrotum
Ovarian ligament, round ligament of uterus	Gubernaculum	Gubernaculum testes
—	Processus vaginalis	Tunica vaginalis

[a] Italics indicates vestigial structure.

Directions: *Each of the numbered items or incomplete statements in this section is followed by answers or by completions of the statement. Select the **one** lettered answer or completion that is **best** in each case.*

1. One day a 9-year-old girl surprisingly announces to her mother, "Guess what, mommy, I'm not a girl; I'm a boy." The mother is shocked but does not act on the comment. During the next few years, the mother notices some tomboyish behavior and difficulty in social adjustment at school. When the girl is 12 years old, puberty starts with a striking virilization of the external genitalia. The mother is extremely concerned and seeks medical attention. What is the most likely cause?

(A) Male pseudointersexuality
(B) Female pseudointersexuality
(C) Congenital adrenal hyperplasia
(D) Testicular feminization
(E) Illegal use of anabolic steroids

2. The most common cause of female pseudointersexuality is

(A) a 46,XO genotype
(B) a 47,XXY genotype
(C) lack of androgen receptors
(D) congenital adrenal hyperplasia
(E) inadequate production of testosterone and müllerian-inhibiting factor (MIF)

3. The most common cause of male pseudointersexuality is

(A) a 45,XO genotype
(B) a 47,XXY genotype
(C) inadequate production of testosterone and MIF
(D) congenital adrenal hyperplasia
(E) lack of androgen receptors

4. The most common cause of testicular feminization syndrome is

(A) a 45,XO genotype
(B) a 47,XXY genotype
(C) inadequate production of testosterone and MIF
(D) congenital adrenal hyperplasia
(E) lack of androgen receptors

5. In the male, failure of the urethral folds to fuse completely results in

(A) hypospadias
(B) epispadias
(C) cryptorchidism
(D) congenital inguinal hernia
(E) hydrocele

6. The Y chromosome carries a gene on its short arm that codes for

(A) testosterone
(B) MIF
(C) testes-determining factor (TDF)
(D) progesterone
(E) estrogen

7. Bilateral cryptorchidism usually results in

(A) impotence
(B) sterility
(C) male pseudointersexuality
(D) female pseudointersexuality
(E) testicular feminization syndrome

8. A 17-year-old girl presents with a complaint of amenorrhea. Physical examination reveals good breast development and normal amount of pubic hair. A rudimentary vagina and a mobile mass within both the right and left labia majora are found on pelvic examination. Ultrasound reveals the absence of a uterus. What is the diagnosis?

(A) Testicular feminization syndrome
(B) Gonadal dysgenesis
(C) Cryptorchidism
(D) Female pseudointersexuality
(E) Hypospadias

ANSWERS AND EXPLANATIONS

1. A. Reduced levels of androgens during fetal development of an XY male fetus cause feminization of the male external genitalia such that the baby can be phenotypically mistaken for female. Parents raise the XY male baby as a girl until puberty or other medical problems bring the child to medical attention.

2. D. Female pseudointersex individuals have a 46,XX genotype. This condition is most commonly caused by congenital adrenal hyperplasia, in which the fetus produces excessive amounts of androgens. The high androgen level masculinizes the female genitalia.

3. C. Male pseudointersex individuals have a 46,XY genotype. This condition is most commonly caused by inadequate production of testosterone and MIF by the fetal testes. The low testosterone and MIF levels stunt the development of the male genitalia.

4. E. The most common cause of testicular feminization syndrome is the lack of androgen receptors in the urogenital folds and labioscrotal swellings. Because these tissues lack androgen receptors, they are blind or unresponsive to androgens. Consequently, these tissues develop into female external genitalia even though the fetus has a 46,XY genotype.

5. A. Failure of the urethral folds to fuse completely results in the external urethral orifice opening onto the ventral surface of the penis, a condition known as hypospadias.

6. C. The gene product that is coded on the short arm of the Y chromosome is called the testes-determining factor (TDF).

7. B. Sterility is a common result of bilateral cryptorchidism. When both testes fail to descend into the scrotum, the increased temperature they are exposed to in the abdominal cavity inhibits spermatogenesis.

8. A. This is a classic case of testicular feminization syndrome. A karyotype analysis would reveal that this normal-appearing 17-year-old girl actually has a 46,XY genotype. The mobile masses within the right and left labia majora are the testes and should be surgically removed because this tissue has a propensity toward malignant tumor formation. The most common cause of this syndrome is a lack of androgen receptors in the phallus, urogenital folds, and labioscrotal swellings.

Integumentary System

I. Skin

The skin consists of two layers: the outer layer (or **epidermis**) and the deeper connective tissue layer (or **dermis**). Skin functions as a barrier against infection, serves thermoregulation, and protects the body against dehydration.

A. **Epidermis** The epidermis is derived from the ectoderm.
1. **Early development.** Initially, the epidermis consists of a single layer of ectodermal cells that gives rise to an overlying **periderm** layer. The epidermis soon becomes a three-layered structure consisting of the **stratum basale** (mitotically active), the **intermediate layer** (progeny of stratum basale), and the **periderm**. Peridermal cells are eventually desquamated and form part of the **vernix caseosa**, a greasy substance of peridermal cells and sebum from the sebaceous glands that protects the embryo's skin.
2. **Later development.** The definitive adult layers are formed through the inductive influence of the dermis. The ectodermal cells give rise to five cell layers:
a. **Stratum basale (stratum germinativum)**
b. **Stratum spinosum**
c. **Stratum granulosum**
d. **Stratum lucidum**
e. **Stratum corneum.** This layer is associated with the expression of **56 kDa keratin, 67 kDa keratin,** and **filaggrin** (a binding protein).
3. **Other cells of the epidermis**
a. **Melanoblasts** are derived from **neural crest cells** that migrate into the stratum basal of the epidermis. They differentiate into melanocytes by mid-pregnancy when pigment granules called **melanosomes** are observed.
b. **Langerhans cells** are derived from the **bone marrow (mesoderm)** and migrate into the epidermis. They are involved in antigen presentation.
c. **Merkel cells** are of uncertain origin. They are associated with free nerve endings and probably function as mechanoreceptors.

B. **Dermis** The dermis is derived from both the somatic mesoderm located just beneath the ectoderm and mesoderm of the dermatomes of the body. In the head and neck region, the dermis is derived from neural crest cells.
1. **Early development.** The dermis is initially composed of loosely aggregated mesodermal cells frequently referred to as **mesenchymal cells (or mesenchyme).** The mesenchymal cells secrete a watery-type extracellular matrix rich in glycogen and hyaluronic acid.
2. **Later development.** The mesenchymal cells differentiate into fibroblasts, which secrete increasing amounts of collagen and elastic fibers into the extracellular matrix. Vascularization occurs. Sensory nerves grow into the dermis. The dermis forms projections into the epidermis called **dermal papillae,** which contain tactile sensory receptors (e.g., Meissner's corpuscles).

C. **Clinical considerations**   (Figure 16-1)
 1. **Oculocutaneous albinism (OCA)**
     a. **Type I OCA (tyrosinase negative; classic type)** is an autosomal recessive disorder in which melanocytes **fail to produce melanin pigment.** The cause is a complete absence of the enzyme **tyrosinase** due to mutations in both copies of tyrosinase gene located on **chromosome 11q14-q21.** These individuals have pink skin, gray-blue eyes, and white hair at birth and throughout life.
     b. **Type II OCA (tyrosinase positive)** is an autosomal recessive disorder in which melanocytes **produce some melanin pigment**. The cause is a complete absence of the **P protein** (localizes to the melanosome membrane; function unknown) due to mutations in both copies of the P gene located on **chromosome 15q11-13.** These individuals have pink skin, gray-blue eyes, and dark hair at birth, but the pigment of the skin, eyes, and hair increases as the patient ages.
     c. **Piebaldism,** an autosomal dominant disorder, is a localized albinism in which there is a lack of melanin in isolated patches of skin and/or hair. In general, albinism predisposes to basal cell carcinoma, squamous cell carcinoma, and malignant melanoma.
 2. **Ichthyosis** is excessive keratinization of the skin characterized by dryness, scaling, and cracks in the skin, which may form deep fissures. In severe cases, a **harlequin fetus** may result. It is usually inherited as an autosomal recessive trait but may also be X-linked.
 3. **Psoriasis** is a skin disease characterized by **excess cell proliferation** in the stratum basale and in the stratum spinosum. This results in thickening of the epidermis and shorter regeneration time of the epidermis.
 4. **Ehlers-Danlos syndrome** is an autosomal dominant genetic disorder involving the gene for **peptidyl lysine hydroxylase,** which is an enzyme necessary for the hydroxylation of lysine residues of collagen. It affects mainly **Type I and Type III collagen.** It is characterized by extremely stretchable and fragile skin, hypermobile joints, aneurysms of blood vessels, and rupture of the bowel.
 5. **Hemangiomas** are vascular malformations, that is, benign tumors of endothelial cells. They produce "birthmarks" on the skin. A port-wine stain is a birthmark covering the area of distribution of the trigeminal nerve (CN V) that is frequently associated with an hemangioma of the meninges called **Sturge-Weber syndrome.**
 6. **Junctional epidermolysis bullosa (JEB)** refers to a group of autosomal recessive disorders characterized by bulla (blister) formation. The cause is a mutation in the gene for **laminin 5,** which alters adhesion of stratum basale to the basement membrane. The epidermis is intact but is separated from the underlying dermis. This disease is usually fatal by the time the child reaches 3 to 4 years of age owing to hypoproteinemia, anemia, and infection.

Figure 16-1.   (A) Type I oculocutaneous albinism (OCA). (B) Type II OCA in a black female child. (C) ▶ Piebaldism in a black female child. (D) Harlequin fetus. (E and F) Ehlers-Danlos syndrome. Note the extremely stretchable skin and the cigarette-paper scars over the knees (*arrows*). (G) Hemangiomas located in the scalp, back, and thigh regions of a young infant. (H) An aggressive hemangioma of the face covering the distribution of the trigeminal nerve. (I) Sturge-Weber syndrome. Radiograph shows tram-track calcification of cerebral cortex closely following the cerebral convolutions (or gyri). Calcification of meningeal arteries may also be prominent. (J and K) Epidermolysis bullosa in a young infant shows widespread bullae (blisters) and erosion of the skin. Light micrograph shows a pathologic cleft (*) between the epidermis (*E*) and dermis (*D*). There is also some scarring in the dermis.

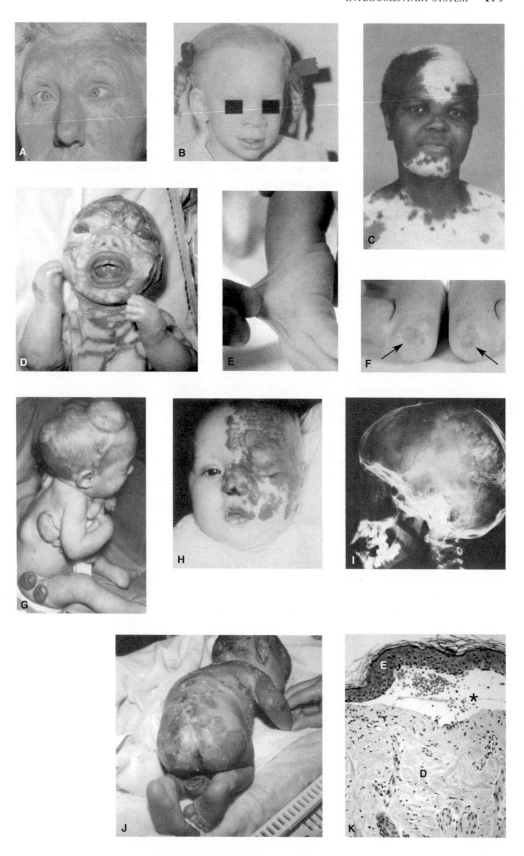

II.   Hair and Nails

Hair and nails are derived from the ectoderm.

A. Hair   At week 12, cells from the stratum basale grow into the underlying dermis and form the **hair follicle**. The deepest part of the hair follicle soon becomes club-shaped to form the **hair bulb**. The hair bulbs are invaginated by mesoderm called the **hair papillae**, which are rapidly infiltrated by blood vessels and nerve endings. The epithelial cells within the hair bulb differentiate into the **germinal matrix** in which cells proliferate, grow toward the surface, keratinize, and form the **hair shaft**. These cells also form the **internal root sheath**. Other epithelial cells of the hair follicle form the **external root sheath**, which is continuous with the epidermis and has a prominent subjacent basement membrane called the **glassy membrane**. Mesodermal cells of the dermis that surround the invaginating hair follicle form the **dermal root sheath** and the **arrector pili muscle**. The first fine hairs, called **lanugo hairs**, are sloughed off at birth. BMP-2 (bone morphogenetic protein), **FGF-2** (fibroblast growth factor), **sonic hedgehog**, and *Msx* (a homeobox gene) appear to be important in hair development.

B. Nails develop from the epidermis. The nails first develop on the tips of the digits, then migrate to the dorsal surface, taking their innervation with them; this is why the median nerve innervates the dorsal surface of three and one-half digits (I-IV).

C. Clinical considerations   (Figure 16-2)
1. **Alopecia** is baldness resulting from an absence or faulty development of the hair follicles.
2. **Hypertrichosis** is an overgrowth of hair. It is frequently associated with spina bifida occulta, which is seen as a patch of hair overlying the defect.
3. **Pili torti** is a familial disorder characterized by **twisted hairs**. It is seen in **Menkes (kinky-hair) disease**, an X-linked recessive neurologic disorder involving a defect in intestinal copper transport.
4. **Trichorrhexis nodosa** is **brittle hair** that breaks easily and is usually associated with metabolic disorders such as **argininosuccinic aciduria**. Argininosuccinic aciduria is an autosomal recessive genetic disorder, which causes a deficiency in the enzyme argininosuccinase of the urea cycle.
5. **Beaded hair** is characterized by elliptical nodes along the hair, which breaks easily at the internodes and is usually associated with **monilethrix**. Monilethrix is an autosomal dominant genetic disorder.
6. **Trichothiodystrophy** is a very rare autosomal recessive genetic disorder characterized by short, brittle hair, with alternating light and dark bands called **tiger-tail hair**.
7. **Uncombable hair syndrome (spun-glass hair)** is an autosomal dominant genetic disorder characterized by blonde, dry, shiny hair that is unable to comb into place. The hair has a triangular shape with a canal-like groove called pili trianguli et canaliculi.

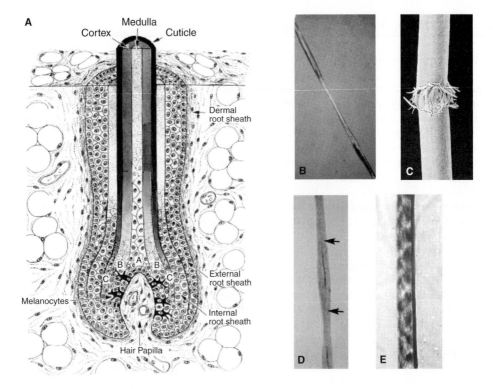

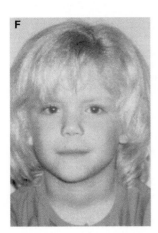

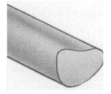

Figure 16-2. (A) Diagram of a hair and its follicle. The expanded lower end of the follicle contains a hair papilla. Formation and growth of the hair depend on the continuous proliferation (note cells in mitosis) and differentiation of cells around the tip of the hair papilla. Cells in region A give rise to the hair medulla. Cells in region B give rise to the hair cortex. Cells in region C give rise to the hair cuticle. Other peripheral cells give rise to the internal and external root sheath. Melanocytes contribute to hair color. (B) Pili torti or twisted hairs. (C) Trichorrhexis nodosa or brittle hair. (D) Beaded hair. The elliptical nodes are shown at the arrows. (E) Tiger-tail hair. (F) Uncombable hair syndrome. Note the triangular-shaped hair with canal-like groove.

III. Mammary, Sweat, and Sebaceous Glands

All are derived from the surface ectoderm.

A. Mammary glands develop from the **mammary ridge**, a downgrowth of the epidermis (ectoderm) into the underlying dermis (mesoderm). Canalization of these epithelial downgrowths results in formation of **alveoli** and **lactiferous ducts**. The lactiferous ducts drain into an epithelial pit, the future **nipple**.

B. Eccrine and **apocrine sweat glands** develop from downgrowths of the epidermis into the underlying dermis.

C. Sebaceous glands develop from the epithelial wall of the hair follicle and elaborate **sebum** into the hair follicles. The tarsal (meibomian) glands of the eyelids do not communicate with hair follicles.

D. Clinical considerations (Figure 16-3)
1. **Gynecomastia** is a condition in which there is excessive development of the male mammary glands. It is frequently associated with Klinefelter's syndrome (47,XXY).
2. **Breast hypertrophy** may occur early in infancy.
3. **Breast hypoplasia** generally occurs asymmetrically when one breast fails to develop completely.
4. **Polythelia** is a condition in which supernumerary nipples occur along the mammary ridge.
5. **Polymastia** is a condition in which supernumerary breasts occur along the mammary ridge.

IV. Teeth (Figure 16-4)

Teeth develop from ectoderm and an underlying layer of neural crest cells.

A. The **dental lamina** develops from the oral epithelium (ectoderm) as a downgrowth into the underlying neural crest layer. The dental lamina gives rise to **tooth buds**, which develop into the **enamel organs**.

B. The **enamel organs** are derived from ectoderm and develop first for the 20 deciduous teeth, then for the 32 permanent teeth. The enamel organs give rise to **ameloblasts**, which produce **enamel**.

C. The **dental papillae** are formed by neural crest cells that underlie the enamel organs. The dental papillae give rise to the **odontoblasts** (which produce **predentin** and **dentin**) and **dental pulp**.

D. The **dental sacs** are formed by a condensation of neural crest cells that surrounds the dental papillae. The dental sacs give rise to **cementoblasts** (which produce **cementum**) and the **periodontal ligaments**.

E. Clinical considerations
1. **Defective enamel formation (amelogenesis imperfecta)** is an autosomal dominant trait.
2. **Defective dentin formation (dentinogenesis imperfecta)** is an autosomal dominant trait.
3. **Vitamin A deficiency.** If vitamin A deficiency is severe, ameloblast cells will atrophy, which results in the absence of enamel. In less severe cases, there is **enamel hypoplasia**.
4. **Vitamin D deficiency.** Severe vitamin D deficiency in children results in rickets, a condition characterized by insufficient deposition of calcium in bony tissue. In teeth, vitamin D deficiency is manifested by **enamel and dentin hypoplasia**.
5. **Tetracycline discoloration.** If tetracycline antibiotics are administered to a pregnant woman, permanent **brown-gray staining** of the teeth result in the child. Tetracycline is deposited in bone and teeth during mineralization.

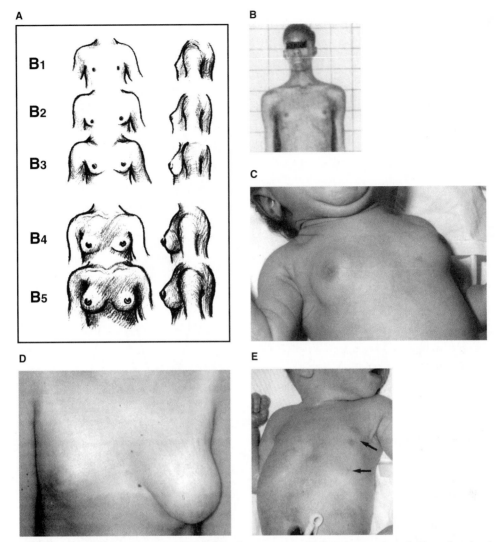

Figure 16-3. **(A)** The Tanner stages of breast development are guidelines in assessing whether a female adolescent is developing normally. In Stage B1 (preadolescent), there is elevation of the papilla only. In Stage B2 (breast bud stage), there is elevation of the breast and papilla as a small mound and enlargement of the areolar diameter. In Stage B3, there is further enlargement of the breast and areola with no separation of their contours. In Stage B4, there is further enlargement with projection of the areola and papilla to form a secondary mound above the level of the breast. In Stage B5 (mature stage), there is projection of the papilla only due to a recession of the areola to the general contour of the breast. **(B)** Gynecomastia in a male with Klinefelter syndrome (47,XXY). **(C)** Breast hypertrophy in a 1-month-old female infant. **(D)** Breast hypoplasia of the right breast in a 16-year-old female. **(E)** Polythelia is shown in which two rudimentary nipples (*arrows*) are located along the left mammary line.

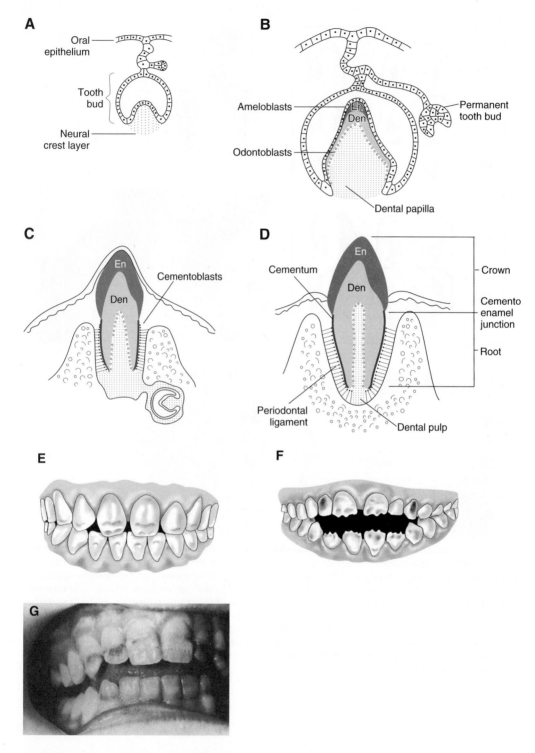

Figure 16-4. (A–D) Diagram of successive stages in the development of a tooth. (A) At week 8. (B) At week 28, note the formation of enamel (*En*) by ameloblasts and dentin (*Den*) by odontoblasts. (C) At postnatal month 6, note the early tooth eruption. (D) At postnatal month 18, note the fully erupted deciduous tooth. Ameloblasts are no longer present, which means further enamel formation is not possible. (E) Clinical appearance of teeth in vitamin A deficiency. (F) Clinical appearance of teeth in vitamin D deficiency. (G) Clinical appearance of teeth in tetracycline staining.

STUDY QUESTIONS FOR CHAPTER 16

*Directions: Each of the numbered items or incomplete statements in this section is followed by answers or by completions of the statement. Select the **one** lettered answer or completion that is **best** in each case.*

1. Melanocytes are found in which epidermal layer?

(A) Stratum basale
(B) Stratum corneum
(C) Stratum granulosum
(D) Stratum lucidum
(E) Stratum spinosum

2. A young black girl shows isolated patches of skin and hair that lack melanin pigment. In addition, other skin lesions are observed that look suspiciously like a malignant melanoma. What is the most likely diagnosis?

(A) Type I oculocutaneous albinism
(B) Type II oculocutaneous albinism
(C) Piebaldism
(D) Ichthyosis
(E) Psoriasis

3. A young infant shows extremely stretchable and fragile skin, hypermobile joints, and cigarette-paper scars over the knees. What is the most likely diagnosis?

(A) Ehlers-Danlos syndrome
(B) Junctional epidermolysis bullosa
(C) Psoriasis
(D) Ichthyosis
(E) Piebaldism

4. A young infant shows skin blisters over the entire body with generalized skin erosion. Pathology indicates a cleft between the epidermis and dermis. What is the most likely diagnosis?

(A) Psoriasis
(B) Junctional epidermolysis bullosa
(C) Ichthyosis
(D) Ehlers-Danlos syndrome
(E) Type II oculocutaneous albinism

5. The administration of which of the following agents may result in discoloration of both deciduous and permanent teeth?

(A) Cephalosporin
(B) Chloramphenicol
(C) Erythromycin
(D) Penicillin
(E) Tetracycline

 ANSWERS AND EXPLANATIONS

1. **A.** Melanocytes are found in the stratum basale, the deepest layer of the epidermis, at the dermoepidermal junction.

2. **C.** Piebaldism is an autosomal dominant disorder and is basically a localized albinism.

3. **A.** Ehlers-Danlos syndrome is an autosomal dominant disorder involving the gene for peptidyl lysine hydroxylase.

4. **B.** Junctional epidermolysis bullosa refers to a group of autosomal recessive disorders caused by a mutation in the gene for laminin 5.

5. **E.** Tetracyclines are bound to calcium in newly formed teeth both in utero and in young children. They may cause discoloration and enamel dysplasia.

Skeletal System

I.   Skull (Figure 17-1)

The skull can be divided into two parts: the neurocranium and the viscerocranium.

A. Neurocranium   The neurocranium consists of the flat bones of the skull (cranial vault) and the base of the skull. The neurocranium develops from neural crest cells except for the basilar part of the occipital bone, which forms from mesoderm of the occipital sclerotomes.

B. Viscerocranium   The viscerocranium consists of the bones of the face involving the pharyngeal arches. The viscerocranium develops from neural crest cells except for the laryngeal cartilages, which forms from mesoderm within pharyngeal arches 4 and 6.

C. Sutures
1. During fetal life and infancy, the flat bones of the skull are separated by dense connective tissue (fibrous joints) called **sutures**. There are five sutures: **frontal suture, sagittal suture, lambdoid suture, coronal suture,** and **squamous suture**.
2. Sutures allow the flat bones of the skull to deform during childbirth (called **molding**) and to expand during childhood as the brain grows. Molding may exert considerable tension at the "obstetrical hinge" (junction of the squamous and lateral parts of the occipital bone) such that the **great cerebral vein (of Galen)** is ruptured during childbirth.

D. Fontanelles are large fibrous areas where several sutures meet.
There are six fontanelles: **anterior fontanelle, posterior fontanelle, two sphenoid fontanelles,** and **two mastoid fontanelles**.
1. The anterior fontanelle is the largest fontanelle and readily palpable in the infant. It pulsates because of the underlying cerebral arteries and can be used to obtain a blood sample from the underlying **superior sagittal sinus**.
2. The **anterior fontanelle and the mastoid fontanelles** close at about **2 years of age** when the main growth of the brain ceases.
3. The **posterior fontanelle and the sphenoid fontanelles** close at about **6 months of age**.

E. Clinical considerations
1. **Abnormalities in skull shape** may result from failure of cranial sutures to form or from premature closure of sutures (**craniosynostoses**).
   a. **Microcephaly** results from failure of the brain to grow; usually associated with mental retardation.
   b. **Oxycephaly (turricephaly or acrocephaly)** is a **tower-like skull** caused by premature closure of the **lambdoid and coronal sutures**. It should be differentiated from **Crouzon syndrome,** which is a dominant genetic condition with a presentation quite similar to that of oxycephaly but is accompanied by malformations of the face, teeth, and ears.

c. **Plagiocephaly** is an asymmetric skull caused by premature closure of the **lambdoid and coronal sutures** on one side of the skull.

d. **Brachycephaly** is a short, square-shaped skull caused by premature closure of the **coronal sutures**.

e. **Scaphocephaly** is a long skull (in the anterior/posterior plane) caused by premature closure of the **sagittal suture**.

f. **Kleeblattschädel** is a cloverleaf skull caused by premature closure of **all sutures** forcing the brain growth through the anterior and sphenoid fontanelles.

g. **Crouzon syndrome** is an autosomal dominant genetic disorder characterized by premature craniosynostosis, midface hypoplasia with shallow orbits, and ocular proptosis. This syndrome is caused by a mutation in the gene for fibroblast growth factor receptor 2 (FGFR2) located on chromosome 10q25-q26.

h. **Apert syndrome** is an autosomal dominant genetic disorder characterized by craniosynostosis leading to turribrachycephaly, syndactyly of hands and feet, various ankyloses, progressive synostoses of the hands, feet, and cervical spine, and mental retardation. This syndrome is caused by a mutation in the gene for fibroblast growth factor receptor 2 (FGFR2) located on chromosome 10q25-q26, exclusively of paternal origin.

i. **Pfeiffer syndrome** is an autosomal dominant genetic disorder characterized by craniosynostosis leading to turribrachycephaly, syndactyly of hands and feet, and broad thumbs and great toes. This syndrome is caused by a mutation in the gene for fibroblast growth factor receptor 2 (FGFR2) located on chromosome 10q25-q26.

2. **Temporal bone formation**
   a. **Mastoid process.** This portion of the temporal bone is absent at birth, which leaves the **facial nerve (CN VII)** relatively unprotected as it emerges from the stylomastoid foramen. In a difficult delivery, forceps may damage CN VII. The mastoid process forms by 2 years of age
   b. **Petrosquamous fissure.** The petrous and squamous portions of the temporal bone are separated by the petrosquamous fissure, which opens directly into the mastoid antrum of the middle ear. This fissure, which may remain open until 20 years of age, provides a route for the spread of infection from the middle ear to the meninges.

3. **Spheno-occipital joint** is a site of growth up to about 20 years of age.

II.   Vertebral Column (Figure 17-2)

A. **Vertebrae in general**   Mesodermal cells from the sclerotome migrate and condense around the notochord to form the **centrum**, around the neural tube to form the **vertebral arches**, and in the body wall to form the **costal processes**.

1. The centrum forms the **vertebral body.**
2. The vertebral arches form the **pedicles, laminae, spinous process, articular processes,** and the **transverse processes.**
3. The costal processes form the **ribs.**

B. The **atlas (C1) and axis (C2)** are highly modified vertebrae.

1. The atlas has no vertebral body or spinous process.
2. The axis has an **odontoid process (dens),** which represents the vertebral body of the atlas.

C. **Sacrum** is a large triangular fusion of five sacral vertebrae forming the posterior/superior wall of the pelvic cavity.

D. **Coccyx** is a small triangular fusion of four rudimentary vertebrae.

E. **Intersegmental position of vertebrae**

1. As mesodermal cells from the sclerotome migrate toward the notochord and neural tube, they split into a **cranial portion** and a **caudal portion**. The caudal portion of each sclero-

tome fuses with the cranial portion of the succeeding sclerotome, which results in the intersegmental position of the vertebra. The splitting of the sclerotome is important because it allows the developing spinal nerve a route of access to the myotome, which it must innervate.

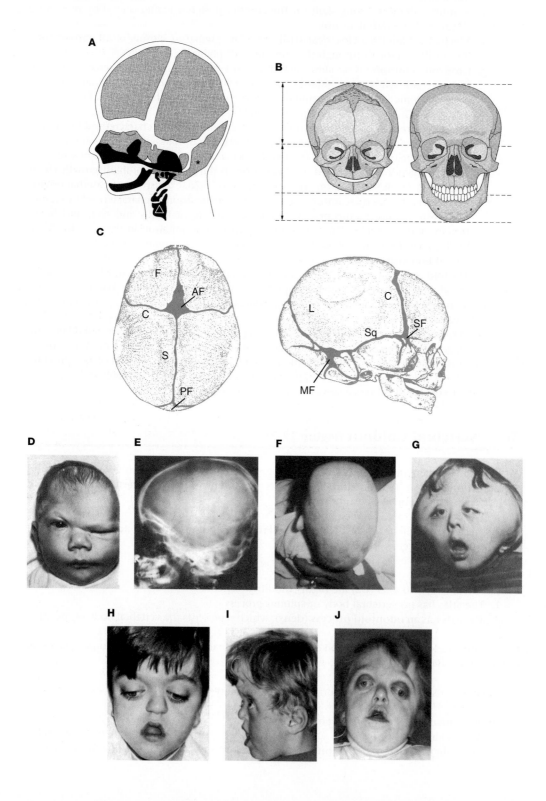

2. In the cervical region, the caudal portion of the fourth occipital sclerotome (O4) fuses with the cranial portion of the first cervical (C1) sclerotome to form the base of the occipital bone. This allows C1 spinal nerve to exit between the base of the occipital bone and C1 vertebrae.

F. **Curves**
   1. The **primary curves** are **thoracic** and **sacral curvatures** that form during the fetal period.
   2. The **secondary curves** are **cervical** and **lumbar curvatures** that form after birth as a result of lifting the head and walking, respectively.

G. **Joints of the vertebral column**
   1. **Synovial joints**
      a. The **atlanto-occipital joint** lies between C1 (atlas) and the occipital condyles.
      b. The **atlantoaxial joint** between C1 (atlas) and C2 (axis).
      c. Facets (**zygapophyseal**) are joints between the inferior and superior articular facets.
   2. **Secondary cartilaginous joints (symphyses)** are the joints between the vertebral bodies in which the **intervertebral disks** play a role. An intervertebral disk consists of the following:
      a. **Nucleus pulposus.** This is a remnant of the embryonic **notochord**. By 20 years of age, all notochordal cells have degenerated such that all notochordal vestiges in the adult are limited to just a noncellular matrix.
      b. **Annulus fibrosus.** This is an outer rim of fibrocartilage derived from mesoderm found between the vertebral bodies.

H. **Clinical considerations**
   1. **Congenital brevicollis (Klippel-Feil syndrome)** results from fusion and shortening of the cervical vertebrae. It is associated with shortness of neck, low hairline, and limited motion of head and neck.
   2. **Intervertebral disk herniation** involves the prolapse of the nucleus pulposus through the defective annulus fibrosis into the vertebral canal. The nucleus pulposus impinges on spinal roots and results in root pain, radiculopathy.
   3. **Spina bifida occulta** results from failure of the vertebral arches to form or fuse.
   4. **Spondylolisthesis** occurs when the pedicles of the vertebral arches fail to fuse with the vertebral body. This allows the vertebral body to move anterior with respect to the vertebrae below it causing **lordosis. Congenital spondylolisthesis** usually occurs at the L5-S1 vertebral level.
   5. **Hemivertebrae** occurs when wedges of vertebrae appear that are usually situated laterally between two other vertebrae.
   6. **Vertebral bar** occurs when there is a localized failure of segmentation on one side of the column usually in a posterolateral site.
   7. **Block vertebra** occurs when there is a lack of separation between two or more vertebrae usually occurring in the lumbar region.

◀ **Figure 17-1.**   **(A)** A diagram of the newborn skull indicating the neurocranium (*shaded area*) and the viscerocranium (*black area*). The bones of the neurocranium and viscerocranium are derived almost entirely from neural crest cells, except for the basilar part of the occipital bone (*), which forms from mesoderm of the occipital sclerotomes, and the laryngeal cartilages (*), which form from mesoderm within pharyngeal arches 4 and 6. **(B)** A diagram depicting the postnatal growth of the skull. After birth, the skull continues ossification toward the sutures. However, the face is relatively underdeveloped and undergoes dramatic changes during childhood and adolescence with the eruption of teeth, formation of sinuses, and elongation of the maxilla and mandible. Note that the profound postnatal changes of the skull are due to the development of the viscerocranium. **(C)** Diagram of the sutures and fontanelles. *AF* = anterior fontanelle; *C* = coronal suture; *F* = frontal suture; *L* = lambdoid suture; *MF* = mastoid fontanelle; *PF* = posterior fontanelle; *SF* = sphenoid fontanelle; *Sq* = squamous suture; *S* = sagittal suture. **(D)** Plagiocephaly. **(E)** Brachiocephaly. **(F)** Scaphocephaly. **(G)** Kleeblattschädel. **(H)** Crouzon syndrome. **(I)** Apert syndrome. **(J)** Pfeiffer syndrome.

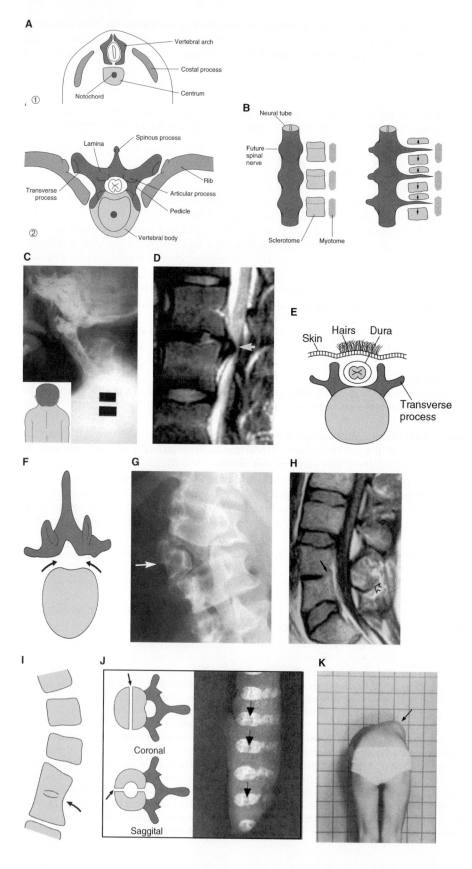

A

① Vertebral arch — Costal process — Notochord — Centrum

② Lamina — Spinous process — Transverse process — Rib — Articular process — Pedicle — Vertebral body

B Neural tube — Future spinal nerve — Sclerotome — Myotome

C

D

E Skin — Hairs — Dura — Transverse process

F

G

H

I

J Coronal — Saggital

K

8. **Cleft vertebra** occurs when a cleft develops in the vertebra usually in a coronal or sagittal plane in the lumbar region.
9. **Idiopathic scoliosis** is a lateral deviation of the vertebral column that involves both deviation and rotation of vertebral bodies.

III.   Ribs

A. Development in general   Ribs develop from costal processes that form at all vertebral levels. However, only in the thoracic region do the costal processes grow into ribs.

B. Clinical considerations
   1. **Accessory lumbar ribs** are the most common.
   2. **Accessory cervical ribs** are attached to the C7 vertebrae and may end either freely or attached to the thoracic cage. Accessory cervical ribs may put pressure on the lower trunk of the brachial plexus and subclavian artery causing superior **thoracic outlet syndrome**.

IV.   Sternum

A. Development in general   The sternum develops from two sternal bars that form in the ventral body wall independent of the ribs and clavicle. The sternal bars fuse with each other in a cranial-caudal direction to form the **manubrium, body**, and **xiphoid process** by week 8.

B. Clinical considerations
   1. **Sternal cleft** occurs when the sternal bars do not fuse completely. It is fairly common and, if small, is generally of no clinical significance.
   2. **Pectus excavatum (funnel chest)** is the most common chest anomaly consisting of a depression of the chest wall, which may extend from the manubrium to the xiphoid process. In addition to the cosmetic appearance, these individuals demonstrate cardiopulmonary restriction, drooped shoulders, protuberant abdomen, and scoliosis such that early surgical intervention is generally recommended.

V.   Bones of the Limbs and Limb Girdles

A. Development in general   The bones of the limb and limb girdles develop from condensations of lateral plate mesoderm within the limb buds. The limb buds are visible at week 4 of devel-

◀ **Figure 17-2.**   (A) Diagram indicating the development of a typical thoracic vertebra. (*1*) At about 5–7 weeks. Mesodermal cells from the sclerotome demonstrate three distinct condensations: centrum, vertebral arch, and costal process. At birth, three ossification centers are present: one in the centrum and one in each vertebral arch. From 3 to 5 years of age the vertebral arches fuse with each other and to the centrum. Ossification ends at about 25 years of age. (*2*) Adult vertebra. Each condensation develops into distinct components of the adult vertebrae as indicated by the shading. (**B**) Diagram depicting the splitting of the sclerotome (*S*) into caudal and cranial portions as the spinal nerves grow out to innervate the myotome. The *dotted lines* indicate where the sclerotome splits, thus allowing the growing spinal nerve to reach the myotome. (**C**) Congenital brevicollis. Radiograph shows congenital fusion of cervical vertebrae. (**D**) Intervertebral disk herniation. MRI shows the protrusion of the L2 disk, causing extradural compression of cauda equina nerve roots (*arrow*). (**E**) Spina bifida occulta. (**F**) Spondylolisthesis. *Arrows* indicate the congenital absence of the pedicles. (**G**) Radiograph indicates hemivertebrae (*arrow*). (**H**) Vertebral bar. MRI shows partial fusion (*solid arrow*) of the L4-L5 vertebral bodies posteriorly. Note also the single fused spinous process (*open arrow*). (**I**) Block vertebra. (**J**) Coronal and sagittal cleft vertebrae. Radiograph shows coronal clefts in vertebrae L1, L2, and L4 (*arrows*). (**K**) Scoliosis. The forward-bending examination will reveal even very small curvatures. The prominence (*arrow*) is produced by chest wall asymmetry.

opment; the upper limb appears first. The limbs are well differentiated at week 8. The limb tip contains the **apical ectodermal ridge**, which exerts an inductive influence on limb growth and development.

B. Clinical considerations

1. **Amelia** (an absence of one or two extremities) may result from the use of the teratogen **thalidomide**.

2. **Polydactyly** is an autosomal dominant disorder that is characterized by the presence of extra digits on the hands and feet.

3. **Syndactyly** (webbed fingers or toes), the most common limb anomaly, results from failure of the hand or foot webs to degenerate between the digits.

4. **Holt-Oram syndrome (heart-hand syndrome)** is an autosomal dominant disorder associated with chromosome 12 that causes anomalies of the upper limb and heart.

VI.   Osteogenesis

Osteogenesis occurs through the conversion of preexisting connective tissue into bone. This process is called **ossification**. During development, two types of ossifications occur.

A. Intramembranous ossification occurs in the embryo when mesoderm or neural crest cells condense into sheets of highly vascular connective tissue, which then **directly** forms a primary ossification center. **Bones that form via intramembranous ossification are** frontal bone, parietal bones, intraparietal part of occipital bone, maxilla, zygomatic bone, squamous part of temporal bone, palatine, vomer, and mandible.

B. Endochondral ossification occurs in the embryo when mesoderm or neural crest cells first form a hyaline cartilage model, which then develops a primary ossification center at the diaphysis. **Bones that form via endochondral ossification are** ethmoid bone, sphenoid bone, petrous and mastoid parts of the temporal bone, basilar part of the occipital bone, incus, malleus, stapes, styloid process, hyoid bone, bones of the limbs, limb girdles, vertebrae, sternum, and ribs.

VII.   General Skeletal Abnormalities (Figure 17-3)

A. Achondroplasia (AC) is the most prevalent form of dwarfism. AC is an autosomal dominant genetic disorder caused by a mutation in the gene for **fibroblast growth factor receptor 3 (FGFR3)** on chromosome 4p16. Pathologic changes are observed at the epiphyseal growth plate where the zones of proliferation and hypertrophy are narrow and disorganized. Horizontal struts of bone eventually grow into the growth plate and "seal" the bone, thereby preventing bone growth. Affected persons are short in stature with shortening of the arms and legs along with a disproportionately long trunk. Mental function is not affected. Chances of AC increase with increasing paternal age.

Figure 17-3.   (A) A boy with achondroplasia. Note the short stature, short limbs and fingers, disproportion- ▶ ate trunk, bowed legs, relatively large head, prominent forehead, and deep nasal bridge. (B and C) A man and a woman with achondroplasia. Note the lordotic curve. (D) Girl with Marfan syndrome. Note the unusually tall stature, exceptionally long limbs, and arachnodactyly (elongated hands and feet with very slender digits). (E) Boy with Marfan syndrome. Note the deformities of the sternum and spine. (F) Infant with osteogenesis imperfecta (OI). This newborn died immediately after birth from respiratory insufficiency. Note the lack of calcified calvaria whereby the finger can easily indent the skull. Note the short, bowed upper and lower limbs. (G) Radiograph of an infant with OI. Note the multiple bone fractures of the upper and lower limb resulting in an accordion-like shortening of the limbs. (H) Man with OI showing the severe crippling deformities. (I) Photograph of a 22-year-old man before he developed telltale signs of acromegaly. (J) The same man at 39 years old with distinct facial appearance of acromegaly.

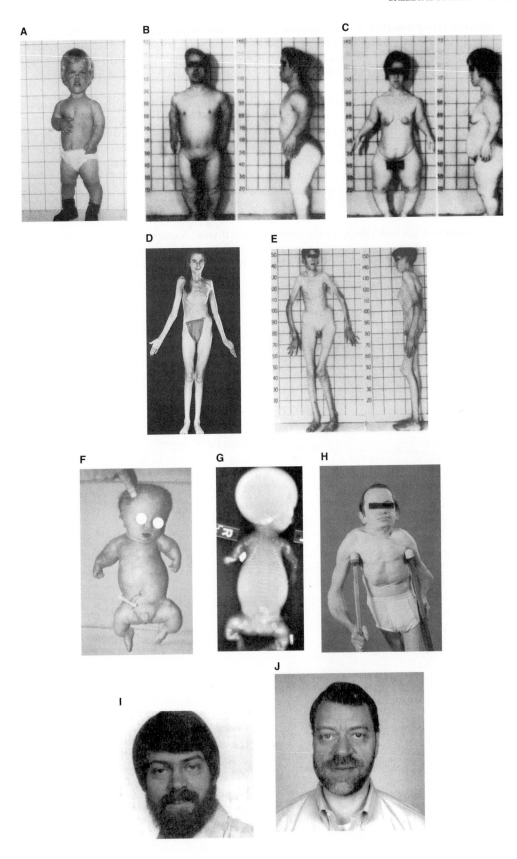

B. Marfan syndrome (MS) is an autosomal dominant genetic disorder caused by a mutation in the gene for the protein **fibrillin** on chromosome 15q21.1, which is an essential component of **elastic fibers**. These individuals are unusually tall, have exceptionally long, thin limbs, and have ectopia lentis (dislocation of the lens), severe near-sightedness, and heart valve incompetence.

C. Osteogenesis imperfecta (OI) is an autosomal dominant (Types I–IV) or recessive (Types II and III) genetic disorder caused by a mutation in the gene for **Type I collagen** on chromosome 7q22 or 17q22. OI is characterized by extreme bone fragility, with spontaneous fractures occurring when the fetus is still in the womb, and blue sclera of the eye. Severe forms of OI are fatal in utero or during the early neonatal period. Milder forms of OI may be confused with child abuse.

D. Acromegaly results from hyperpituitarism. It is characterized by a large jaw, hands, and feet, and sometimes by gigantism.

E. Cretinism occurs when there is a deficiency in fetal thyroid hormone (T3 and T4) and/or thyroid agenesis. Cretinism results in growth retardation, skeletal abnormalities, mental retardation, and neurologic disorders. It is rare except in areas where the water and soil lack iodine.

Directions: *Each of the numbered items or incomplete statements in this section is followed by answers or by completions of the statement. Select the **one** lettered answer or completion that is **best** in each case.*

1. Accessory ribs are most commonly found attached to the

(A) cervical vertebrae
(B) thoracic vertebrae
(C) lumbar vertebrae
(D) manubrium
(E) sternebrae

2. The anterior fontanelle is usually closed by

(A) birth
(B) age 6 months
(C) age 18 months
(D) age 2 years
(E) age 5 years

3. The condition in which the pedicles of the vertebral arches fail to fuse with the vertebral body is called

(A) block vertebrae
(B) cleft vertebrae
(C) hemivertebrae
(D) spondylolisthesis
(E) spina bifida occulta

4. During ultrasound examination, numerous fractures of the long bones of the fetus are observed. This condition is called

(A) achondroplasia
(B) osteogenesis imperfecta
(C) Marfan syndrome
(D) cretinism
(E) acromegaly

5. A female newborn presents with a square-shaped skull with a short occipitofrontal diameter. Premature closure of which of the following sutures is the most likely cause of this finding?

(A) Sphenofrontal
(B) Sphenoparietal
(C) Lambdoidal
(D) Sagittal
(E) Coronal

 ANSWERS AND EXPLANATIONS

1. **C.** Accessory ribs are most commonly attached to lumbar vertebrae. When present (incidence 0.5%–1%), a cervical rib is usually attached to the seventh cervical vertebra. Cervical ribs may compress the brachial plexus and subclavian vessels and cause superior thoracic outlet syndrome.

2. **D.** The anterior fontanelle is usually closed by 2 years of age; the posterior and sphenoid fontanelles are usually closed by 6 months of age.

3. **D.** When the pedicles fail to fuse with the vertebral body a condition called spondylolisthesis results. This allows the vertebral body to move anterior with respect to the vertebrae below it causing lordosis.

4. **B.** Osteogenesis imperfecta is a deficiency of Type I collagen and results in spontaneous fractures of fetal bones and blue sclera of the eye.

5. **B.** Brachycephaly is the premature closure of the coronal sutures, which leads to square-shaped skull with a short occipitofrontal diameter.

Muscular System

I.　Skeletal Muscle

A. Molecular events　Mesodermal (mesenchymal) cells within somites become committed to a muscle-forming cell line through a poorly understood mechanism to form **myogenic cells**. Myogenic cells enter the cell cycle (i.e., undergo mitosis), which is stimulated by **FGF** (fibroblast growth factor) and **TGF-β** (transforming growth factor). **Pax-3** and **myf-5** stimulate myogenic cells to begin expression of **MyoD** (a helix-loop-helix transcription factor). MyoD binds to the **E box** (CANNTG) on DNA, which removes the myogenic cells from the cell cycle (i.e., mitosis stops) and switches on **muscle-specific genes** to form **postmitotic myoblasts**. Myoblasts begin to synthesize **actin** and **myosin** while they fuse with each other to form multinucleated **myotubes**. Myotubes synthesize **actin, myosin, troponin, tropomyosin,** and **other muscle proteins**. These proteins aggregate into **myofibrils** at which stage the cells are called **muscle fibers**. Because muscle fibers are postmitotic, further growth is accomplished by means of **satellite cells**, which operate by poorly understood mechanisms.

B. Paraxial mesoderm is a thick plate of mesoderm on each side of the midline. The paraxial mesoderm becomes organized into segments known as **somitomeres**, which form in a craniocaudal sequence. **Somitomeres 1–7** do not form somites but contribute mesoderm to the head and neck region (pharyngeal arches). **The remaining somitomeres** further condense in a craniocaudal sequence to form 42–44 pairs of somites of the trunk region. The somites closest to the caudal end eventually disappear to give a final count of approximately **35 pairs of somites**. Somites further differentiate into the sclerotome (cartilage and bone component), myotome (muscle component),and dermatome (dermis of skin component).

C. Head and neck musculature is derived from somitomeres 1–7 of the head and neck region, which participate in the formation of the pharyngeal arches.
  1. **Extraocular muscles** are derived from somitomeres 1, 2, 3, and 5. Somitomeres 1, 2, and 3 are called **preotic myotomes**. The extraocular muscles are innervated by CN III, CN IV, and CN VI.
  2. **Tongue muscles** are derived from **occipital myotomes**. The tongue muscles are innervated by CN XII.

D. Trunk musculature (Figure 18-1) is derived from myotomes in the trunk region. Each myotome partitions into a dorsal **epimere** and a ventral **hypomere**.
  1. The **epimere** develops into the extensor muscles of the neck and vertebral column (e.g., erector spinae). The epimere is innervated by **dorsal rami of spinal nerves**.
  2. The **hypomere** develops into the scalene, prevertebral, geniohyoid, infrahyoid, intercostal, abdominal muscles, lateral and ventral flexors of the vertebral column, quadratus lumborum, and pelvic diaphragm. The hypomere is innervated by **ventral rami of spinal nerves**.

E. **Limb musculature** is derived from myotomes (somites) in the upper limb bud region and lower limb bud region. This mesoderm migrates into the limb bud and forms a **posterior condensation** and an **anterior condensation**.

1. The posterior condensation develops into the **extensor and supinator musculature of the upper limb** and the **extensor and abductor musculature of the lower limb**.

2. The anterior condensation develops into the **flexor and pronator musculature of the upper limb** and the **flexor and adductor musculature of the lower limb**.

II.   Smooth Muscle

The smooth muscle of the gastrointestinal tract and the tunica media of blood vessels is derived from mesoderm.

III.   Cardiac Muscle

Cardiac muscle is derived from mesoderm that surrounds the primitive heart tube and becomes the myocardium.

IV.   Clinical Considerations (Figure 18-1)

A. **Prune-belly syndrome** occurs when the **abdominal musculature** is absent or very hypoplastic, most likely involving cells of the hypomere.

B. **Poland syndrome** is a relatively uncommon chest anomaly characterized by the **partial or complete absence of the pectoralis major muscle**. In addition, affected individuals may demonstrate partial agenesis of the ribs and sternum, mammary gland aplasia, or absence of the latissimus dorsi and serratus anterior muscles.

C. **Congenital torticollis (wryneck)** occurs when the **sternocleidomastoid muscle** is abnormally shortened, causing rotation and tilting of the head. It may be caused by injury to the sternocleidomastoid muscle during childbirth, formation of a hematoma, and eventual fibrosis of the muscle.

D. **Duchenne muscular dystrophy (DMD)**   DMD is an **X-linked recessive disorder** caused by a mutation in the gene for **dystrophin** on the short arm of chromosome X (Xp21). X-linked recessive inheritance means that males who inherit only one defective copy of the DMD gene from the mother have the disease. Dystrophin anchors the cytoskeleton (actin) of skeletal muscle cells to the extracellular matrix through a transmembrane protein (α-dystroglycan and β-dystroglycan) and stabilizes the cell membrane. A mutation of the DMD gene destroys the ability of dystrophin to anchor actin to the extracellular matrix. The characteristic dysfunction in DMD is **progressive muscle weakness and wasting**. Death occurs as a result of cardiac or respiratory failure, usually in late teens or 20s.

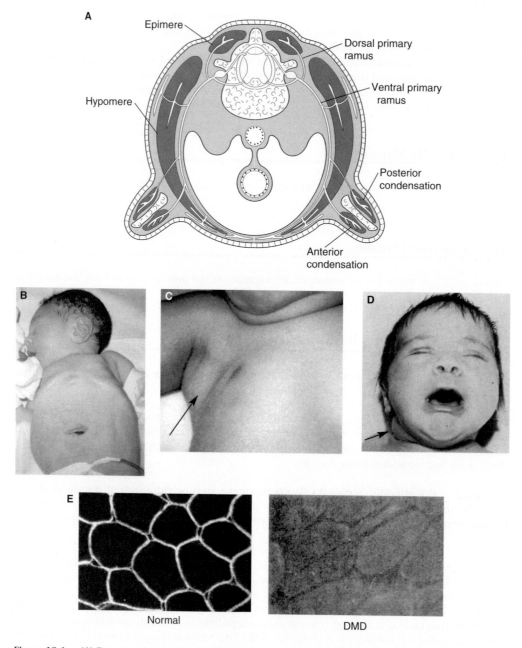

Figure 18-1. **(A)** Drawing of transverse section through the thorax and limb bud, showing the muscles of the epimere, hypomere, and limb bud. The limb bud musculature develops from mesoderm of various myotomes. The epimeric muscles are innervated by dorsal primary rami, and the hypomeric and limb muscles are innervated by ventral primary rami of spinal nerves. **(B)** Prune-belly syndrome. The absence of the abdominal musculature is apparent, causing a widening of the flanks. **(C)** Poland syndrome. The absence of the right pectoralis major muscle (*arrow*) and loss of the right anterior axillary fold are apparent. **(D)** Congenital torticollis (wryneck). A fibrous mass in the right sternocleidomastoid muscle is apparent (*arrow*). **(E)** Duchenne muscular dystrophy (DMD). Immunofluorescent staining for dystrophin shows intense staining at the periphery of skeletal muscle cells in normal individuals and complete absence of staining in the DMD patient.

*Directions: Each of the numbered items or incomplete statements in this section is followed by answers or by completions of the statement. Select the **one** lettered answer or completion that is **best** in each case.*

1. The extrinsic eye muscles develop from which of the following?

(A) Cervical somites
(B) Epimere
(C) Hypomere
(D) Occipital somites
(E) Preotic somites

2. The tongue muscles develop from which of the following?

(A) Cervical somites
(B) Epimere
(C) Hypomere
(D) Occipital somites
(E) Preotic somites

3. The biceps brachii muscle develops from which of the following?

(A) Hypomere
(B) Epimere
(C) Anterior condensation
(D) Posterior condensation
(E) Preotic somites

4. The biceps femoris muscle develops from which of the following?

(A) Hypomere
(B) Epimere
(C) Anterior condensation
(D) Posterior condensation
(E) Preotic somites

ANSWERS AND EXPLANATIONS

1. **E.** The extrinsic eye muscles arise from the preotic somites (myotomes) found near the prochordal plate. Recent research indicates that the extrinsic eye muscles are derived from somitomeres 1, 2, 3, and 5.

2. **D.** The tongue muscles (intrinsic and extrinsic) arise from the occipital somites (myotomes).

3. **C.** Because the biceps brachii muscle is a flexor of the antebrachium (forearm), it develops from the anterior condensation of myotomic mesoderm.

4. **C.** Because the biceps femoris muscle is a flexor of the leg, it develops from the anterior condensation of myotomic mesoderm.

CHAPTER
19

Upper Limb

I. Overview of Development

Lateral plate mesoderm migrates into the limb bud and condenses along the central axis to eventually form the **vasculature** and **skeletal** components of the upper limb. **Mesoderm from the somites** migrates into the limb bud and condenses to eventually form the **musculature** component of the upper limb.

A. Apical ectodermal ridge (AER) is a ridge of thickened ectoderm at the apex of the limb bud. The AER produces **FGF** (fibroblast growth factor), which interacts with the underlying mesoderm to promote outgrowth of the limb by stimulating mitosis and preventing terminal differentiation of the underlying mesoderm. The AER expresses the ***Wnt7*** gene that directs the organization of the limb bud along the dorsal-ventral axis.

B. Zone of polarizing activity (ZPA) consists of mesodermal cells located at the base of the limb bud. The ZPA produces **sonic hedgehog** (a diffusible protein encoded by a segment polarity gene), which directs the organization of the limb bud along the anterior-posterior polar axis and patterning of the digits. Sonic hedgehog activates the gene for **BMP** (bone morphogenetic protein) and the ***Hoxd-9, Hoxd-10, Hoxd-11, Hoxd-12***, and ***Hoxd-13*** genes. **Retinoic acid** also plays a significant role in limb polarization.

C. Digit formation occurs as a result of selected **apoptosis (cell death)** within the AER such that five separate regions of AER remain at the tips of the future digits. The exact mechanism is poorly understood, although **BMP**, ***Msx-1***, and **retinoic acid receptor** may play a role.

II. Vasculature (Figure 19-1)

The **aortic arch 4** forms the proximal part of the right subclavian artery. The **7th intersegmental artery** forms the distal part of the right subclavian artery and the entire left subclavian artery. The **subclavian artery (right and left)** continues into the limb bud as the **axis artery**, which ends in a **terminal plexus** near the tip of the limb bud. The **terminal plexus** participates in the formation of the **deep palmar arch** and the **superficial palmar arch**. The **axis artery** initially sprouts the **posterior interosseous artery** and the **median artery** (which is reduced to an unnamed vessel in the adult). The axis artery later sprouts the **radial artery** and **ulnar artery**. The axis artery persists in the adult as the **axillary artery, brachial artery, anterior interosseous artery,** and **deep palmar arch**.

III. Musculature (Figure 19-1)

The upper limb bud site lies opposite somites C4, C5, C6, C7, C8, T1, and T2. During week 5, mesoderm from these somites (myotomes) migrates into the limb bud and forms a **posterior condensation** and an **anterior condensation**. The mesoderm of these condensations differentiates into myoblasts and then a splitting of the condensations occurs into anatomically recognizable muscles of the upper limb although little is known about this process.

A. The **posterior condensation** gives rise to the following muscles: deltoid, supraspinatus, infraspinatus, teres minor, teres major, subscapularis, triceps brachii, anconeus, brachioradialis, extensor carpi radialis longus, extensor carpi radialis brevis, extensor digitorum, extensor digiti minimi, extensor carpi ulnaris, supinator, abductor pollicis longus, extensor pollicis brevis, extensor pollicis longus, and extensor indicis. In general, the posterior condensation gives rise to the **extensor and supinator musculature**.

B. The **anterior condensation** gives rise to the following muscles: biceps brachii, brachialis, coracobrachialis, pronator teres, flexor carpi radialis, palmaris longus, flexor carpi ulnaris, flexor digitorum superficialis, flexor digitorum profundus, flexor pollicis brevis, flexor pollicis longus, pronator quadratus, abductor pollicis brevis, opponens pollicis, adductor pollicis, abductor digiti minimi, flexor digiti minimi brevis, opponens digiti minimi, lumbricales, dorsal and palmar interossei. In general, the anterior condensation gives rise to the **flexor and pronator musculature**.

IV. Nerves (Brachial Plexus) (Figure 19-1)

Local molecular messages produced at the base of the limb bud guide the early nerve fibers into the limb bud. The muscles themselves do not provide any specific target messages to the ingrowing nerve fibers. **Ventral primary rami from C5, C6, C7, C8, and T1** arrive at the base of the limb bud and join in a specific pattern to form the **upper trunk, middle trunk**, and **lower trunk**. Each trunk divides into **posterior divisions** and **anterior divisions**. Posterior divisions grow into the posterior condensation of mesoderm and join to form the **posterior cord**. Anterior divisions grow into the anterior condensation of mesoderm and join to form the **medial cord** and **lateral cord**.

A. With further development of the limb musculature, the posterior cord branches into the **axillary nerve (C5, C6)** and **radial nerve (C5, C6, C7, C8, T1)**, thereby innervating all the muscles that form from the posterior condensation.

B. With further development of the limb musculature, the medial cord and lateral cord branch into the **musculocutaneous nerve (C5, C6, C7)**, **ulnar nerve (C8, T1)**, and **median nerve (C5, C6, C7, C8, T1)**, thereby innervating all the muscles that form from the anterior condensation.

V. Rotation of the Upper Limb (Figure 19-1)

The upper limb buds appear at week 4 as small bulges oriented in a **coronal plane**. The upper limb buds undergo a horizontal movement in week 6 so that they are now oriented in a **sagittal plane**. The upper limbs **rotate laterally 90°** during weeks 6–8 such that the elbow points posteriorly, the extensor compartment lies posterior, and the flexor compartment lies anterior. This rotation causes the originally straight segmental pattern of innervation (dermatomes) to be somewhat modified in the adult.

VI. Skeletal (Figure 19-2)

The **lateral plate mesoderm** forms the **scapula, clavicle, humerus, radius, ulna, carpals, metacarpals**, and **phalanges**. All the bones of the upper limb undergo endochondral ossification. However, the clavicle undergoes both membranous and endochondral ossification. The **timing of bone formation** follows this time course:

A. Week 5 Lateral plate mesoderm within the limb bud condenses.

B. Week 6 Condensed mesoderm chondrifies to form a hyaline cartilage model of the upper limb bones.

C. Week 7 Primary ossification centers are seen in the clavicle, humerus, radius, and ulnar bones. The clavicle is the first bone in the entire body to ossify.

D. Week 9 to birth Primary ossification centers are seen in the scapula, metacarpals, and phalanges.

E. Childhood Secondary ossification centers form in the epiphyseal ends. All carpal bones begin ossification.

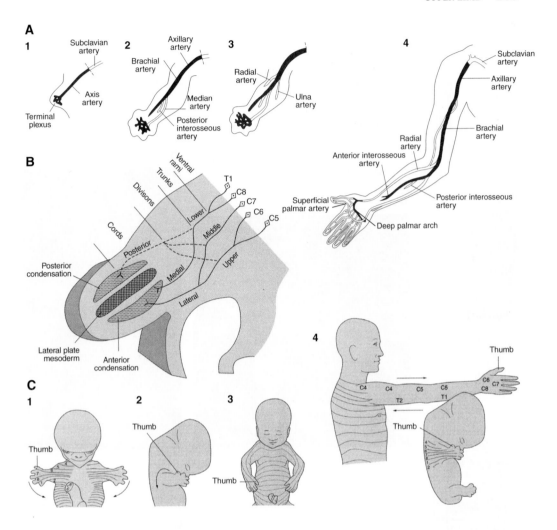

Figure 19-1. **(A)** Diagram depicting the development of arteries of the upper limb. (*1, 2, 3*) Early limb bud. The earliest arterial supply of the upper limb bud is the axis artery (*black*) and terminal plexus (*black*). The first branches of the axis artery are the posterior interosseous artery and the median artery. The last branches of the axis artery are the radial artery and ulnar artery. (*4*) Adult upper limb. The axis artery persists as the axillary artery, brachial artery, anterior interosseous artery, and deep palmar arch (*black*). **(B)** Diagram of the muscle and nerve development of the upper limb. Lateral plate mesoderm (*hatched area*) forms down the central axis of the limb bud and is responsible for the formation of the blood vessels and bones of the upper limb. Mesoderm from the somites (myotomes) migrates into the limb bud and forms a posterior and anterior condensation (*dotted areas*). Ventral primary rami from C5 to T1 leave the neural tube and undergo extensive rearrangement into upper, middle, and lower trunks. Each trunk divides into posterior (*dotted lines*) and anterior (*solid lines*) divisions. The posterior divisions selectively grow into the posterior condensation and form the posterior cord. The anterior divisions selectively grow into the anterior condensation and form the medial and lateral cords. **(C)** Rotation of the upper limb. (*1*) Ventral view of a week 4 embryo. Upper limb buds are oriented in a coronal plane. Note the segmental pattern of innervation from C4 to T2. In week 6, the upper limb buds undergo a horizontal movement (*curved arrows*) such that the upper limb buds become oriented in a sagittal plane (as shown in 2). (*2*) Side view of a week 6 embryo. Note the upper limb bud oriented in the sagittal plane. During weeks 6–8, the upper limb buds rotate 90° laterally (*curved arrow*). (*3*) Ventral view of a week 8 embryo. Note the position of the upper limb with elbows pointing posterior. (*4*) Dermatome pattern in the adult upper limb and limb bud. The 90° lateral rotation of the upper limb bud causes the originally straight segmental pattern of innervation in the embryo to be somewhat modified ("twisted in a spiral") such that the dermatome pattern in the adult is altered. However, an orderly dermatome pattern can still be recognized in the adult if the upper limb is positioned in the sagittal plane with the thumb pointing superiorly (as shown). The dermatomes from C4 can be counted distally down the superior border of the upper limb (*arrow*) to C7 at the middle finger and then back proximally up the inferior border of the upper limb (*arrow*) to T2. Note the position of the thumb in *1, 2, 3,* and *4*.

A

Week 5   Week 6

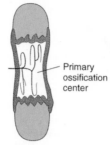

Primary
ossification
center

Weeks 7–9

B

At birth

C

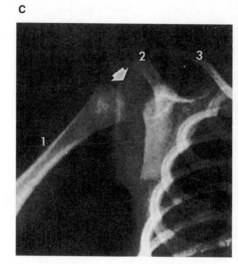

D

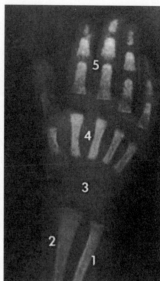

E

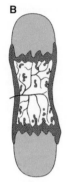

Childhood

F

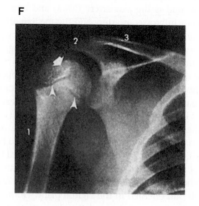

G

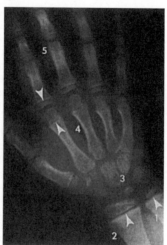

◄**Figure 19-2.** Bone formation in the upper limb. **(A)** Week 5, lateral plate mesoderm condenses (*hatched*). Week 6, hyaline cartilage (*light shading*) model of future bones forms. Weeks 7–9, primary ossification centers within the diaphysis appear such that bone (*dark shading*) forms (osteogenesis). **(B)** At birth, the diaphysis consists of bone (*dark shading*), whereas the epiphysis remains hyaline cartilage (*light shading*). This is important to note when interpreting radiographs of newborns. **(C)** Radiograph of a newborn at the shoulder region (*1* = humerus; *2* = acromion; *3* = clavicle) shows the portion of the hyaline cartilage model that has been replaced by radiodense bone (*white*). Note that the epiphyseal end of the humerus (*white arrow*) is still hyaline cartilage at birth and therefore appears radiolucent (*dark*). **(D)** Radiograph of a newborn arm and hand shows the portion of the hyaline cartilage model that has been replaced by radiodense bone (*white*) in the ulna (*1*), radius (*2*), metacarpals (*4*), and phalanges (*5*). Note the epiphyseal ends of these bones (*1, 2, 4, 5*) and all of the carpal bones (*3*) are still hyaline cartilage and therefore radiolucent (*dark*). The carpal bones of the wrist begin to ossify much later in childhood. **(E)** During childhood, secondary ossification centers form in the epiphyseal ends of the bones. During childhood and adolescence, the growth in length of long bones occurs at the epiphyseal growth plate. **(F)** Note the radiograph of a 6-year-old child at the shoulder region (*1* = humerus; *2* = acromion; *3* = clavicle). Since secondary ossification centers are present within the epiphyseal ends of the humerus, the head of the humerus is now radiodense (*white arrow*), and the epiphyseal growth plate (*arrowheads*) where hyaline cartilage is present remains radiolucent (*dark*). This is not to be confused with a bone fracture. **(G)** The radiograph of a 6-year-old child at the wrist and hand demonstrates the radiodense bone (*white*) within the diaphyseal and epiphyseal portions of the ulnar bone (*1*) and radius bone (*2*) as well as the radiolucent (*dark*) epiphyseal growth plates (*arrowheads*), which are hyaline cartilage. The diaphyseal and epiphyseal portions of the metacarpals (*4*) and phalanges (*5*) as well as their epiphyseal growth plates (*arrowheads*) can also be observed. Note that the carpal bones (*3*) have begun to ossify.

STUDY QUESTIONS FOR CHAPTER 19

*Directions: Each of the numbered items or incomplete statements in this section is followed by answers or by completions of the statement. Select the **one** lettered answer or completion that is **best** in each case.*

1. Which of the following arteries is one of the first branches to form from the axis artery?

(A) Radial artery
(B) Ulnar artery
(C) Axillary artery
(D) Median artery
(E) Brachial artery

2. The humerus develops from which of the following?

(A) Somite mesoderm
(B) Lateral plate mesoderm
(C) Intermediate mesoderm
(D) Extraembryonic mesoderm
(E) Sclerotome mesoderm

3. The long head of the triceps muscle develops from which of the following?

(A) Posterior condensation
(B) Anterior condensation
(C) Lateral plate mesoderm
(D) Extraembryonic mesoderm
(E) Sclerotome mesoderm

4. Which of the following muscles will the lateral cord of the brachial plexus innervate?

(A) Triceps
(B) Supinator
(C) Extensor carpi ulnaris
(D) Extensor digitorum
(E) Biceps brachii

5. During weeks 6–8, the upper limb will rotate

(A) medially 90°
(B) laterally 90°
(C) medially 180°
(D) laterally 180°
(E) no rotation

ANSWERS AND EXPLANATIONS

1. **D.** The median artery is one of the first branches to form from the axis artery. In the adult, the median artery does not persist and is probably reduced to a small, unnamed vessel. This is why the median nerve does not have an accompanying artery in the adult like the ulnar nerve (ulnar artery) and radial nerve (radial artery).

2. **B.** All bones of the upper limb form from lateral plate mesoderm that condenses along the central axis of the upper limb bud.

3. **A.** Somite mesoderm migrates into the limb bud and forms two condensations. The posterior condensation of the upper limb gives rise to the extensors of the upper limb, which attain a posterior location in the adult because of the lateral rotation of 90°.

4. **E.** One of the nerves that forms from the lateral cord of the brachial plexus is the musculocutaneous nerve. The musculocutaneous nerve will innervate muscles derived from the anterior condensation (flexors). Biceps brachii muscle is a flexor at the elbow joint. Note that the biceps brachii muscle and the musculocutaneous nerve are related embryologically to the anterior condensation and anterior divisions (which form the lateral cord) and in the adult are located anterior. This occurs because of the lateral rotation of 90°.

5. **B.** The upper limb rotates laterally 90° so that the elbows point posteriorly.

Lower Limb

I. Overview of Development

Lateral plate mesoderm migrates into the limb bud and condenses along the central axis to eventually form the **vasculature** and **skeletal** components of the upper limb. **Mesoderm from the somites** migrates into the limb bud and condenses to eventually form the **musculature** component of the upper limb.

A. Apical ectodermal ridge (AER) is a ridge of thickened ectoderm at the apex of the limb bud. The AER produces **FGF** (fibroblast growth factor) that interacts with the underlying mesoderm to promote outgrowth of the limb by stimulating mitosis and preventing terminal differentiation of the underlying mesoderm. The AER expresses the **Wnt7** gene that directs the organization of the limb bud along the dorsal-ventral axis.

B. Zone of polarizing activity (ZPA) consists of mesodermal cells located at the base of the limb bud. The ZPA produces **sonic hedgehog** (a diffusible protein encoded by a segment polarity gene) that directs the organization of the limb bud along the anterior-posterior polar axis and patterning of the digits. Sonic hedgehog activates the gene for **BMP** (bone morphogenetic protein) and the **Hoxd-9, Hoxd-10, Hoxd-11, Hoxd-12,** and **Hoxd-13** genes. **Retinoic acid** also plays a significant role in limb polarization.

C. Digit formation occurs as a result of selected **apoptosis (cell death)** within the AER such that five separate regions of AER remain at the tips of the future digits. The exact mechanism is poorly understood, although **BMP, Msx-1, and retinoic acid receptor** may play a role.

II. Vasculature (Figure 20-1)

The **umbilical artery** gives rise to the **axis artery** of the lower limb, which ends in a **terminal plexus** near the tip of the limb bud. The **terminal plexus** participates in the formation of the **deep plantar arch**. The **axis artery** sprouts the **anterior tibial artery** (which continues as the **dorsalis pedis artery**) and **posterior tibial artery** (which terminates as the **medial plantar artery** and **lateral plantar artery**). Although most of the axis artery regresses, the axis artery ultimately persists in the adult as the **inferior gluteal artery, sciatic artery** (accompanying the sciatic nerve), proximal part of the **popliteal artery**, and distal part of the **peroneal artery**. The **external iliac artery** gives rise to the **femoral artery** of the lower limb, which constitutes a separate second arterial channel into the lower limb that connects to the axis artery. The femoral artery sprouts the **profunda femoris artery**.

III. Musculature (see Figure 20-1)

The lower limb bud site lies opposite somites L1, L2, L3, L4, L5, S1, and S2. During week 5, mesoderm from these somites (myotomes) migrates into the limb bud and forms a **posterior condensation** and an **anterior condensation**. The mesoderm of these condensations differentiates into myoblasts and then a splitting of the condensations occurs into anatomically recognizable muscles of the lower limb although little is known about this process.

A. The **posterior condensation** gives rise to the following muscles: gluteus maximus, gluteus medius, gluteus minimus, piriformis, pectineus, iliacus, tensor fascia lata, sartorius, rectus femoris, vastus lateralis, vastus medialis, vastus intermedius, short head of biceps femoris, tibialis anterior, extensor hallucis longus, extensor digitorum longus, peroneus tertius, peroneus longus, peroneus brevis, extensor digitorum brevis, extensor hallucis brevis. In general, the posterior condensation gives rise to the **extensor and abductor musculature**.

B. The **anterior condensation** gives rise to following muscles: adductor longus, adductor brevis, adductor magnus, gracilis, obturator externus, obturator internus, superior and inferior gemelli, quadratus femoris, semitendinosus, semimembranosus, long head of biceps femoris, gastrocnemius, soleus, plantaris, popliteus, flexor hallucis longus, flexor digitorum longus, tibialis posterior, abductor hallucis, flexor digitorum brevis, abductor digiti minimi, quadratus plantae, lumbricales, flexor hallucis brevis, adductor hallucis, flexor digiti minimi brevis, dorsal and plantar interossei. In general, the anterior condensation gives rise to the **flexor and adductor musculature**.

IV. Nerves (Lumbosacral Plexus) (see Figure 20-1)

Local cell biological messages produced at the base of the limb bud guide the early nerve fibers into the limb bud; the muscle themselves do not provide any specific target messages to the ingrowing nerve fibers. **Ventral primary rami from L2, L3, L4, L5, S1, S2, and S3** arrive at the base of the limb bud and divide into **posterior divisions** and **anterior divisions**. Posterior divisions grow into the posterior condensation of mesoderm. Anterior divisions grow into the anterior condensation of mesoderm.

A. With further development of the limb musculature, the posterior divisions branch into the **superior gluteal nerve (L4, L5, S1)**, **inferior gluteal nerve (L5, S1, S2)**, **femoral nerve (L2, L3, L4)**, and **common peroneal nerve (L4, L5, S1, S2)**, thereby innervating all the muscles that form from the posterior condensation.

B. With further development of the limb musculature, the anterior divisions branch into the **tibial nerve (L4, L5, S1, S2, S3)** and **obturator nerve (L2, L3, L4)**, thereby innervating all the muscles that form from the anterior condensation.

V. Rotation of the Lower Limb (see Figure 20-1)

The lower limb buds appear in week 4 (about 4 days after the upper limb bud) as small bulges oriented in a **coronal plane**. The lower limb buds undergo a horizontal movement in week 6 so that they are now oriented in a **sagittal plane**. The lower limbs **rotate medially 90°** during weeks 6–8 such that the knee points anteriorly, the extensor compartment lies anterior, and the flexor compartment lies posterior. This rotation causes the originally straight segmental pattern of innervation (dermatomes) to be somewhat modified in the adult. Note that the upper limbs rotate laterally 90°, whereas the lower limbs rotate medially 90°, which sets up the following anatomic situations:

A. Flexor compartment of upper limb is anterior, whereas flexor compartment of lower limb is posterior.

B. Extensor compartment of upper limb is posterior, whereas extensor compartment of lower limb is anterior.

C. Flexion at the wrist joint is analogous to plantar flexion at the ankle joint.

D. Extension at the wrist joint is analogous to dorsiflexion at the ankle joint.

VI. Skeletal (see Figure 20-2)

The **lateral plate mesoderm** forms the **ilium, ischium, pubis, femur, tibia, fibula, tarsals, metatarsals,** and **phalanges**. All bones of the lower limb undergo endochondral ossification. The **timing of bone formation** follows this time course:

A. Week 5   Lateral plate mesoderm within the limb bud condenses.

B. Week 6   Condensed mesoderm chondrifies to form a hyaline cartilage model of all the lower limb bones.

C. Week 7   Primary ossification centers are seen in the femur and tibia.

D. Week 9 to birth   Primary ossification centers are seen in the ilium, ischium, pubis, fibula, calcaneus, talus, metatarsals, and phalanges. The ossification of the calcaneus (weeks 16–20) is used medicolegally to establish maturity.

E. Childhood   Secondary ossification centers form in the epiphyseal ends. The remaining tarsal bones begin ossification.

Figure 20-1.   **(A)** Diagram depicting the development of arteries of the lower limb. *(1, 2, 3, 4)* Early limb bud. ▶ The earliest arterial supply of the lower limb bud is the axis artery (*black*) and terminal plexus (*black*), which arises from the umbilical artery. The axis artery gives off branches forming the anterior tibial artery and posterior tibial artery and undergoes regression and some remodeling in selected areas. The external iliac artery gives rise to the femoral artery, which constitutes a separate second arterial channel in the lower limb. *(5)* Adult lower limb. The axis artery persists as the inferior gluteal artery, sciatic artery, proximal part of the popliteal artery, and distal part of the peroneal artery. The *Xs* indicate areas of regression. **(B)** Diagram of the muscle and nerve development of the lower limb. Lateral plate mesoderm (*hatched area*) forms down the central axis of the limb bud and is responsible for the formation of the blood vessels and bones of the lower limb. Mesoderm from somites (myotomes) migrates into the limb bud and forms a posterior and anterior condensation (*dotted areas*). Ventral primary rami from L2 to S3 leave the neural tube and divide into posterior (*dotted lines*) and anterior (*solid lines*) divisions. The posterior divisions selectively grow into the posterior condensation. The anterior divisions selectively grow into the anterior condensation. **(C)** Rotation of the lower limb. *(1)* Ventral view of a week 4 embryo. Lower limb buds are oriented in a coronal plane. Note the segmental pattern of innervation from L1 to S2. In week 6, the lower limbs undergo a horizontal movement (*curved arrows*) such that the lower limb buds become oriented in a sagittal plane (as shown in 2). *(2)* Side view of a week 6 embryo. Note the lower limb oriented in a parasagittal plane. During weeks 6–8, the lower limb buds rotate 90° medially (*curved arrow*). *(3)* Ventral view of a week 8 embryo. Note the position of the lower limb with knees pointing anterior. *(4)* Dermatome pattern in the adult lower limb and limb bud. The 90° medial rotation of the lower limb bud causes the originally straight segmental pattern of innervation in the embryo to be somewhat modified ("twisted in a spiral") such that the dermatome pattern in the adult is altered. However, an orderly dermatome pattern can still be recognized in the adult if the lower limb is positioned in a parasagittal plane with the big toe pointing superiorly (as shown). The dermatomes from L1 can be counted distally down the superior border of the lower limb (*arrow*) to L5 and then back proximally up the inferior border of the lower limb (*arrow*) to S2. Note the position of the big toes in *1, 2, 3,* and *4*.

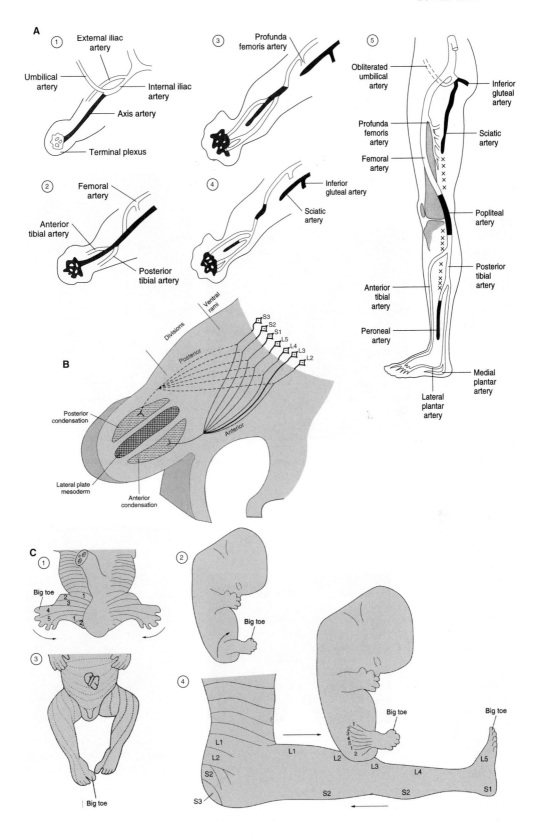

A

Week 5

Week 6

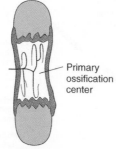
Primary
ossification
center

Weeks 7–9

B

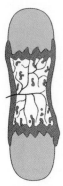
At birth

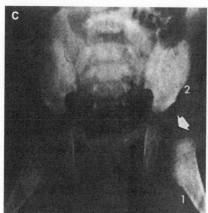
C

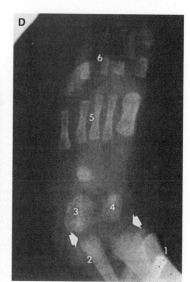
D

E

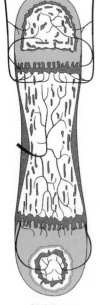
Childhood

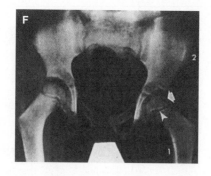
F

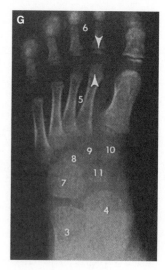
G

◀ **Figure 20-2.** Bone formation in the lower limb. **(A)** Week 5, lateral plate mesoderm condenses (*hatched*). Week 6, hyaline cartilage (*light shading*) model of future bones forms. Weeks 7–9, primary ossification centers within the diaphysis appear such that bone (*dark shading*) forms (osteogenesis). **(B)** At birth, the diaphysis consists of bone (*dark shading*), whereas the epiphysis remains hyaline cartilage. This is important to note when interpreting radiographs of newborns. **(C)** The radiograph of a newborn at the hip region (*1* = femur; *2* = ilium) shows the portions of the hyaline cartilage model that have been replaced by radiodense bone (*white*). Note that the epiphyseal end of the femur (*white arrow*) is still hyaline cartilage at birth and therefore appears radiolucent (*dark*). **(D)** The radiograph of a newborn at the ankle and foot shows the portions of the hyaline cartilage model that have been replaced by radiodense bone (*white*) in the tibia (*1*), fibula (*2*), calcaneus (*3*), talus (*4*), metatarsals (*5*), and phalanges (*6*). Note that the epiphyseal ends of the tibia and fibula are still cartilage and therefore radiolucent (*white arrows*). **(E)** During childhood, secondary ossification centers form in the epiphyseal ends of the bones. During childhood and adolescence, the growth in length of long bones occurs at the epiphyseal growth plate. **(F)** Note the radiograph of a 6-year-old child at the hip region (*1* = femur; *2* = ilium). Since secondary ossification centers are present within the epiphyseal ends, the head of the femur is now radiodense (*white arrow*), and the epiphyseal growth plate (*arrowhead*) where hyaline cartilage is present remains radiolucent (*dark*). This is not to be confused with a bone fracture. **(G)** On the radiograph of a 6-year-old child at the foot, the diaphyseal and epiphyseal portions of the metatarsals (*5*) and phalanges (*6*) as well as their epiphyseal growth plates (*arrowheads*) can be observed. The remaining tarsal bones have begun to ossify (*7* = cuboid; *8* = lateral cuneiform; *9* = intermediate cuneiform; *10* = medial cuneiform; *11* = navicular). *3* = calcaneus; *4* = talus.

STUDY QUESTIONS FOR CHAPTER 20

Directions: *Each of the numbered items or incomplete statements in this section is followed by answers or by completions of the statement. Select the **one** lettered answer or completion that is **best** in each case.*

1. Which of the following arteries gives rise to the axis artery of the lower limb?

(A) External iliac artery
(B) Femoral artery
(C) Profound femoral artery
(D) Umbilical artery
(E) Inferior gluteal artery

2. The femur develops from which of the following?

(A) Somite mesoderm
(B) Lateral plate mesoderm
(C) Intermediate mesoderm
(D) Extraembryonic mesoderm
(E) Sclerotome mesoderm

3. The rectus femoris muscle develops from which of the following?

(A) Posterior condensation
(B) Anterior condensation
(C) Lateral plate mesoderm
(D) Extraembryonic mesoderm
(E) Sclerotome mesoderm

4. Which of the following muscles will the posterior divisions of the lumbosacral plexus innervate?

(A) Semitendinosus
(B) Semimembranosus
(C) Long head of biceps femoris
(D) Rectus femoris
(E) Gastrocnemius

5. During weeks 6–8, the lower limb bud will rotate

(A) medially 90°
(B) laterally 90°
(C) medially 180°
(D) laterally 180°
(E) no rotation

ANSWERS AND EXPLANATIONS

1. D. Early in development, the umbilical artery gives rise to the axis artery.

2. B. All bones of the lower limb form from lateral plate mesoderm that condenses along the central axis of the lower limb bud.

3. A. Somite mesoderm migrates into the limb bud and forms two condensations. The posterior condensation of the lower limb gives rise to the extensors of the lower limb, which attain an anterior location in the adult because of the medial rotation of 90°.

4. D. One of the nerves that forms from the posterior divisions of the lumbosacral plexus is the femoral nerve. Posterior divisions of the lumbosacral plexus will innervate muscles derived from the posterior condensation (extensors). The rectus femoris muscle is an extensor at the knee joint. Note that the rectus femoris muscle and the femoral nerve are related embryologically to the posterior condensation and posterior divisions even though in the adult they are located anteriorly. This occurs because of the medial rotation of 90°.

5. A. The lower limb bud will rotate medially 90° so that the knee points anteriorly.

Body Cavities

I. Formation of the Intraembryonic Coelom (Figure 21-1)

The formation of the intraembryonic coelom begins when spaces coalesce within the lateral mesoderm and form a horseshoe-shaped space that opens into the chorionic cavity (extraembryonic coelom) on the right and left side. The intraembryonic coelom is remodeled due to the craniocaudal folding and lateral folding of the embryo. The intraembryonic coelom can best be visualized as a balloon whose walls are visceral mesoderm (closest to the viscera) and somatic mesoderm (closest to the body wall). The intraembryonic coelom provides the needed room for growth of various organs.

II. Partitioning of the Intraembryonic Coelom

The intraembryonic coelom is initially one continuous space. To form the definitive adult pericardial, pleural, and peritoneal cavities, two partitions must develop. The two partitions are the **paired pleuropericardial membranes** and the **diaphragm.**

A. The **paired pleuropericardial membranes** are sheets of somatic mesoderm that separate the **pericardial cavity** from the **pleural cavities** (see Figure 21-1). The formation of these membranes appears to be aided by lung buds invading the lateral body wall and by tension on the common cardinal veins resulting from rapid longitudinal growth. These membranes develop into the definitive **fibrous pericardium** surrounding the heart.

B. The **diaphragm** separates the **pleural cavities** from the **peritoneal cavity** (see Figure 21-1). The diaphragm is formed through the fusion of tissue from four different sources:
1. The **septum transversum** is a thick mass of mesoderm located between the primitive heart tube and the developing liver. The septum transversum is the primordium of the **central tendon of the diaphragm** in the adult.
2. The **paired pleuroperitoneal membranes** are sheets of somatic mesoderm that appear to develop from the dorsal and dorsolateral body wall by an unknown mechanism.
3. The **dorsal mesentery of the esophagus** is invaded by myoblasts and forms the **crura of the diaphragm** in the adult.
4. The **body wall** contributes muscle to the peripheral portions of the definitive diaphragm.

III. Positional Changes of the Diaphragm

During week 4 of development, the developing diaphragm becomes innervated by the **phrenic nerves**, which originate from C3, C4, and C5 and pass through the pleuropericardial membranes (this explains the definitive location of the phrenic nerves associated with the fibrous pericardium). By week 8, there is an apparent **descent of the diaphragm to L1** because of the

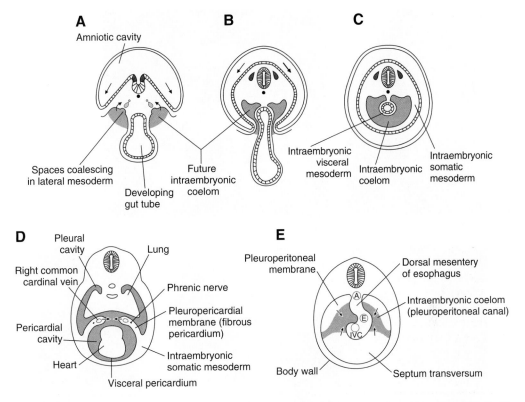

Figure 21-1. Diagram illustrating the formation and partitioning of the intraembryonic coelom (IC). **(A–C)** Cross sections show various stages of IC formation while the embryo undergoes lateral folding. **(D)** Cross section shows two folds of intraembryonic somatic mesoderm carrying the phrenic nerves and common cardinal veins. The two folds fuse in the midline (*arrows*) to form the pleuropericardial membrane. This separates the pericardial cavity (*shaded*) from the pleural cavity (*shaded*). **(E)** Cross section of an embryo at week 5 shows the four components that fuse (*arrows*) to form the diaphragm, which closes off the IC between the pleural and peritoneal cavities. The portions of the IC that connect the pleural and pericardial cavities in the embryo are called the pleuroperitoneal canals (*shaded*). *A* = aorta; *E* = esophagus; *IVC* = inferior vena cava.

rapid growth of the neural tube. The phrenic nerves are carried along with the "descending diaphragm," which explains their unusually long length in the adult.

IV.   Clinical Considerations (Figure 21-2)

A. Congenital diaphragmatic hernia is a herniation of abdominal contents into the pleural cavity caused by a **failure of the pleuroperitoneal membrane** to develop or fuse with the other components of the diaphragm. A congenital diaphragmatic hernia is most commonly found on the **left posterolateral side** and is usually life-threatening because abdominal contents compress the lung buds, causing **pulmonary hypoplasia**. Clinical signs in the newborn include an unusually flat abdomen, breathlessness, severe dyspnea, peristaltic bowel sounds over the left chest, and cyanosis. It can be detected prenatally using ultrasonography.

B. Esophageal hiatal hernia is a herniation of the stomach through the esophageal hiatus into the pleural cavity caused by an abnormally large esophageal hiatus. An esophageal hiatal hernia renders the **esophagogastric sphincter** incompetent so that stomach contents reflux into the esophagus. Clinical signs in the newborn include vomiting (frequently projectile) when the infant is laid on its back after feeding.

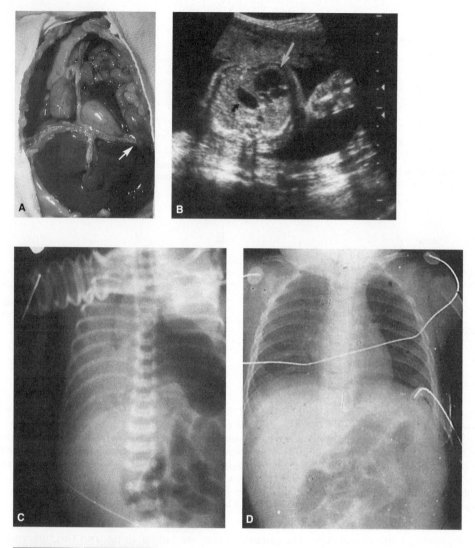

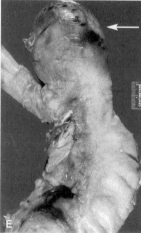

Figure 21-2. **(A)** Photograph of a congenital diaphragmatic hernia. Note the defect (*arrow*) in the diaphragm that allows loops of intestine and a portion of the liver to enter the pleural cavity. There is attendant pulmonary hypoplasia. **(B)** A sonogram of a congenital diaphragmatic hernia. Note the heart (*white arrow*) shifted to the right by a herniated fluid-filled stomach (*black arrow*). **(C)** Radiograph of a congenital diaphragmatic hernia. Note the loops of intestine within the pleural cavity as indicated by the bowel gas above and below the diaphragm and the mediastinal shift to the right. **(D)** Radiograph after surgical repair of a congenital diaphragmatic hernia. Note the bowel gas present only below the diaphragm and the mediastinal shift back to the midline. **(E)** Photograph of an esophageal hiatal hernia. Note the large saccular, discolored, ischemic portion of the stomach (*arrow*) and the deviation of the esophagus to the right.

STUDY QUESTIONS FOR CHAPTER 21

*Directions: Each of the numbered items or incomplete statements in this section is followed by answers or by completions of the statement. Select the **one** lettered answer or completion that is **best** in each case.*

1. A congenital diaphragmatic hernia may result from failure of the

(A) septum transversum to develop
(B) pleuroperitoneal membranes to fuse in a normal fashion
(C) pleuropericardial membrane to develop completely
(D) dorsal mesentery of the esophagus to develop
(E) body wall to form the peripheral part of the diaphragm

2. A congenital diaphragmatic hernia most commonly occurs

(A) on the right anteromedial side
(B) on the right posterolateral side
(C) on the left anteromedial side
(D) on the left posterolateral side
(E) anywhere on the left side

3. A congenital diaphragmatic hernia is usually life-threatening because it is associated with

(A) pulmonary hypoplasia
(B) pulmonary hyperplasia
(C) physiologic umbilical hernia
(D) liver hypoplasia
(E) liver agenesis

4. An 8-day-old boy presents with a history of complete loss of breath at times and of turning blue on a number of occasions. If the baby is placed in an upright or sitting position, his breathing improves. Physical examination reveals an unusually flat stomach when the newborn is lying down; auscultation demonstrates no breath sounds on the left side of the thorax. What is the diagnosis?

(A) Physiologic umbilical herniation
(B) Esophageal hiatal hernia
(C) Tetralogy of Fallot
(D) Congenital diaphragmatic hernia
(E) Tricuspid atresia

5. During week 4, the developing diaphragm is located at

(A) C3, C4, C5
(B) T3, T4, T5
(C) T8, T9, T10
(D) L1, L2, L3
(E) L4, L5, L6

6. An apparently healthy newborn with a hearty appetite has begun feedings with formula. When she is laid down in the crib after feeding, she experiences projectile vomiting. Which of the following conditions is a probable cause of this vomiting?

(A) Physiologic umbilical herniation
(B) Esophageal hiatal hernia
(C) Tetralogy of Fallot
(D) Congenital diaphragmatic hernia
(E) Tracheoesophageal fistula

ANSWERS AND EXPLANATIONS

1. B. The formation of the diaphragm occurs through the fusion of tissue from four different sources. The pleuroperitoneal membranes normally fuse with the three other components during week 6 of development. Abnormal development or fusion of one or both of the pleuroperitoneal membranes causes a patent opening between the thorax and abdomen through which abdominal viscera may herniate.

2. D. Congenital diaphragmatic hernias occur most commonly on the left posterolateral side. The pleuroperitoneal membrane on the right side closes before the left for reasons that are not clear. Consequently, the patency on the left side remains unclosed for a longer time. The portion of the diaphragm formed by the pleuroperitoneal membrane in the newborn is located posterolateral.

3. A. The herniation of abdominal contents into the pleural cavity compresses the developing lung bud, resulting in pulmonary hypoplasia. Lung development on the ipsilateral (left) side of the herniation is most commonly affected, but lung development on the contralateral (right) side can also be compromised. The lungs may achieve normal size and function after surgical reduction of the hernia and repair of the diaphragm. However, mortality is high owing to pulmonary hypoplasia.

4. D. Loss of breath and cyanosis result from pulmonary hypoplasia associated with congenital diaphragmatic hernia. Placing the baby in an upright position reduces the hernia somewhat and eases the pressure on the lungs, thereby increasing the baby's comfort. The baby's stomach is flat (instead of the plump belly of a normal newborn) because the abdominal viscera have herniated into the thorax. Auscultation reveals no breath sounds on the left side because of pulmonary hypoplasia.

5. A. Although it may seem unusual, the adult diaphragm has its embryologic beginning at the cervical level (C3, C4, C5). Nerve roots from C3, C4, and C5 enter the developing diaphragm, bringing both motor and sensory innervation. With the subsequent rapid growth of the neural tube, there is an apparent descent of the diaphragm to its adult levels (thoracic and lumbar). However, the diaphragm retains its innervation from C3, C4, and C5, which explains the unusually long phrenic nerves.

6. B. An esophageal hiatal hernia is a herniation of the stomach through the esophageal hiatus into the pleural cavity. This compromises the esophagogastric sphincter so that stomach contents can easily reflux into the esophagus. The combination of a full stomach after feeding and lying down in the crib will cause vomiting in this newborn.

Pregnancy

I. Endocrinology of Pregnancy

A. **Human chorionic gonadotropin (hCG)**

1. **Definition.** hCG is a glycoprotein hormone produced by the **syncytiotrophoblast** that stimulates the production of progesterone by the corpus luteum (i.e., maintains corpus luteum function). hCG can be assayed in **maternal blood at day 8** or **maternal urine at day 10** using a radioimmunoassay with antibodies directed against the β-subunit of hCG. This is the basis of the early pregnancy test kits purchased over the counter.

2. **Quantitative hCG dating of pregnancy.** During weeks 1–6 of a normal pregnancy, hCG levels increase by about 70% every 48 hours.

Number of Weeks Pregnant	hCG Level
0–2 weeks	0–250 mIU/mL
2–4 weeks	100–5000 mIU/mL
1–2 months	4000–200,000 mIU/mL
2–3 months	8000–100,000 mIU/mL
2nd trimester	4000–75,000 mIU/mL
3rd trimester	1000–5000 mIU/mL

3. **Other tests using hCG.** Low hCG levels may predict a spontaneous abortion or indicate an ectopic pregnancy. Elevated hCG levels may indicate a multiple pregnancy, hydatidiform mole, or gestational trophoblastic neoplasia.

B. **Human placental lactogen (hPL)** is a protein hormone produced by the **placenta,** which induces lipolysis thereby elevating free fatty acid levels in the mother. It is considered the "growth hormone" of the latter half of pregnancy. hPL can be assayed in **maternal blood at week 6.** hPL levels vary with placental mass (i.e., may indicate a multiple pregnancy) and rapidly disappear from maternal blood after delivery.

C. **Prolactin (PRL)** is a protein hormone produced by the **maternal adenohypophysis, fetal adenohypophysis,** and **decidual tissue of the uterus,** which prepares the mammary glands for lactation. PRL can be assayed in **maternal blood throughout pregnancy** or later in **amniotic fluid.** Near term, PRL levels rise to a maximum of about 100 ng/mL (normal nonpregnant PRL levels range between 8–25 ng/mL).

D. Progesterone (PG) is a steroid hormone produced by the **corpus luteum** until week 8 and then by the **placenta** until birth. PG does the following:

    a. Prepares the endometrium for implantation (nidation) and maintains the endometrium.

    b. Is used by the fetal adrenal cortex as a precursor for corticosteroid and mineralocorticoid synthesis.

    c. Is used by the fetal testes as a precursor for testosterone synthesis.

E. Estrone, estradiol, and estriol

    1. Little is known about the specific function of these steroid hormones in the mother or fetus during pregnancy. These hormones are produced by a complex series of steps involving the **maternal liver, placenta,** and **fetal adrenal gland** and **fetal liver** as indicated below:

        a. Cholesterol from the maternal liver is converted to pregnenolone by the placenta.

        b. Pregnenolone is converted to pregnenolone sulfate.

        c. Pregnenolone sulfate is converted to dehydroepiandrosterone sulfate (DHEA-SO$_4$) by the fetal adrenal gland.

        d. DHEA-SO$_4$ is converted to estrone and estradiol by the placenta.

        e. DHEA-SO$_4$ is also converted to 16α-hydroxy DHEA-SO$_4$ by the fetal liver.

        f. 16α-hydroxy DHEA-SO$_4$ is converted to estriol by the placenta.

    2. Estrone is a fairly weak estrogen.

    3. Estradiol is the most potent estrogen.

    4. Estriol is a very weak estrogen but is produced in very high amounts during pregnancy. Estriol can be assayed in **maternal blood** (shows a distinct diurnal variation with peak amounts early in the morning) and **maternal urine** (24-hour urine sample shows no diurnal variation). Significant amounts of estriol are produced at month 3 (i.e., early 2nd trimester) and continue to rise until birth. Maternal urinary levels of estriol have long been recognized as a **reliable index of fetal-placental function** because estriol production is dependent on a normal functioning fetal adrenal cortex, fetal liver, and placenta.

II. Pregnancy Dating

The **estimated date of confinement (EDC)** is based on the assumption that a woman has a 28-day cycle with ovulation on day 14 or day 15. In general, the duration of a normal pregnancy is **280 days (40 weeks) from the first day of the last menstrual period (LMP)**. A common method of determining the EDC (Naegele's rule) is to count back 3 months from the first day of the LMP and then add 1 year and 7 days; this method is reasonably accurate in women with regular menstrual cycles.

III. Pregnancy Milestones

A. The **first trimester** extends from the LMP through week 12. Important events are:

    1. At days 8–10, a positive pregnancy test is obtained by hCG assay.

    2. At week 12, the uterine fundus is palpable at the pubic symphysis; Doppler fetal heart rate is first audible.

B. The **second trimester** extends from the end of the first trimester through week 27. Important events are:

    1. At weeks 14–18, amniocentesis is performed when suspicion of fetal chromosomal abnormalities exists.

    2. At week 16, the uterine fundus is palpable midway between the pubic symphysis and umbilicus.

    3. At weeks 16–18, the first fetal movements occur (**quickening**) in a woman pregnant for the second time or more.

4. At weeks 17–20, fetal heart rate is audible with fetoscope.
5. At week 18, female and male external genitalia can be distinguished by ultrasound (i.e., sex determination).
6. At weeks 18–20, the first fetal movements occur (**quickening**) in a woman's first pregnancy.
7. At week 20, the uterine fundus is palpable at the umbilicus.
8. At weeks 25–27, the lungs become capable of respiration; surfactant is produced by Type II pneumocytes. There is a 70%–80% chance of survival in infants born at the end of the second trimester. If death occurs, it is generally as a result of lung immaturity and resulting respiratory distress syndrome (hyaline membrane disease).
9. At week 27, the fetus weighs about 1000 grams (a little more than 2 pounds).

C. The **third trimester** extends from the end of the second trimester until term or week 40. Important events that occur during the third trimester are:
   1. Pupillary light reflex is present.
   2. Descent of the fetal head to the pelvic inlet (called **lightening**) occurs.
   3. Rupture of the amniochorionic membrane occurs with labor usually beginning about 24 hours later.
   4. The fetus weighs about 3300 grams (about 7–7.5 pounds).

IV. Prenatal Diagnostic Procedures

Prenatal diagnosis is indicated in about **8%** of all pregnancies. Prenatal diagnostic procedures include the following:

A. **Ultrasonography** is commonly used to date a pregnancy, to diagnose a multiple pregnancy, to assess fetal growth, to determine placenta location, to determine the position and lie of the fetus, to detect certain congenital anomalies, and to monitor needle or catheter insertion during amniocentesis and chorionic villus biopsy. In obstetric ultrasonography, 2.25–5.0 MHz frequencies are used for good tissue differentiation. The term **anechoic** refers to tissues with few or no echoes (e.g., bladder, brain, cavities, amniotic fluid). **Echogenic** refers to tissues with a high capacity to reflect ultrasound. **B-scan ultrasonography** consists of an **A-mode** and an **M-mode** (which provide precise measurements) and **time position scan** with a permanent record of cinephotography. **Real-time ultrasonography** provides an easy, immediate, and definitive demonstration of fetal life.

B. **Amniocentesis** is a transabdominal sampling of **amniotic fluid** and **fetal cells**. Amniocentesis is performed at weeks 14–18 and is indicated in the following situations: the woman is over 35 years of age; a previous child has a chromosomal anomaly; one parent is a known carrier of a translocation or inversion; one or both parents are known carriers of an X-linked recessive or autosomal recessive trait; or there is a history of neural tube defects. The sample obtained is used in the following studies:
   1. **α-Fetoprotein assay** is used to diagnose neural tube defects.
   2. **Spectrophotometric assay of bilirubin** is used to diagnose hemolytic disease of the neworn (i.e., erythroblastosis fetalis) due to Rh-incompatibility.
   3. **Lecithin-sphingomyelin (L/S) ratio** and **phosphatidylglycerol assay** are used to determine lung maturity of the fetus.
   4. **DNA analysis.** A wide variety of DNA methodologies are available (e.g., karyotype analysis, Southern blotting, and RFLP analysis [restriction fragment length polymorphism]) to diagnose chromosomal abnormalities and single-gene defects.

C. **Chorionic villus biopsy** is a transabdominal or transcervical sampling of the chorionic villi to obtain a large amount of **fetal cells** for DNA analysis. Chorionic villus biopsy is performed at weeks 6–11 (i.e., much earlier than amniocentesis), thereby providing an early source of fetal cells for DNA analysis.

D. Percutaneous umbilical blood sampling (PUBS) is a sampling of **fetal blood** from the umbilical cord.

V.   Fetal Distress During Labor (Intrapartum)

Defined in terms of **fetal hypoxia** and measured by changes in either **fetal heart rate (FHR)** or **fetal scalp capillary pH**. The normal baseline FHR is 120–160 beats/min. However, fetal hypoxia causes a decrease in FHR (or **fetal bradycardia**), that is, **FHR of <120 beats/min**. The normal fetal scalp capillary pH is 7.25–7.35. However, fetal hypoxia causes a decrease in pH, that is, a **pH of <7.20**.

VI.   The APGAR Score (Table 22-1)

Assesses five characteristics (**a**ppearance, **p**ulse, **g**rimace, **a**ctivity, **r**espiratory effort) in the newborn infant to determine which infants need resuscitation. The APGAR score is calculated at 1 minute and 5 minutes after birth. To obtain an APGAR score, score 0, 1, or 2 for the five characteristics and add them together.

A.   APGAR score of 0–3 indicates a life-threatening situation.

B.   APGAR score of 4–6 indicates temperature and ventilation support is needed.

C.   APGAR score of 7–10 indicates a normal situation.

TABLE 22-1	*Assessing the APGAR Score*			
		Score		
Characteristic	0	1	2	Example[a]
Appearance, color	Blue, pale	Body pink, extremities blue	Completely pink	1
Pulse, heart rate	Absent	<100 bpm	>100 bpm	2
Grimace, reflex, irritability	No response	Grimace	Vigorous crying	0
Activity, muscle tone	Flaccid	Some flexion of extremities	Active motion, Flexed extremities	0
Respiratory effort	None	Weak, irregular	Good, crying	1
APGAR score				4

[a]Clinical example: A newborn infant at 5 minutes after birth has a pink body but blue extremities (score 1), a heart rate of 125 bpm (score 2), no grimace or reflex (score 0), a flaccid muscle tone (score 0), and weak irregular breathing (score 1). The total APGAR score is 4. This infant needs ventilation and temperature support.

VII.   Puerperium

Extends from immediately after delivery of the baby until the reproductive tract returns to the nonpregnant state in approximately 4–6 weeks. Important events that occur during puerperium are:

A.   Involution of the uterus.

B.   Afterpains due to uterine contractions.

C.   Uterine discharge (lochia).

D. In nonlactating women, menstrual flow returns within 6–8 weeks postpartum and ovulation returns within 2–4 weeks postpartum.

E. In lactating women, ovulation may return within 10 weeks postpartum. Birth control protection afforded by lactation is ensured for only 6 weeks after which time pregnancy is possible.

VIII. Lactation

A. During pregnancy, hPL, PRL, progesterone, estrogens, cortisol, and insulin stimulate the growth of **lactiferous ducts** and proliferation of epithelial cells to form **alveoli**; alveoli secrete **colostrum**.

B. After delivery of the baby, lactation is initiated by a decrease in progesterone and estrogens along with the release of PRL from the adenohypophysis. This initiates **milk production.**

C. During suckling, a stimulus from the breast inhibits the release of PRL-inhibiting factor from the hypothalamus, thereby causing a **surge in PRL,** which increases milk production. In addition, stimulation of the nipples during suckling causes a **surge of oxytocin,** which causes the expulsion of accumulated milk ("milk letdown") by stimulating myoepithelial cells.

IX.   Small for Gestational Age Infant (SGA)

SGA, fetal growth restriction (FGR), intrauterine growth restriction (IUGR), and low birth weight are all terms used to describe a small baby or a fetus that has not reach its growth potential. Although the definition is controversial, the most common definition of SGA is a body weight **below the 10th percentile for gestational age.** The clinical features of a SGA infant include: thin, loose peeling skin, decreased skeletal muscle mass, decreased subcutaneous adipose tissue, the face has a shrunken or "wizened" appearance, thin umbilical cord, and meconium staining. The methods to clinically estimate gestation age include: measurement of the fundal height, which is the distance between the upper edge of the pubic symphysis and the top of the uterine fundus using a tape measure; ultrasound measurement of the fetal abdominal circumference; and ultrasound measurement of fetal weight. SGA may be caused by **maternal, fetal, or placental factors.** **Maternal factors include:** severe maternal starvation, maternal hypoxemia, preeclampsia, maternal viral or parasitic infections, maternal substance abuse, toxic exposures (e.g., warfarin, anticonvulsants, antineoplastic drugs, folic acid antagonists), high altitude, demographic factors (e.g., race, maternal age at first birth, pregnancy at the extremes of reproductive life). **Fetal factors include:** karyotype abnormalities (e.g., trisomies, autosomal deletions, mosaicism), genetic syndromes (e.g., Bloom syndrome, dwarfism, Russell-Silver syndrome), major congenital anomalies, multiple gestation (e.g., twins, triplets, quintuplets). **Placental factors include:** abnormal uteroplacental vasculature, abruptio placentae, gross placental anomalies (e.g., single umbilical artery, velamentous umbilical cord insertion, placental hemangioma). SGA infants have a wide variety of clinical problems, which include: difficult cardiopulmonary transition; meconium aspiration; persistent pulmonary hypertension; greater rates of neonatal death, necrotizing enterocolitis, and respiratory distress; impaired thermoregulation; hypoglycemia; polycythemia; hyperviscosity; impaired immune function; and increased fetal, neonatal, and perinatal mortality.

X.   Collection and Storage of Umbilical Cord Blood

Umbilical cord blood (UCB) is the blood that remains in the umbilical cord and placenta following the birth of an infant. Collection and storage of UCB are important because UCB contains **hematopoietic stem cells,** which can be used to reconstitute the bone marrow in patients with a wide variety of malignant and nonmalignant diseases (e.g., acute and chronic leukemia, lymphoma, aplastic anemia, sickle cell anemia, thalassemia major). As commonly known, the engraftment and survival rates following hematopoietic cell transplantation in the above-mentioned patients is enhanced when the donor and recipient are genetically matched. In this regard, hematopoietic cell transplantation using UCB has a lower rate of both acute and chronic graft-versus-host disease when compared to bone marrow or peripheral blood sources. The efficacy of UCB in hematopoietic cell transplantation is related to the total number of nucleated cells (ideally $>4 \times 10^7$ nucleated cell per kilogram of recipient body weight) and the number of CD34+ cells present in a UCB unit. The *in utero* collection of UCB involves the following steps: after delivery of the infant, the umbilical cord is clamped and cut in the usual manner; before expulsion of the placenta, a 16-gauge needle is inserted into the umbilical vein located within the umbilical cord; UCB is allowed to drain into a collection bag containing an anticoagulant solution; collection time is usually 2–4 minutes and ideally 40–60 mL of UCB is collected.

STUDY QUESTIONS FOR CHAPTER 22

*Directions: Each of the numbered items or incomplete statements in this section is followed by answers or by completions of the statement. Select the **one** lettered answer or completion that is **best** in each case.*

1. Human chorionic gonadotropin (hCG) is produced by which of the following?

(A) Ectoderm
(B) Cytotrophoblast
(C) Decidua basalis
(D) Syncytiotrophoblast
(E) Mesoderm

2. A reliable index of fetal-placenta function is maternal urinary levels of

(A) estrone
(B) human placental lactogen (hPL)
(C) prolactin (PRL)
(D) progesterone
(E) estriol

3. The first fetal movements occur in which of the following trimesters?

(A) First trimester
(B) Second trimester
(C) Third trimester

4. The Doppler fetal heart rate is first audible in which of the following trimesters?

(A) First trimester
(B) Second trimester
(C) Third trimester

5. The lungs become capable of respiration in which of the following trimesters?

(A) First trimester
(B) Second trimester
(C) Third trimester

6. Which of the following structures produces progesterone late in pregnancy?

(A) Placenta
(B) Corpus luteum
(C) Syncytiotrophoblast
(D) Fetal adenohypophysis
(E) Maternal liver

ANSWERS AND EXPLANATIONS

1. D. The syncytiotrophoblast produces hCG.

2. E. Maternal urinary levels of estriol have long been recognized as a reliable index of fetal-placental function because estriol production is dependent on a normal-functioning fetal adrenal cortex, fetal liver, and placenta.

3. B. The first fetal movements occur in the second trimester.

4. A. The fetal heart rate is first audible in the first trimester at around week 12.

5. B. The lungs become capable of respiration at weeks 25–27 in the second trimester.

6. A. Progesterone is a steroid hormone that is produced by the placenta up until birth. The corpus luteum also produces progesterone, but only until week 8 of pregnancy.

CHAPTER

23

Numerical Chromosomal Anomalies

I.   Polyploidy

Polyploidy is the addition of an extra haploid set or sets of chromosomes (i.e., 23) to the normal diploid set of chromosomes (i.e., 46).

A. Triploidy is a condition in which cells contain **69 chromosomes**. It results in spontaneous abortion of the conceptus or brief survival of the liveborn infant after birth. Triploidy occurs as a result of either a **failure of meiosis in a germ cell** (e.g., fertilization of a diploid egg by a haploid sperm) or **dispermy** (two sperm that fertilize one egg).

B. Tetraploidy is a condition in which cells contain **92 chromosomes**. It results in spontaneous abortion of the conceptus. Tetraploidy occurs as a result of **failure of the first cleavage division**.

II.   Aneuploidy (Figure 23-1)

Aneuploidy is the addition of one chromosome (**trisomy**) or loss of one chromosome (**monosomy**). Trisomy results in spontaneous abortion of the conceptus. However, trisomy 13 (Patau syndrome), trisomy 18 (Edwards syndrome), trisomy 21 (Down syndrome), and Klinefelter syndrome (47,XXY) are found in the liveborn population. Monosomy results in spontaneous abortion of the conceptus. However, monosomy X chromosome (45,X; Turner syndrome) is found in the liveborn population. Aneuploidy occurs as a result of **nondisjunction during meiosis**.

A. Trisomy 13 (Patau syndrome) is characterized by profound mental retardation (is the leading cause of inherited mental retardation), congenital heart defects, cleft lip and palate, omphalocele, and polydactyly. Infants usually die soon after birth

B. Trisomy 18 (Edwards syndrome) is characterized by mental retardation congenital heart defects, small facies and prominent occiput, overlapping fingers, and rocker-bottom heels. Infants usually die soon after birth.

C. Trisomy 21 (Down syndrome) is characterized by moderate mental retardation (is the leading cause of inherited mental retardation), microcephaly, microphthalmia, colobomata, cataracts and glaucoma, flat nasal bridge, epicanthic folds, protruding tongue, simian crease in hand, increased nuchal skin folds, appearance of an "X" across the face when the baby cries because the upward slanted palpebral fissures run in a line with the nasolabial folds, and congenital heart defects. Alzheimer neurofibrillary tangles and plaques are found in Down syndrome patients over 30 years of age. Acute megakaryocytic leukemia is frequently present.

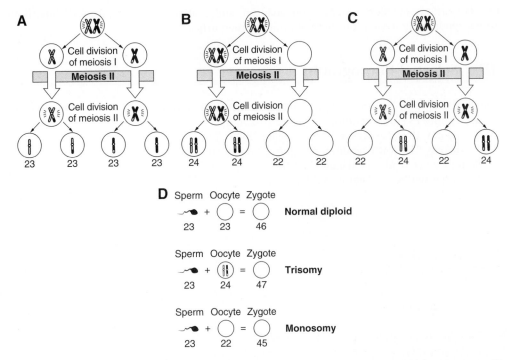

Figure 23-1. (A) Normal meiotic divisions (I and II) producing gametes with 23 chromosomes. (B) Nondisjunction occurring in meiosis I producing gametes with 24 and 22 chromosomes. (C) Nondisjunction occurring in meiosis II producing gametes with 24 and 22 chromosomes. (D) Although nondisjunction may occur in either spermatogenesis or oogenesis, there is a higher frequency of nondisjunction in oogenesis. This schematic drawing depicts nondisjunction in oogenesis. If an abnormal oocyte (24 chromosomes) is fertilized by a normal sperm (23 chromosomes), a zygote with 47 chromosomes is produced (i.e., trisomy). If an abnormal oocyte (22 chromosomes) is fertilized by a normal sperm (23 chromosomes), a zygote with 45 chromosomes is produced (i.e., monosomy).

1. Trisomy 21 is the most common type of trisomy; its frequency increases with **advanced maternal age**.
2. Trisomy 21 is associated with **low α-fetoprotein levels** in amniotic fluid or maternal serum.
3. A specific region on chromosome 21 seems to be markedly associated with numerous features of trisomy 21. This region is called **DSCR (Down syndrome critical region)**. The following genes have been mapped to the DSCR (although their role is far from clear): carbonyl reductase, SIM2 (a transcription factor), p60 subunit of chromatin assembly factor, holocarboxylase synthetase, ERG (a proto-oncogene), GIRK2 (a K^+ ion channel), and PEP19 (a Ca^{2+}-dependent signal transducer).
4. Trisomy 21 may also be caused by a chromosomal translocation (see Chapter 24) between chromosomes 14 and 21 [i.e., t(14;21)].

D. Klinefelter syndrome (47,XXY) is a trisomic condition **found only in males** and characterized by varicose veins, arterial and venous leg ulcers, scant body and pubic hair, male hypogonadism, sterility with fibrosus of seminiferous tubules, marked decrease in testosterone levels, elevated gonadotropin levels, gynecomastia, dull mentality, antisocial behavior, delayed speech as a child, and eunuchoid habitus.

E. Turner syndrome (monosomy X; 45,X) is a monosomic condition **found only in females** and characterized by short stature, low-set ears, ocular hypertelorism, ptosis, low posterior hairline, webbed neck due to a remnant of a fetal cystic hygroma, congenital hypoplasia of lymphatics causing peripheral edema of hands and feet, shield chest, pinpoint nipples, congenital heart defects, aortic coarctation, female hypogonadism, and ovarian fibrous streaks (i.e., infertility). Turner syndrome is a common cause of primary amenorrhea.

III. Selected Photographs

The photographs in Figure 23-2 illustrate the chromosomal anomalies discussed in this chapter.
  A. Trisomy 13 (Patau syndrome) (Figure 23-2 *A, B*)
  B. Trisomy 18 (Edwards syndrome) (Figure 23-2 *C, D*)
  C. Trisomy 21 (Down syndrome) (Figure 23-2 *E, F, G*)
  D. Klinefelter syndrome (Figure 23-2 *H*)
  E. Turner syndrome (Figure 23-2 *I, J*)

Figure 23-2. **(A and B)** Trisomy 13 (Patau syndrome). Key features are microcephaly with sloping forehead, ▶ scalp defects, microphthalmia, cleft lip and palate, polydactyly, fingers flexed and overlapping, and cardiac malformations. **(C and D)** Trisomy 18 (Edwards syndrome). Key features are low birth weight, lack of subcutaneous fat, prominent occiput, narrow forehead, small palpebral fissures, low-set and malformed ears, micrognathia, short sternum, and cardiac malformations. **(E)** Trisomy 21 (Down syndrome). Photograph of a young child with Down syndrome. Note the flat nasal bridge, prominent epicanthic folds, oblique palpebral fissures, low-set and shell-like ears, and protruding tongue. From Bickley LS, Szilagyi P. *Bates' Guide to Physical Examination and History Taking,* 4th ed. Philadelphia: Lippincott Williams and Wilkins, 2003. **(F)** Photograph of hand in infant with Down syndrome showing the simian crease. **(G)** Radiograph of hand showing the curved fifth digit and malformation of the middle phalanx of the fifth digit in Down syndrome. **(H)** Photograph of 14-year-old boy with Klinefelter syndrome (47,XXY). Note the hypogonadism and eunuchoid habitus. **(I)** Turner syndrome (45,X). Photograph of a 3-year-old girl with Turner syndrome. Note the webbed neck resulting from delayed maturation of lymphatics, short stature, and broad shield chest. **(J)** Photograph of 14-year-old girl with Turner syndrome (45,X). Note the webbed neck due to delayed maturation of lymphatics.

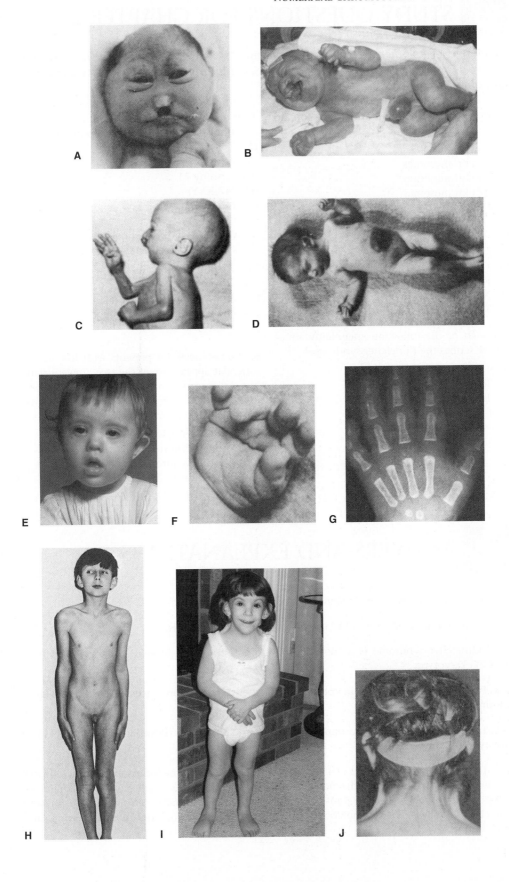

STUDY QUESTIONS FOR CHAPTER 23

*Directions: Each of the numbered items or incomplete statements in this section is followed by answers or by completions of the statement. Select the **one** lettered answer or completion that is **best** in each case.*

1. Triploidy is a condition in which cells contain

(A) 46 chromosomes
(B) 69 chromosomes
(C) 23 chromosomes
(D) 45 chromosomes
(E) 47 chromosomes

2. Aneuploidy occurs as a result of which of the following?

(A) Dispermy
(B) Failure of meiosis in a germ cell
(C) Failure of the first cleavage division
(D) Nondisjunction during meiosis
(E) Trispermy

3. Which of the following aneuploidy situations describes the Klinefelter syndrome?

(A) Trisomy 13
(B) Trisomy 18
(C) Trisomy 21
(D) (47,XXY)
(E) (45,X)

4. Which of the following aneuploidy situations describes the Patau syndrome?

(A) Trisomy 13
(B) Trisomy 18
(C) Trisomy 21
(D) (47,XXY)
(E) (45,X)

5. Which of the following aneuploidy situations describes the Turner syndrome?

(A) Trisomy 13
(B) Trisomy 18
(C) Trisomy 21
(D) (47,XXY)
(E) (45,X)

6. A male newborn presents with low muscle tone, flat appearance of the face, upward slanting eye creases, small ears, extremely flexible joints, and a large tongue. What diagnosis will most likely be confirmed by karyotype analysis?

A) Marfan syndrome
(B) Noonan syndrome
(C) Edwards syndrome
(D) Klinefelter syndrome
(E) Down syndrome

 # ANSWERS AND EXPLANATIONS

1. **B.** Triploidy is a condition in which cells contain 69 chromosomes.

2. **D.** Aneuploidy occurs as result of nondisjunction during meiosis.

3. **D.** Klinefelter syndrome is a trisomic condition found only in males characterized by a (47,XXY) karyotype.

4. **A.** Patau syndrome is a trisomic condition characterized by the presence of an additional chromosome 13.

5. **E.** Turner syndrome is a monosomic condition found only in females characterized by a (45,X) karyotype.

6. **E.** The physical characteristics of a newborn with Down syndrome (or trisomy 21) include low muscle tone, flat appearance of the face, upward slanting eye creases, small ears, single skin crease in the palm, extremely flexible joints, large tongue, and other traits. Although these physical characteristics may not be very obvious, the diagnosis can be made (or confirmed) following karyotype testing.

Structural Chromosomal Abnormalities

I.   Deletions

A deletion is a loss of chromatin from a chromosome. The following are clinical examples caused by deletions.

A. Chromosome 4p deletion (Wolf-Hirschhorn syndrome) is caused by a deletion in the short arm of **chromosome 4 (4p16)**. This deletion is characterized by a prominent forehead and broad nasal root ("Greek warrior helmet"), short philtrum, down-turned mouth, congenital heart defects, growth retardation, and severe mental retardation.

B. Chromosome 5p deletion (cri du chat or cat's cry syndrome) is caused by a deletion in the short arm of **chromosome 5 (5p15)**. This deletion is characterized by a round facies, a catlike cry, congenital heart defects, microcephaly, and mental retardation.

C. Ring chromosome 14 is caused when **chromosome 14** forms a ring structure with breakpoints at **14p11** and **14q32**. This deletion is characterized by mild dysmorphic features, frequent seizures, and variable mental retardation.

II.   Microdeletions

Microdeletions are a loss of chromatin from a chromosome that can be detected only by high-resolution banding. The following are clinical examples caused by microdeletions.

A. Prader-Willi syndrome (PW) is caused by a microdeletion in the long arm of **chromosome 15 (15q11-13)** derived from the **father**. PW is characterized by hyperphagia (insatiable appetite), hypogonadism, hypotonia, obesity, short stature, small hands and feet, behavior problems (rage, violence), and mild-to-moderate mental retardation. PW illustrates the phenomenon of **genomic imprinting**, which is the differential expression of genes depending on the parent of origin. Clearly, both paternal and maternal genes are necessary and complementary for normal development to occur. This is consistent with the view that some genes are differentially activated or inactivated (i.e., imprinted) during gametogenesis. The mechanism of inactivation (or genomic imprinting) involves **DNA methylation of cytosine nucleotides** using methylating enzymes during gametogenesis, resulting in transcriptional inactivation. Other examples that highlight the role of genomic imprinting include **hydatidiform moles** and **Beckwith-Wiedemann syndrome**. The counterpart of PW is **Angelman syndrome**.

B. Angelman syndrome (AS; happy puppet syndrome) is caused by a microdeletion in the long arm of **chromosome 15 (15q11-13)** derived from the **mother**. AS is characterized by gait ataxia (stiff, jerky, unsteady, upheld arms), seizures, happy disposition with inappropriate laughter, and severe mental retardation (only 5- to 10-word vocabulary. AS is an example of **genomic imprinting** (see above). The counterpart of AS is **Prader-Willi syndrome**.

C. DiGeorge syndrome (DS) is caused by a microdeletion in the long arm of **chromosome 22 (22q11)**, which is also called the **DiGeorge chromosomal region (DGCR)**. DS is characterized by congenital heart defects in the conotruncal region, immunodeficiency due to absence of the thymus gland, hypocalcemia due to absence of parathyroid glands, hypertelorism, low-set prominent ears, and micrognathia. DS has a phenotypic and genotypic similarity to **velocardiofacial syndrome (VCFS)**; that is, both DS and VCFS are manifestations of a microdeletion at 22q11. The following genes have been mapped to 22q11 or DGCR (although their role is far from clear): catechol-*O*-methyltransferase (COMT; an enzyme used in catecholamine metabolism), GpIbb (receptor for von Willebrand factor), DGCR3 (a leucine zipper transcription factor), and citrate transport protein (CTP).

D. Miller-Dieker syndrome (MD; agyria; lissencephaly) is caused by a microdeletion in the short arm of **chromosome 17p13.3.** MD is characterized by lissencephaly (smooth brain, i.e., no gyri), microcephaly, and a high and furrowing forehead. Death occurs early. Lissencephaly should not be mistakenly diagnosed in premature infants, whose brains have not yet developed an adult pattern of gyri (gyri begin to appear normally at about week 28).

E. WAGR syndrome is caused by a microdeletion in the short arm of **chromosome 11p13** where the WT1 gene (Wilms' tumor gene 1) is located. WT1 encodes for a zinc finger DNA-binding protein that is required by normal embryologic development of the genitourinary system. WT1 isoforms synergize with **SF-1 (steroidogenic factor-1)**, which is a nuclear receptor that regulates the transcription of a number of genes involved in reproduction, steroidogenesis, and male sexual development. WAGR is characterized by: **W**ilms' tumor, **a**niridia (absence of the iris), **g**enitourinary abnormalities (e.g., gonadoblastoma), and mental **r**etardation. Since the WAGR syndrome involves the deletion of a series of adjacent genes, it is a good example of a **contiguous gene syndrome**.

F. Williams syndrome (WS) is caused by a microdeletion in the long arm of **chromosome 7q11.23** where the **ELN gene (elastin gene)** and **LIMK1 gene** are located. The ELN gene encodes for elastin protein, which is an important component of elastic fibers of connective tissue. The LIMK1 gene encodes for a brain-expressed kinase that seems to be involved in visual-spatial cognition. WS is characterized by: facial dysmorphology (e.g., prominent lips, wide mouth, periorbital fullness of subcutaneous tissues, short palpebral tissues, short upturned nose, long philtrum), congenital heart defects (e.g., supravalvular aortic stenosis, pulmonic valvular stenosis, septal defects), renal abnormalities, hoarse voice, and mild mental deficiency with uneven cognitive disabilities.

III.   Translocations

Translocations result from breakage and exchange of segments between chromosomes. The following are clinical examples caused by translocations.

A. Robertsonian translocation t(13q14q) is caused by a translocation between the long arms (q) of chromosomes 13 and 14 where the breakpoint is near the centromere. The short arms (p) of chromosomes 13 and 14 are generally lost. Carriers of this robertsonian translocation are **clinically normal** because 13p and 14p, which are lost, contain only inert DNA and some rRNA (ribosomal RNA) genes, which occur in multiple copies on other chromosomes. Robertsonian translocation t(13q14q) is the **most common translocation found in humans**.

B. Robertsonian translocation t(14q21q) is caused by a translocation between the long arms (q) of chromosomes 14 and 21 where the breakpoint is near the centromere. The short arms (p) of chromosomes 14 and 21 are generally lost. Carriers of this robertsonian translocation are **clinically normal**. The clinical issue in this robertsonian translocation occurs when the carriers produce gametes by meiosis and reproduce. Depending on how the chromosomes segregate during meiosis, conception can produce offspring with trisomy 21 (livebirth), trisomy 14 (early miscarriage), monosomy 14 or 21 (early miscarriage), normal chromosome complement (live birth), or a t(14q21q) carrier (live birth). Consequently, a couple whose one member is a t(14q21q) carrier may have a baby with trisomy 21 (Down syndrome) or recurrent miscarriages.

C. **Acute promyelocytic leukemia t(15;17)(q21;q21)** is caused by a reciprocal translocation between band q21 on chromosome 15 and band q21 on chromosome 17. This results in a fusion of the **promyelocyte gene (PML gene)** on chromosome 15q21 with the **retinoic acid receptor gene (RARα gene)** on chromosome 17q21, thereby forming the *pml/rarα* oncogene. The **PML/RARα oncoprotein** (a transcription factor) blocks the differentiation of promyelocytes to mature granulocytes such that there is continued proliferation of promyelocytes. This leukemia is characterized by coagulopathy and severe bleeding.

D. **Chronic myeloid leukemia t(9;22)(q34;q11)** is caused by a reciprocal translocation between band q34 on chromosome 9 and band q11 on chromosome 22. This is referred to as the **Philadelphia chromosome**. It results in a fusion of the *ABL* gene on chromosome 9q34 with the *BCR* gene on chromosome 22q11, thereby forming the *abl/bcr* oncogene. The **ABL/BCR oncoprotein** (a tyrosine kinase) has enhanced tyrosine kinase activity that transforms hematopoietic precursor cells. This leukemia is characterized by an increased number of granulocytes in all stages of maturation and many mature neutrophils.

IV.   Unstable Expanding Repeat Mutations (Dynamic Mutations)

Dynamic mutations are mutations that involve the **insertion of a repeat sequence** either outside or inside the gene. Dynamic mutations demonstrate a **threshold length**. **Below a certain threshold length**, the repeat sequence is stable, does not cause disease, and is propagated to successive generations without change in length. **Above a certain threshold length**, the repeat sequence is unstable, causes disease, and is propagated to successive generations in expanding lengths. The exact mechanism by which expansion of the repeat sequences occurs is not known. One of the hallmarks of diseases caused by these mutations is **anticipation**, which means the age of onset is lower and degree of severity is worsened in successive generations. Dynamic mutations are divided into two categories:

A. **Highly expanded repeats outside the gene.** In this category of dynamic mutation, various repeat sequences (e.g., CGG, CCG, GAA, CTG, CCTG, ATTCT, CCCCGCCCCGCG) undergo very large expansions. Below threshold length expansions are $\approx$5–50 repeats. Above threshold length expansions are $\approx$100–1000 repeats. This category of dynamic mutations is characterized by the following clinical conditions.

1. **Fragile X syndrome (Martin-Bell syndrome).** Fragile X syndrome involves two mutation sites. Fragile X site A involves a 200–1000+ unstable repeat sequence of (CGG)n located in a 5′ UTR of the FMR 1 gene (fragile X mental retardation 1 gene) on chromosome Xq27.3. Fragile X site B involves a 200+ unstable repeat sequence of (CCG)n located in a promoter region of the FMR 1 gene on chromosome Xq28. **Fragile X syndrome** is an X-linked recessive genetic disorder caused by a fragile site on chromosome Xq27 or Xq28. The fragile site is observed when cells are cultured in a **folate–depleted** medium. The fragile site is produced by a CGG repeat mutation near the **FMR1 gene**. The FMR1 gene encodes for a protein called **FMRP**, whose exact function is not known but has RNA-binding capability. Fragile X syndrome is the second leading cause of inherited mental retardation. (Down syndrome is the number one cause.) Fragile X syndrome is characterized by: mental retardation (most severe in males), macroorchidism, speech delay, behavioral problems (e.g., hyperactivity, attention deficit), prominent jaw, and large, dysmorphic ears.

2. **Friedreich ataxia (FA).** FA involves a 200–1700 unstable repeat sequence of (GAA)n located in intron 1 of the frataxin gene on chromosome 9q13–a21.1. FA is an autosomal-recessive genetic disorder caused by the unstable repeat sequence on chromosome 9q13–a21.1. The frataxin gene encodes for a protein called **frataxin,** which is a mitochondrial protein whose precise function is unknown but appears to play a role in antioxidation. A longstanding hypothesis is that FA is a result of mitochondrial accumulation of iron, which may promote oxidative stress injury. FA is characterized by: degeneration of the posterior columns and spinocerebellar tracts; loss of sensory neurons in the dorsal root ganglion; ataxia of all four limbs; optic atrophy; swallowing dysfunction; pyramidal tract disease; cardiomyopathy (arrhythmias); and diabetes.

3. **Myotonic dystrophy (DM).** DM involves two mutation sites.
   a. **DM1** involves a 50–4000 unstable repeat sequence of $(CTG)_n$ located in a 3′ UTR of the DM1 gene on chromosome 19q13. Myotonic dystrophy Type 1 (DM1) is an autosomal-dominant genetic disorder caused by the unstable repeat sequence on chromosome 19q13. The DM1 gene encodes for a **serine threonine protein kinase.** DM1 is characterized by: myotonia (delayed muscle relaxation after contraction), cataracts, cardiomyopathy with conduction defects, multiple endocrinopathies, and low intelligence or dementia.
   b. **DM2** involves a 75–11,000 unstable repeat sequence of $(CCTG)_n$ located in intron 1 of the DM2 gene on chromosome 3q21. Myotonic dystrophy Type 2 (DM2 or proximal myotonic myopathy) is an autosomal-dominant genetic disorder caused by the unstable repeat sequence on chromosome 3q21. The DM2 gene encodes for **zinc finger protein 9.** DM2 is characterized by: myalgia and painful muscle cramps, fluctuating weakness and stiffness, calf pseudohypertrophy, diabetes, hypothyroidism, cardiac conduction defects, deafness, and gastrointestinal symptoms.

4. **Spinocerebellar ataxia (SCA).** Numerous classification systems have been proposed for the autosomal-dominant ataxias. Using a system based on genetic loci, numerous SCAs have been classified (SCA1-26; numbers continue to grow). SCA involves multiple mutation sites.
   a. **SCA8** involves a 110–500+ unstable repeat sequence of $(CTG)_n$ located in a RNA-coding gene (antisense RNA) on chromosome 13q21. SCA Type 8 is an autosomal-dominant genetic disorder caused by the unstable repeat sequence on chromosome 13q21. The SCA 8 gene probably encodes for an **antisense RNA** that regulates a brain-specific actin-binding protein. SCA 8 is characterized by: slow, progressive cerebellar ataxia affecting gait, speech, swallowing, limb movements, and eye movements; and cerebral atrophy.
   b. **SCA11** involves a 1000+ unstable repeat sequence of $(ATTCT)_n$ located in an intron sequence of the SCA11 gene on chromosome 15q14—q21. SCA Type 11 is an autosomal-dominant genetic disorder caused by the unstable repeat sequence on chromosome 15q13-q21. The SCA 11 gene encodes for an **unknown protein or RNA.** SCA Type 11 is characterized by: a relatively mild, pure cerebellar ataxia.

5. **Juvenile myoclonus epilepsy (JME).** JME involves a 40–80 unstable repeat sequence of $(CCCCGCCCCGCG)_n$ located in a promoter region of the GABRA 1 gene (α1 subunit of the gamma-aminobutyric acid receptor subtype A) on chromosome 21q22.3. JME is an autosomal-recessive genetic disorder caused by the unstable repeat sequence on chromosome 21q22.3. The GABRA 1 gene encodes for the **α1 subunit of the gamma-aminobutyric acid receptor subtype A.** JME is characterized by: myoclonic jerks (often upon awakening in the morning), absence seizures, and generalized tonic-clonic seizures typically seen in a healthy young teenager.

B. **Moderately expanded CAG repeats with the gene.** In this category of dynamic mutation, a CAG repeat sequence undergoes moderate expansions. Below threshold length expansions are ≈10–30 repeats. Above threshold length expansions are ≈40–200 repeats. Since CAG codes for the amino acid **glutamine,** a long tract of glutamines (polyglutamine tract) will be inserted into the amino acid sequence of the protein and causes the protein to aggregate within certain cells. This category of dynamic mutations is characterized by the following clinical conditions.

1. **Huntington disease (HD).** HD involves a 26–100+ unstable repeat sequence of $(CAG)_n$ located in an exon (or coding) sequence of the HD gene on chromosome 4p16.3. HD is an autosomal-dominant genetic disorder caused by the CAG repeat sequence on chromosome 4p16.3. The HD gene encodes for a protein called **huntingtin**, which is a cytoplasmic protein present in neurons within the striatum, cerebral cortex, and **cerebellum**, although its precise function is unknown. HD is characterized by: a primary manifestation is movement jerkiness most apparent at movement termination; chorea; memory deficits; affective disturbances; personality changes; diffuse and marked atrophy (neuronal loss) of the neostriatum; and neuronal intranuclear aggregates.

2. **Kennedy syndrome (KS; spinobulbar muscular atrophy).** KS involves a 38–62 unstable repeat sequence of $(CAG)_n$ located in an exon (or coding) sequence of the AR gene (androgen receptor gene) on chromosome Xq21. KS is an X-linked recessive genetic disorder caused by the CAG repeat sequence on chromosome Xq21. The KS gene encodes for the **androgen receptor protein,** which is a member of the steroid-thyroid-retinoid superfamily of nuclear receptors. The CAG repeat mutation in the AR gene seems to be a gain of function mutation because there is a well-known syndrome called Complete Androgen Insensitivity that is caused by a loss of function mutation in the AR gene. KS is characterized by: progressive loss of anterior motor neurons, late onset gynecomastia, defective spermatogenesis, and a hormonal profile consistent with androgen resistance. How this CAG repeat mutation causes the neurological deficits is unknown.

3. **Spinocerebellar ataxia (SCA).** Numerous classification systems have been proposed for the autosomal-dominant ataxias. Using a system based on genetic loci, numerous SCAs have been classified (SCA1-26; numbers continue to grow). SCA involves multiple mutation sites.

   a. **SCA1** involves a 39–83 unstable repeat sequence of $(CAG)_n$ located in an exon (or coding) sequence of the SCA 1 gene on chromosome 6p23. SCA Type 1 is an autosomal-dominant genetic disorder caused by the CAG repeat sequence on chromosome 6p23. The SCA 1 gene encodes for **ataxin-1**, whose function is not known. Ataxin-1 is phosphorylated on serine 776 by Akt kinase, and this serine is crucial in mediating the pathogenesis of SCA Type 1. SCA Type 1 is characterized by: progressive cerebellar ataxia, dysarthria, bulbar dysfunction, and intranuclear aggregates.

   b. **SCA2** involves a 32–77 unstable repeat sequence of $(CAG)_n$ located in an exon (or coding) sequence of the SCA2 gene on chromosome 12q24. SCA Type 2 is an autosomal dominant genetic disorder caused by the CAG repeat sequence on chromosome 12q24. The SCA 2 gene encodes for **ataxin-2**, which functions in RNA splicing. SCA Type 2 is characterized by: progressive cerebellar ataxia, dysarthria, bulbar dysfunction, slow saccadic eye movements, and intracytoplasmic aggregates.

   c. **SCA3 (Machado-Joseph disease; MJD)** involves a 62–86 unstable repeat sequence of $(CAG)_n$ located in an exon (or coding) sequence of the SCA3/MJD gene on chromosome 14q32.1. SCA Type 3 is an autosomal-dominant genetic disorder caused by the CAG repeat sequence on chromosome 14q32.1. The SCA3/MJD gene encodes for **ataxin-3**, whose function is unknown. SCA Type 3 is characterized by: progressive cerebellar ataxia, dysarthria, bulbar dysfunction, extrapyramidal features including rigidity and dystonia, upper and lower motor neuron signs, cognitive impairments, and intranuclear aggregates.

   d. **SCA6** involves a 21–30 unstable repeat sequence of $(CAG)_n$ located in an exon (or coding) sequence of the SCA6 gene on chromosome 19p13. SCA Type 6 is an autosomal-dominant genetic disorder caused by the CAG repeat sequence on chromosome 19q13. The SCA6 gene encodes for the **α-1A subunit of P/Q type calcium channel protein.** SAC Type 6 is characterized by: progressive cerebellar ataxia, cerebellar atrophy, horizontal and vertical nystagmus, abnormal vestibulo-ocular reflex, and intracytoplasmic aggregates.

   e. **SCA7** involves a 37–200 unstable repeat sequence of $(CAG)_n$ located in an exon (or coding) sequence of the SCA7 gene on chromosome 3p12-p21.1. SCA Type 7 is an autosomal-dominant genetic disorder caused by the CAG repeat sequence on chromosome

3p12-p21.1. The SCA7 gene encodes for **ataxin-7,** whose function is unknown. SCA Type 7 is characterized by: progressive cerebellar ataxia, seizures, myoclonus, cardiac involvement, and vision loss.

   f. SCA17 involves a 47–63 unstable repeat sequence of $(CAG)_n$ located in an exon (or coding) sequence on the TBP gene (TATA-binding protein gene) on chromosome 6q27. SCA Type 17 is an autosomal-dominant genetic disorder caused by the CAG repeat sequence on chromosome 6q27. The SCA 17 gene encodes for **TATA-binding protein,** which is a general transcription factor. SCA Type 17 is characterized by: progressive cerebellar ataxia, dementia, eventually leading over the years to bradykinesia, dysmetria, dysdiadochokinesis, hyperreflexia, and paucity of movement.

C. Trinucleotide repeat expansions. In addition to the above-mentioned dynamic mutations, there is another category of mutation that involves short, stable trinucleotide repeat expansions (not considered a dynamic mutation). This category of mutation is characterized by the following clinical conditions.

    a. Oropharyngeal muscular dystrophy (PABP2 gene)

    b. Pseudoachondroplasia (COMP gene)

    c. Synpolydactyly (HOXD 13 gene)

V.   Isochromosomes

Isochromosomes occur when the centromere divides transversely (instead of longitudinally) such that one of the chromosome arms is duplicated and the other arm is lost.

   Isochromosome Xq is a clinical example caused by an isochromosome. **Isochromosome Xq** is caused by a duplication of the long arm (q) and loss of short arm (p) of chromosome X. This isochromosome is found in 20% of females with **Turner syndrome**. The occurrence of isochromosomes within any of the autosomes is generally a lethal situation.

VI.   Inversions

Inversions are the reversal of the order of DNA between two breaks in a chromosomes. **Pericentric inversions** occur on both sides of the centromere. **Paracentric inversions** occur on the same side of the centromere. Carriers of inversions are normal. The diagnosis of an inversion is generally a coincidental finding during prenatal testing or the repeated occurrence of spontaneous abortions or stillbirths.

VII.   Breakage

Breakages are breaks in chromosomes resulting from sunlight (or ultraviolet) irradiation, ionizing irradiation, DNA cross-linking agents, or DNA damaging agents. These insults may cause **depurination of DNA, deamination of cytosine to uracil,** or **pyrimidine dimerization,** which must be repaired by DNA repair enzymes. The clinical importance of DNA repair enzymes is illustrated by some rare inherited diseases that involve genetic defects in DNA repair enzymes such as the following.

A. Xeroderma pigmentosum (XP) is an autosomal-recessive genetic disorder in which the affected individuals are hypersensitive to **sunlight (UV radiation).** XP is characterized by: acute sun sensitivity with sunburn-like reaction, severe skin lesions around the eyes and eyelids, and malignant skin cancers (basal and squamous cell carcinomas and melanomas) whereby most individuals die by 30 years of age. XP is caused by the inability to remove pyrimidine dimers because of a genetic defect in one or more of the **nucleotide excision repair**

enzymes. There are seven complementation groups in XP **(XPA–XPG).** The seven genes involved in the cause of XP include: XPA gene located on chromosome 9q22.3, which encodes for a DNA repair enzyme; **ERCC3 gene** located on chromosome 2q21, which encodes for TFIIH basal transcription factor complex helicase; **XPC gene** located on chromosome 3p25, which encodes for a DNA repair enzyme; **ERCC2 gene** located on chromosome 19q13.2, which encodes for TFIIH basal transcription factor complex helicase; **DDB2 gene** located on chromosome 11p12, which encodes for DNA damage binding protein 2; **ERCC4 gene** located on chromosome 16p13.3, which encodes for a DNA repair enzyme; **ERCC5 gene** located on chromosome 13q33, which encodes for DNA repair enzyme. There is an XP variant gene **(XPV gene or hRAD30 gene),** which encodes for DNA polymerase eta that is involved in error-free replication of DNA damaged by UV radiation.

B. Ataxia-telangiectasia (AT) is an autosomal-recessive genetic disorder involving a gene locus on chromosome 11q22-q23 in which the affected individuals are hypersensitive to **ionizing radiation.** AT is characterized by: cerebellar ataxia with depletion of Purkinje cells, progressive nystagmus, slurred speech, oculocutaneous telangiectasia initially in the bulbar conjunctiva followed by ear, eyelid, cheeks, and neck, immunodeficiency, and death in the second decade of life. AT is caused by genetic defects in **DNA recombination repair enzymes.** The **ATM gene (AT mutated)** is involved in the cause of AT. The ATM gene located on chromosome 11q22 encodes for a protein where one region resembles a **PI-3 kinase** (phosphatidylinositol-3 kinase) and another region resembles a **DNA repair enzyme/cell cycle checkpoint protein.**

C. Fanconi anemia (FA; most common form of congenital aplastic anemia) is an autosomal-recessive genetic disorder involving gene loci on chromosomes 16q24, 9q22, and 3p26 in which affected individuals are hypersensitive to **DNA cross-linking agents.** FA is characterized by: short stature, hypopigmented spots, café-au-lait spots, hypogonadism, microcephaly, hypoplastic or aplastic thumbs, renal malformation including unilateral aplasia or horseshoe kidney, acute leukemia, progressive aplastic anemia, head and neck tumors, and medulloblastoma. FA is caused by genetic defects in **DNA recombination repair enzymes** used to repair chromosome defects that occur during homologous recombination. There are eleven complementation groups in FA **(FA-A to FA-L).** To date, eight of the genes have been cloned. The **FA-A gene** (involved in 65% of FA cases) located on chromosome 16q24 encodes for a protein that normalizes cell growth, corrects sensitivity to chromosomal breakage in the presence of mitomycin C, and generally promotes genomic stability. Several of the FA genes form a nuclear-protein complex that interacts with **BRCA1 and BRCA2** (breast cancer susceptibility genes 1 and 2) as the final common pathway. In this regard, BRCA2 has been found to be identical to FANC-D1.

D. Bloom syndrome (BS) is an autosomal-recessive genetic disorder involving a gene locus on chromosome 15q26 in which affected individuals are hypersensitive to a **wide variety of DNA-damaging agents.** BS is characterized by: long, narrow face, erythema with telangiectasias in butterfly distribution over the nose and cheeks, high-pitched voice, small stature, small mandible, immunodeficiency with decreased IgA, IgM, and IgG levels, predisposition to several types of cancers, and increased frequency in the Ashkenazi Jewish population. BS is caused by genetic defects in enzymes involved in DNA repair. The **BLM gene** is involved in the cause of BS. The BLM gene located on chromosome 15q26 encodes for a protein that has strong homology to the **RecQ helicases** (a subfamily of DExH box-containing DNA and RNA helicases).

E. Hereditary nonpolyposis colorectal cancer (HNPCC) is an autosomal-dominant genetic disorder that accounts for 3%–5% of all colorectal cancers. HNPCC is characterized by: onset of colorectal cancer at a young age; high frequency of carcinomas proximal to the splenic flexure; multiple synchronous or metachronous colorectal cancers; and presence of extracolonic cancers (e.g., endometrial and ovarian cancer; adenocarcinomas of the stomach, small intestine, and hepatobiliary tract). HNPCC is caused by genetic defects in **DNA mismatch repair enzymes,** which recognize single nucleotide mismatches or loops that occur in microsatellite repeat areas. The **MLH1, MSH2, MSH6, PMS1, and PMS2 genes** are involved in the cause of HPNCC. These genes are the human homologues to the *Escherichia coli* **mutS** and **mutL** genes that code for DNA mismatch repair enzymes.

VIII. Selected Photographs

A. Chromosome 4p deletion (Wolf-Hirschhorn syndrome) and chromosome 5p deletion (cri du chat syndrome) are illustrated in Figure 24-1*A* and *B*.

B. Prader-Willi syndrome, Angelman syndrome, DiGeorge syndrome, and Miller-Dieker syndrome are illustrated in Figure 24-2*A–D*.

C. Robertsonian t(13q14q), robertsonian t(14q21q), acute promyelocytic leukemia t(15;17) (q21;q21), and chronic myeloid leukemia t(9;22)(q34;q11) are illustrated in Figure 24-3*A–D*.

D. Fragile X syndrome, xeroderma pigmentosum, ataxia-telangiectasia, Fanconi's anemia, and Bloom syndrome are illustrated in Figure 24-4*A–E*.

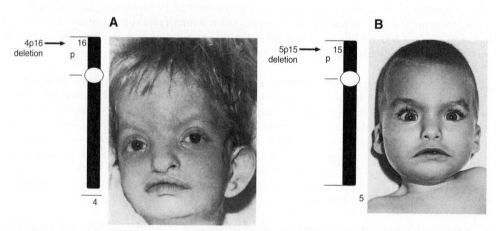

Figure 24-1. Deletion abnormalities. **(A)** Chromosome 4p deletion (Wolf-Hirschhorn syndrome). The deletion at 4p16 is shown on chromosome 4. Photograph of a 5-year-old boy with Wolf-Hirschhorn syndrome shows a prominent forehead and broad nasal root ("Greek warrior helmet"), short philtrum, down-turned mouth, and severe mental retardation (IQ = 20). **(B)** Chromosome 5p deletion (cri du chat [cat's cry] syndrome). The deletion at 5p15 is shown on chromosome 5. Photograph of an infant with cri du chat shows round facies, microcephaly, and mental retardation.

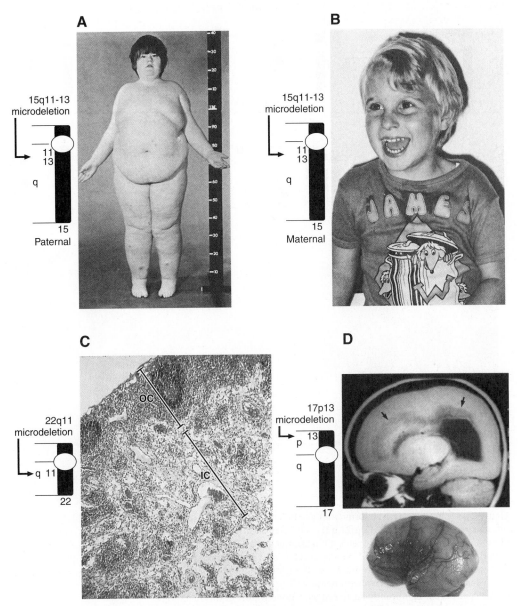

Figure 24-2. Microdeletion abnormalities. **(A)** Prader-Willi syndrome. The microdeletion at 15q11-13 is shown on chromosome 15 inherited from the father (paternal). Photograph of a 10-year-old boy with Prader-Willi syndrome shows hypogonadism, hypotonia, obesity, short stature, and small hands and feet. **(B)** Angelman syndrome (happy puppet syndrome). The microdeletion at 15q11-13 is shown on chromosome 15 inherited from the mother (maternal). Photograph of a 5-year-old boy with Angelman syndrome shows happy disposition with inappropriate laughter and severe mental retardation (only a 5- to 10-word vocabulary). **(C)** DiGeorge syndrome. The microdeletion at 22q11 is shown on chromosome 22. Photomicrograph of a lymph node from a patient with DiGeorge syndrome shows the absence of T lymphocytes within the inner cortex (*IC*; or paracortex; or thymic-dependent zone). The outer cortex (*OC*) shows abundant B lymphocytes within lymphatic follicles. **(D)** Miller-Dieker syndrome (agyria, lissencephaly). The microdeletion at 17p13.3 is shown on chromosome 17. MRI (*top figure*) shows complete absence of gyri in the cerebral hemispheres. The lateral ventricles are indicated by *arrows*. Photograph of a brain at autopsy from an infant with Miller-Dieker syndrome (*bottom figure*) shows complete absence of gyri.

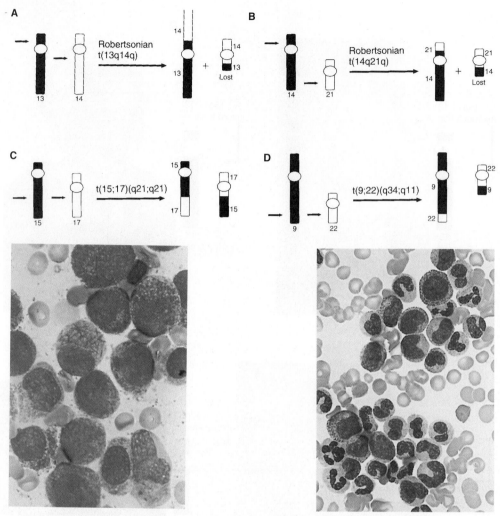

Figure 24-3. Translocation abnormalities. **(A)** Robertsonian t(13q14q). **(B)** Robertsonian t(14q21q). **(C)** Acute promyelocytic leukemia t(15;17)(q21;q21). The translocation between chromosomes 15 and 17 is shown. Photomicrograph of acute promyelocytic leukemia shows abnormal promyelocytes with their characteristic pattern of heavy granulation and bundle of Auer rods. **(D)** Chronic myeloid leukemia t(9;22)(q34;q11). The translocation between chromosomes 9 and 22 is shown. Photomicrograph of chronic myeloid leukemia shows marked granulocytic hyperplasia with neutrophilic precursors at all stages of maturation. Erythroid (red blood cell) precursors are significantly decreased with none shown in this field.

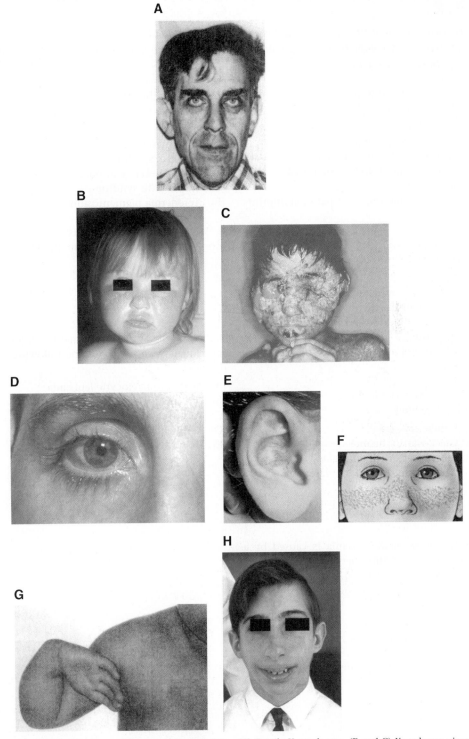

Figure 24-4.   Fragile site and breakage abnormalities. (**A**) Fragile X syndrome. (**B and C**) Xeroderma pigmentosum. (**D–F**) Ataxia-telangiectasia. (**G**) Fanconi syndrome. (**H**) Bloom syndrome.

STUDY QUESTIONS FOR CHAPTER 24

Directions: Each of the numbered items or incomplete statements in this section is followed by answers or by completions of the statement. Select the **one** lettered answer or completion that is **best** in each case.

1. Cri du chat syndrome is characterized by which of the following?

(A) Catlike cry
(B) Greek warrior helmet
(C) Absence of the thymus gland
(D) Chromosome 15q11-13 maternal imprinting
(E) Chromosome 15q11-13 paternal imprinting

2. DiGeorge syndrome is characterized by which of the following?

(A) Catlike cry
(B) Greek warrior helmet
(C) Absence of the thymus gland
(D) Chromosome 15q11-13 maternal imprinting
(E) Chromosome 15q11-13 paternal imprinting

3. Prader-Willi syndrome is characterized by which of the following?

(A) Catlike cry
(B) Greek warrior helmet
(C) Absence of the thymus gland
(D) Chromosome 15q11-13 maternal imprinting
(E) Chromosome 15q11-13 paternal imprinting

4. Chronic myeloid leukemia is caused by a reciprocal translocation between band q34 on chromosome 9 and band q11 on chromosome 22. This is referred to as the

(A) Chicago chromosome
(B) Boston chromosome
(C) St. Louis chromosome
(D) Philadelphia chromosome
(E) Baltimore chromosome

5. Which of the following is due to chromosomal breakage caused by sunlight or UV radiation?

(A) Angelman syndrome
(B) Fragile X syndrome
(C) Miller-Dieker syndrome
(D) Prader-Willi syndrome
(E) Xeroderma pigmentosum

6. Which of the following is the most common translocation found in humans?

(A) t(14q21q)
(B) t(13q14q)
(C) t(15;17)(q21;q21)
(D) t(9;22)(q34;q11)

7. Isochromosome Xq is sometimes found in individuals with which of the following syndromes?

(A) Acute promyelocytic leukemia
(B) Chronic myeloid leukemia
(C) Turner syndrome
(D) Klinefelter syndrome
(E) Down syndrome

ANSWERS AND EXPLANATIONS

1. A. The cri du chat syndrome is also called cat's cry syndrome because affected children demonstrate a catlike cry.

2. C. DiGeorge syndrome is characterized by immunodeficiency due to the absence of the thymus gland and by hypocalcemia due to the absence of the parathyroid glands.

3. E. Prader-Willi syndrome involves a microdeletion in chromosome 15q11-13 derived from the father.

4. D. The reciprocal translocation t(9;22)(q34;q11) is referred to as the Philadelphia chromosome and results in a fusion gene called the *abl/bcr* oncogene.

5. E. Xeroderma pigmentosum is an autosomal recessive genetic disorder in which affected individuals are hypersensitive to sunlight.

6. B. This robertsonian translocation is the most common translocation in humans. Carriers of this translocation are clinically normal.

7. C. Isochromosome Xq is found in 20% of females with Turner syndrome.

Single-Gene Inherited Diseases

I.   Autosomal-Dominant Inheritance

A. In autosomal-dominant inheritance, the disease is observed **in both males and females with equal probability** who **are heterozygous for the mutant gene**. The characteristic pedigree is **vertical** in that the disease is passed from one generation to the next generation. An example of an autosomal-dominant inherited disease is Huntington disease. Other autosomal-dominant inherited disorders are listed in the Appendix.

B. Huntington disease (HD). HD involves a 26–100+ unstable repeat sequence of (CAG)n located in an exon (or coding) sequence of the HD gene on chromosome 4p16.3. HD is an autosomal-dominant genetic disorder caused by the CAG repeat sequence on chromosome 4p16.3. The HD gene encodes for a protein called **huntingtin**, which is a cytoplasmic protein present in neurons within the striatum, cerebral cortex, and cerebellum, although its precise function is unknown. HD is characterized by: a primary manifestation is movement jerkiness most apparent at movement termination; chorea (dancelike movements); memory deficits; affective disturbances; personality changes; diffuse and marked atrophy of the neostriatum because of cell death of cholinergic neurons and GABA-ergic neurons within the striatum (caudate nucleus and putamen), and a relative increase in dopaminergic neuron activity; and neuronal intranuclear aggregates.

II.   Autosomal-Recessive Inheritance

A. In autosomal-recessive inheritance, the disease is observed **in both males and females with equal probability** who are **homozygous for the mutant gene**. The characteristic pedigree is **horizontal** in that affected individuals tend to be limited to a single sibship and the disease is not found in multiple generations. An example of an autosomal-recessive inherited disease is cystic fibrosis. Other autosomal-recessive inherited disorders are listed in the Appendix.

B. Cystic fibrosis (CF)   CF is characterized by the **production of abnormally thick mucus** by epithelial cells lining the respiratory and gastrointestinal tracts. This results clinically in **obstruction of pulmonary airways** and **recurrent respiratory bacterial infections**. CF is caused by **autosomal-recessive** mutation such that an individual must receive two defective copies of the CF gene (one from each parent) to have the disease. The CF gene is located on the **long arm (q arm) of chromosome 7 (7q)** between bands q21 and q31. The CF gene encodes for a protein called **CFTR** (cystic fibrosis transporter), which functions as a Cl⁻ **channel**. A mutation in the CF gene destroys the Cl⁻ transport function of CFTR. In North America, 70% of CF cases are due to a **three-base deletion** that codes for the amino acid **phenylalanine at position #508** such that phenylalanine is missing from CFTR.

III. X-Linked Dominant Inheritance

A. In X-linked dominant inheritance, the disease is observed **in both males and females (with no male-to-male transmission)**. All daughters of an affected man are affected because all receive the X chromosome bearing the mutant gene from their father. All sons of an affected man are normal because they receive only the Y chromosome from the father. An example of an X-linked dominant inherited disease is hypophosphatemic rickets. Other X-linked dominant inherited disorders are listed in the Appendix.

B. Hypophosphatemic rickets (HR)   HR is a vitamin D-resistant rickets characterized by low blood Po_4^{2-} levels, high urinary Po_4^{2-} levels, short stature, and bony deformities.

IV. X-Linked Recessive Inheritance

A. In X-linked recessive inheritance, the disease is **usually** observed **only in males (with no male-to-male transmission)** because males have only one X chromosome; that is, males are **hemizygous** for X-linked genes (i.e., no backup copy of the gene). In X-linked recessive inheritance, heterozygous females are clinically normal but may be detected by subtle clinical features (like intermediate enzyme levels, and so on).

Can the disease ever be observed in females? The answer is yes according to the following mechanism: In females, one of the two X chromosomes is inactivated during the **late blastocyst stage** to form a **Barr body** in a process called **dosage compensation (or lyonization)**. The choice of whether the maternally derived or paternally derived X chromosome gets inactivated is a **random** and **permanent event**. The mechanism of dosage compensation involves **methylation of cytosine nucleotides**. If the X chromosome with the normal gene is inactivated, the female has one X chromosome with the abnormal gene and will therefore be affected by the disease. An example of X-linked recessive inherited disease is Duchenne muscular dystrophy. Other X-linked recessive inherited disorders are listed in the Appendix.

B. Duchenne muscular dystrophy (DMD) is characterized by **progressive muscle weakness and wasting**. This results clinically in **premature death due to cardiac or respiratory failure** in the late teens to twenties. DMD is caused by an **X-linked recessive** mutation such that the male need only receive one defective copy of the DMD gene (from the mother) to have the disease. The DMD gene is located on the **short arm (p arm) of chromosome X in band 21 (Xp21)**. The DMD gene encodes for a protein called **dystrophin**, which anchors the cytoskeleton (actin) of skeletal muscle cells to the extracellular matrix via a transmembrane protein (**α-dystrophin and β-dystrophin**), thereby stabilizing the cell membrane. A mutation of the DMD gene destroys the ability of dystrophin to anchor actin to the extracellular matrix.

V.   Mitochondrial Inheritance

A. In mitochondrial inheritance, the disease is observed in **both males and females who have an affected mother** (not father). Diseases that have mitochondrial inheritance are caused by mutations in the mitochondrial DNA (mtDNA). They are inherited entirely through **maternal transmission** because sperm mitochondria do not pass into the ovum at fertilization. Because mtDNA replicates autonomously from nuclear DNA and mitochondria segregate in daughter cells independently of nuclear chromosomes, the proportion of mitochondria carrying an mtDNA mutation can differ among somatic cells. This heterogeneity is termed **heteroplasmy** and plays a role in the variable phenotype of mitochondrial disease. An example of a mitochondrial inherited disease is Leber hereditary optic neuropathy. Other mitochondrial inherited disorders are listed in the Appendix.

B. Leber hereditary optic neuropathy (LHON) LHON is characterized by a **progressive optic nerve degeneration**. This results clinically in **blindness**. LHON is due to mutations in **mitochondrial DNA (mtDNA)** such that the inheritance is entirely by **maternal transmission.** mtDNA is inherited only from the mother because sperm mitochondria do not pass into the ovum at fertilization. Fifty percent of all cases of LHON involve the *ND4* gene located on mtDNA when a missense mutation changes an **arginine to histidine**. The *ND4* gene encodes for a protein called **subunit 4 of the NADH dehydrogenase complex,** which functions in the **electron transport chain** and the **production of adenosine triphosphate (ATP)**. A mutation of the *ND4* gene decreases the production of ATP so that the demands of a very active neuronal metabolism cannot be met.

VI. The Family Pedigree in Various Inherited Diseases

A family pedigree is a graphic method of charting the family history using various symbols. Figure 25-1 shows a variety of family pedigrees in relation to certain inherited diseases.

Figure 25-1. **(A)** A prototype family pedigree and explanation of the various symbols. Proband = person who ▶ brought the condition to medical attention. **(B)** Pedigree of autosomal dominant inheritance. The disease is observed in both males and females with equal probability who are heterozygous for the mutant gene. The characteristic pedigree is vertical in that the disease is passed from one generation to the next generation. **(C)** Pedigree of autosomal recessive inheritance. The disease is observed in both males and females with equal probability who are homozygous for the mutant gene. The characteristic pedigree is horizontal in that affected individuals tend to be limited to a single sibship and the disease is not found in multiple generations. **(D)** Pedigree of X-linked dominant inheritance. The disease is observed in both males and females (with no male-to-male transmission). All daughters of an affected man are affected because they receive the X chromosome bearing the mutant gene from their father. All sons of an affected man are normal because they receive only the Y chromosome from the father. **(E)** Pedigree of X-linked recessive inheritance. The disease is usually observed only in males (with no male-to-male transmission). **(F)** Pedigree of mitochondrial inheritance. The disease is observed in both males and females who have an affected mother. Note that affected sons and daughters are siblings of an affected mother. And, affected fathers do not produce affected siblings.

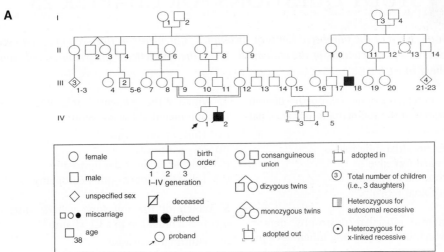

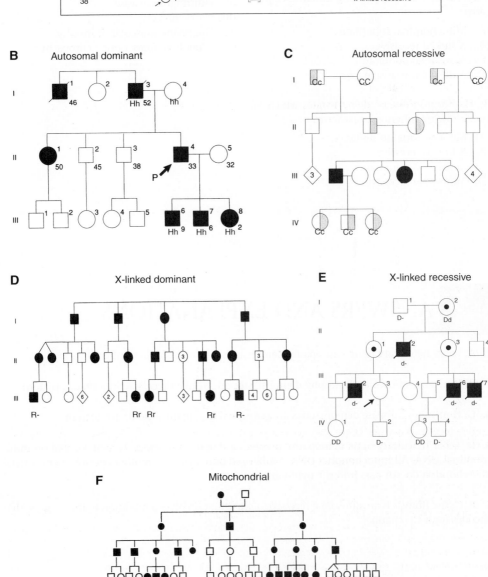

STUDY QUESTIONS FOR CHAPTER 25

*Directions: Each of the numbered items or incomplete statements in this section is followed by answers or by completions of the statement. Select the **one** lettered answer or completion that is **best** in each case.*

1. Leber hereditary optic neuropathy demonstrates which of the following inheritance patterns?

(A) Mitochondrial inheritance
(B) X-linked recessive
(C) Autosomal dominant
(D) Autosomal recessive

2. Duchenne muscular dystrophy demonstrates which of the following inheritance patterns?

(A) Mitochondrial inheritance
(B) X-linked recessive
(C) Autosomal dominant
(D) Autosomal recessive

3. Huntington disease demonstrates which of the following inheritance patterns?

(A) Mitochondrial inheritance
(B) X-linked recessive
(C) Autosomal dominant
(D) Autosomal recessive

4. Which of the following is inherited entirely through maternal transmission?

(A) Huntington disease
(B) Cystic fibrosis
(C) Duchenne muscular dystrophy
(D) Leber hereditary optic neuropathy

5. Which of the following genetic diseases involves a mutation in a Cl^- channel?

(A) Huntington disease
(B) Cystic fibrosis
(C) Duchenne muscular dystrophy
(D) Leber hereditary optic neuropathy

 ANSWERS AND EXPLANATIONS

1. **A.** Leber hereditary optic neuropathy demonstrates a mitochondrial inheritance pattern.

2. **B.** Duchenne muscular dystrophy demonstrates an X-linked recessive inheritance pattern.

3. **C.** Huntington disease demonstrates an autosomal dominant inheritance pattern.

4. **D.** Leber hereditary optic neuropathy involves a mutation in the *ND4* gene located on mitochondrial DNA. All mitochondrial DNA is inherited only from the mother because sperm (male) mitochondria do not pass into the ovum at fertilization.

5. **B.** Cystic fibrosis is an autosomal recessive disease that involves a mutation in the CF gene that encodes for a Cl^- channel.

Multifactorial Inherited Diseases

I. Introduction

Multifactorial inheritance involves many genes that have a small, equal, and additive effect **(genetic component)** as well as an **environmental component.** Both components contribute to a person inheriting the liability to develop a certain disease. If one considers only the genetic component of a multifactorial disease, the term **polygenic** is used. An example of a multifactorial disease is type 1 diabetes. Other multifactorial inherited disorders are listed in the Appendix.

II. Type 1 Diabetes

The characteristic dysfunction in diabetes is a **destruction of pancreatic β cells** that produce insulin. This results clinically in hyperglycemia, ketoacidosis, and exogenous insulin dependence. Long-term clinical effects include neuropathy, retinopathy leading to blindness, and nephropathy leading to kidney failure. Type 1 diabetes demonstrates an association with the highly polymorphic **HLA (human leukocyte antigen) class II genes**, which play a role in immune responsiveness. The specific loci involved in type 1 diabetes are called **HLA-DR3** and **HLA-DR4 loci.** HLA-DR3 and HLA-DR4 loci are located on the **short arm (p arm) of chromosome 6 (p6).** HLA-DR3 and HLA-DR4 loci code for **cell-surface glycoproteins** that are structurally similar to immunoglobulin proteins and are expressed mainly by B lymphocytes and macrophages. It is hypothesized that alleles closely linked to HLA-DR3 and HLA-DR4 loci somehow alter the immune response such that the individual has an immune response to an environmental antigen (e.g., virus). The immune response "spills over" and leads to the destruction of pancreatic β cells. Markers for immune destruction of pancreatic β cells include **autoantibodies to glutamic acid decarboxylase (GAD$_{65}$), insulin,** and **tyrosine phosphatases IA-2 and IA-2β.** At present, it is not known whether the autoantibodies play a causative role in the destruction of the pancreatic β cell or whether the autoantibodies form secondarily after the pancreatic β cells have been destroyed.

STUDY QUESTIONS FOR CHAPTER 26

Directions: *Each of the numbered items or incomplete statements in this section is followed by answers or by completions of the statement. Select the **one** lettered answer or completion that is **best** in each case.*

1. Multifactorial inherited diseases involve which of the following?

(A) Only a genetic component
(B) Only an environmental component
(C) Both a genetic and environmental component
(D) Only one dominant gene
(E) Only one X-linked gene

2. Type I diabetes is a multifactorial disease that involves which of the following?

(A) HLA Class I genes
(B) HLA Class II genes
(C) HLA Class II genes
(D) HLA Class IV genes

 ANSWERS AND EXPLANATIONS

1. **C.** A multifactorial disease involves many genes that have a small, equal, and additive effect as well as an environmental component.

2. **B.** Type I diabetes involves HLA Class II genes. The specific locus is called HLA-DR3 and HLA-DR4.

Teratology

I. Introduction

A teratogen is any infectious agent, drug, chemical, or irradiation that alters fetal morphology or fetal function if the fetus is exposed during a critical stage of development.

A. The **resistant period (week 1 of development)** is the time when the conceptus demonstrates the "all-or-none" phenomenon (i.e., the conceptus either dies as a result of the teratogen or survives unaffected).

B. The **maximum susceptibility period (weeks 3–8; embryonic period)** is the time during which the embryo is most susceptible to teratogens because all organ morphogenesis occurs at this time.

C. The **lowered susceptibility period (weeks 9–38; fetal period)** is the time during which the fetus has a lowered susceptibility to teratogens because all organ systems have already formed. Teratogen exposure generally results in a **functional derangement** of an organ system.

II. Infectious Agents

May be viral or nonviral; however, bacteria appear to be nonteratogenic.

A. Viral infections may reach the fetus via the amniotic fluid after vaginal infection, transplacentally via the bloodstream after maternal viremia, or by direct contact during passage through an infected birth canal.

    1. Rubella virus (German measles; member of TORCH) belongs to the **Togaviridae** family, which are **enveloped, icosahedral positive single-stranded RNA viruses**. The rubella virus is transmitted to the fetus **transplacentally**. The risk of fetal rubella infection is greatest during the **first month of pregnancy** and apparently declines thereafter. Fetal rubella infection results in the classic triad of **cardiac defects** (i.e., patent ductus arteriosus, pulmonary artery stenosis, atrioventricular (AV) septal defects), **cataracts**, and **low birth weight**. With the pandemic of rubella in 1964, the complexity of this syndrome became apparent, and the term **expanded rubella syndrome** became standard. The clinical manifestations include intrauterine growth retardation (most common manifestation), hepatosplenomegaly, generalized adenopathy, hemolytic anemia, hepatitis, jaundice, meningoencephalitis, eye involvement (e.g., cataracts, glaucoma, retinopathy), bluish-purple lesions on yellow jaundiced skin ("blueberry muffin spots"), osteitis (celery-stalk appearance of long bones), and sensorineural deafness. Exposure of pregnant women to rubella requires immediate assessment of their immune status. If the exposed pregnant woman is known to be immune (i.e., with antibodies present), she can be assured of having no risk. Postexposure prophylaxis of pregnant women with immune globulin (IG) is not recommended and should be considered only if abortion is not an option. Control measures for rubella prevention should be placed on immunization of children.

2. **Cytomegalovirus (CMV; member of TORCH)** belongs to the **Herpesviridae** family, which are **large, enveloped, icosahedral, double-stranded DNA viruses.** CMV is a ubiquitous virus and the **most common fetal infection.** It is transmitted to the fetus **transplacentally** or by the **virus ascending from the cervix during a recurrence,** with more severe malformations resulting when infection occurs during the first half of pregnancy. CMV is also transmitted to perinates **during passage through the birth canal or through breast milk** but causes no apparent disease. Both primary and recurrent infections of the mother can result in transmission of CMV to the fetus. In mothers with recurrent infection, the presence of CMV antibodies does not prevent CMV transmission to the fetus but does protect the fetus from major fetal malformations. Consequently, the risk of major fetal malformations is much higher in infants of mothers who had a primary CMV infection during pregnancy compared with mothers who have had recurrent infections. The most common manifestation of CMV fetal infection is **sensorineural deafness. Cytomegalic inclusion disease** (characterized by multiorgan involvement) is the most serious but least common manifestation of CMV infection and results in intrauterine growth retardation, microcephaly, chorioretinitis, hepatosplenomegaly, osteitis (celery-stalk appearance of long bones), discrete cerebral calcifications, mental retardation, heart block, and bluish-purple lesions on yellow jaundiced skin (blueberry muffin spots). **Ganciclovir** treatment of the neonate is being evaluated for symptomatic congenital CMV infection.

3. **Herpes simplex virus (HSV-1; HSV-2; member of TORCH)** belongs to the **Herpesviridae** family, which are **large, enveloped, icosahedral, double-stranded DNA viruses.** Most neonatal infections are caused by HSV-2 (in 75% of cases). HSV-2 is transmitted to the fetus **transplacentally** only occasionally (in 5% of cases). HSV-2 is most commonly transmitted to the fetus by **direct contact during passage through an infected birth canal** (intrapartum; 85% of cases). The risk of neonatal infection is higher with primary maternal HSV infection (30%–50%) than with recurrent maternal HSV infection (3%) because the infant is exposed to large amounts of virus in the absence of neutralizing antibodies. At **10–11 days of age,** some intrapartum HSV-infected infants present with the disease localized to the **skin** (discrete vesicular lesion, large bullae, or denuded skin; hallmark signs), **eye** (keratoconjunctivitis, uveitis, chorioretinitis, cataracts, retinal dysplasia), or **mouth** (ulcerative lesions of the mouth, tongue, or palate). At **15–17 days of age,** some intrapartum HSV-infected infants present with **CNS involvement** (with or without skin, eye, or mouth involvement) due to axonal retrograde transport of HSV to the brain. Clinical manifestations of CNS involvement include lethargy, bulging fontanelles, focal or generalized seizures, opisthotonus, decerebrate posturing, and coma. Untreated disease results in a 40%–50% mortality rate, and most survivors have neurologic sequelae. At **9–11 days of age,** some intrapartum HSV-infected infants present with **disseminated disease.** Clinical manifestations of disseminated disease include CNS, liver, adrenal gland, pancreas, and kidney involvement due to hematogenous spread of HSV. Untreated disease results in an 80% mortality rate, and most survivors have neurologic sequelae. The only intervention shown to prevent neonatal HSV infection is delivery by cesarean section within 4–6 hours of rupture of the amniotic membranes. **Acyclovir suppressive therapy** has been used in women after a first episode of genital HSV infection during pregnancy to prevent a clinical HSV recurrence at delivery. The efficacy of acyclovir and valacyclovir treatment of the neonate is under study.

4. **Varicella-zoster virus (VZV; varicella or chickenpox)** belongs to the **Herpesviridae** family, which are **large, enveloped, icosahedral, double-stranded DNA viruses.** VZV is the cause of two clinical syndromes: a **primary infection** (varicella or chickenpox usually occurring in children) and a **secondary infection** (herpes zoster or shingles usually occurring in adults along a single sensory dermatome). VZV is transmitted to the fetus **transplacentally** in 25% of the cases, but **fetal varicella syndrome** develops only when maternal VZV infection occurs in the first trimester. The clinical manifestations of fetal varicella syndrome include cicatricial (scarring) skin lesions in a dermatomal pattern,

limb and digit hypoplasia, limb paresis/paralysis, hydrocephalus, microcephaly/mental retardation, seizures, chorioretinitis, and cataracts. Neonates whose mothers develop chickenpox 6–21 days before delivery do not show signs of severe chickenpox because maternal antibodies are produced and delivered to the fetus. Neonates whose mothers develop chickenpox earlier than 5 days before delivery or 2 days postpartum develop severe chickenpox with increased mortality and morbidity (i.e., fever, skin lesions, hemorrhagic rash, respiratory distress, and pneumonia). **Acyclovir** treatment of the neonate is recommended. Varicella-zoster immunoglobulin (VZIG) is recommended for neonates whose mothers develop chickenpox earlier than 5 days before delivery or 2 days postpartum. Administration of the live, attenuated VZV vaccine to susceptible women before pregnancy and to their susceptible household members (older than 1 year) is the most effective method of prevention.

5. **Human immunodeficiency virus (HIV)** belongs to the **Retroviridae** family (or **Lentivirus** subfamily), which are **diploid, enveloped positive single-stranded RNA viruses.** HIV is believed by some to be the major cause of **acquired immunodeficiency syndrome (AIDS).** However, others believe that multiple blood transfusions (e.g., hemophiliacs), consumption of megadoses of antibiotics as prophylaxis against sexually transmitted diseases, and continuous use of drugs (e.g., amyl and butyl nitrite) to heighten orgasm may destroy CD4$^+$ T cells and lead to AIDS. The placenta is a highly effective barrier to HIV infection of the fetus. However, HIV is transmitted to the fetus **through blood containing HIV or HIV-infected lymphoid cells** near the time of delivery or after 35 weeks of gestation. Increased exposure of the fetus or neonate to maternal HIV blood increases the risk of HIV transmission. HIV infection does not appear to cause any congenital malformations, but results in chronic multisystem infections. The clinical manifestations of HIV include **fungal infections** (e.g., *Candida* esophagitis, cryptococcal meningitis, histoplasmosis, coccidioidomycosis, *Pneumocystis carinii* pneumonia), **bacterial infections** (e.g., *Mycobacterium tuberculosis*, *Mycobacterium avium-intracellulare* complex, *Streptococcus pneumoniae* infection, gastroenteritis caused by *Salmonella*, *Shigella*, and *Campylobacter*), **viral infections** (e.g., HSV-1, HSV-2, and CMV), and protozoan infections (e.g., *Cryptosporidium, Giardia, Toxoplasma*, and *Entamoeba*). All HIV-infected children younger than 1 year old should receive a regimen of two nucleoside reverse transcriptase (RT) inhibitors (e.g., zidovudine, didanosine, lamivudine, stavudine) and a nonnucleoside RT inhibitory (e.g., nevirapine, efavirenz) or a protease inhibitor (e.g., ritonavir, nelfinavir). Prevention of perinatal HIV transmission is accomplished by zidovudine treatment to the pregnant mother during pregnancy and to the newborn for the first 6 weeks of life.

B. **Nonviral infections**
  1. *Toxoplasma gondii* (TG; member of TORCH) is a **protozoan parasite** whose life cycle is divided into a **sexual phase,** which occurs only in cats **(the definitive host),** and an **asexual phase,** which occurs in intermediate hosts. Generally speaking, mice that eat cat feces contaminate fields, thereby infecting cows, sheep, and pigs. TG is transmitted to humans primarily through ingestion of oocyst-containing water or food or consumption of cyst-containing raw or undercooked meat. In addition, inhalation or ingestion of oocysts from soil, dust, or cat litter box may occur. TG is transmitted to the fetus **transplacentally** in 25%, 54%, and 65% of pregnant women with untreated primary toxoplasmosis during the first, second, and third trimester, respectively. TG infection results in miscarriage, perinatal death, chorioretinitis, microcephaly, hydrocephalus, and encephalomyelitis with cerebral calcification. About 10% of congenitally infected infants who have severe TG infection die, and most surviving infants are left with major neurologic sequelae (e.g., mental retardation, seizures, spasticity, and visual deficits). Acutely infected women who elect to proceed with the pregnancy should be treated with **spiramycin** (a macrolide antibiotic). If prenatal diagnosis indicates that the fetus is infected, then **pyrimethamine** (folic acid antagonist), **sulfadiazine** (folic acid antagonist), and **leucovorin** (folinic acid) are added.
  2. *Treponema pallidum* (TP) is a **spirochete** causing **syphilis** and is transmitted to the fetus **transplacentally** in 10%, 40%, 50%, and 50% of pregnant women with a late latent stage,

early latent stage, primary stage, and secondary stage of syphilis, respectively. Infection acquired at birth through contact with a genital lesion in the birth canal may also occur but is rare. The most important determinant of risk to the fetus is the maternal stage of syphilis. TP infection results in miscarriage; perinatal death; hepatosplenomegaly; hepatitis; joint swelling; vesiculobullous blisters whose fluid contains active spirochetes and is highly infective; nasal discharge with rhinitis; a maculopapular rash located on the extremities that is initially oval and pink but then turns copper brown and desquamate (palms and soles); eye findings that include chorioretinitis, glaucoma, cataracts, and uveitis; anemia; jaundice; focal erosions of the proximal medial tibia (Wimberger sign); osteitis (celery-stalk appearance of long bones); saw-toothed appearance of the metaphysis of long bones; abnormal teeth (Hutchinson teeth); and acute syphilitic leptomeningitis that may present as neck stiffness; and chronic meningovascular syphilis (cranial nerve palsy, hydrocephalus, cerebral infarction).

Early congenital syphilis refers to the clinical manifestations that appear in an infant **within 2 years of age. Late congenital syphilis** refers to clinical manifestations that appear **after a child is 2 years of age.** Some infants may remain asymptomatic until 2–5 years of age. The clinical manifestations of late congenital syphilis result from inflammation of scars caused by early congenital syphilis. Penicillin treatment given to the infected mother usually provides adequate therapy for the fetus. If not, the infant is treated with penicillin. All pregnant women should be tested for syphilis on their first antenatal visit. For high-risk women, additional tests at 28 weeks' gestation and at delivery should be performed.

III. TORCH Infections

TORCH infections are caused by *Toxoplasma* **(T), rubella (R), cytomegalovirus (C), herpesvirus (H),** and **other (O)** bacterial and viral infections that are grouped together because they cause similar clinical and pathologic manifestations. See above discussion for specifics.

IV. Childhood Vaccinations

A general practical guide to childhood vaccinations includes the following:

A. MMR vaccine protects against **m**easles, **m**umps, and **r**ubella; it is given in two doses at 12–15 months and at 4–6 years.

B. Polio vaccine protects against polio; it is given in four doses at 2 months, 4 months, 6–18 months, and 4–6 years.

C. DTaP vaccine protects against **d**iphtheria, **t**etanus, and **p**ertussis; it is given in five doses at 2 months, 4 months, 6 months, 15–18 months, and 4–6 years. A tetanus booster is given at 11 years.

D. Hib vaccine protects against *Haemophilus influenzae* type **b**; it is given in four doses at 2 months, 4 months, 6 months, and 12–15 months.

E. HBV vaccine protects against **h**epatitis **B**; it is given in four doses at birth, 1 month, 4 months, and 6–18 months.

F. Varicella vaccine protects against chickenpox; it is given in one dose at 12–18 months.

G. Pneumococcal vaccine (PCV7) protects against pneumonia, blood infections, and meningitis; it is given in four doses at 2 months, 4 months, 6 months, and 12–25 months.

V. Category X Drugs

Absolute contraindication in pregnancy.

A. Thalidomide is an **antinauseant** drug that was prescribed for pregnant women (no longer used) for "morning sickness." This drug can cause limb reduction (e.g., meromelia, amelia), ear and nasal abnormalities, cardiac defects, lung defects, pyloric or duodenal stenosis, and gastrointestinal atresia. Thalidomide has undergone a resurgence in use for treatment of multiple myeloma.

B. Aminopterin and methotrexate are **folic acid antagonists** used in cancer chemotherapy. These drugs can cause small stature, abnormal cranial ossification, ocular hypertelorism, low-set ears, cleft palate, and myelomeningocele.

C. Busulfan (Myleran), chlorambucil (Leukeran), and cyclophosphamide (Cytoxan) are **alkylating agents** used in cancer chemotherapy. These drugs can cause cleft palate, eye defects, hydronephrosis, renal agenesis, absence of toes, and growth retardation.

D. Phenytoin (Dilantin) is an **antiepileptic** drug. In 30% of cases, this drug causes **fetal hydantoin syndrome**, which results in growth retardation, mental retardation, microcephaly, craniofacial defects, and nail and digit hypoplasia. In most cases, phenytoin causes cleft lip, cleft palate, and congenital heart defects.

E. Triazolam (Halcion) and estazolam (ProSom) are **hypnotic** drugs. These drugs can cause cleft lip and cleft palate, especially if used in the first trimester of pregnancy.

F. Warfarin (Coumadin) is an **anticoagulant** drug that acts by inhibiting vitamin K–dependent coagulation factors. This drug can cause stippled epiphyses, mental retardation, microcephaly, seizures, fetal hemorrhage, and optic atrophy in the fetus. Note that <u>war</u>farin causes WAR on the fetus.

G. Isotretinoin (Accutane) is a **retinoic acid derivative** used in the treatment of **severe acne.** This drug can cause CNS abnormalities, external ear abnormalities, eye abnormalities, facial dysmorphia, and cleft palate (i.e., **vitamin A embryopathy**).

H. Clomiphene (Clomid) is a nonsteroidal **ovulatory stimulant** used in women with ovulatory dysfunction. Although no causative evidence of a deleterious effect of clomiphene on the human fetus has been established, there have been reports of birth anomalies.

I. Diethylstilbestrol is a **synthetic estrogen** that was used to prevent spontaneous abortion in women. This drug can cause cervical hood, T-shaped uterus, hypoplastic uterus, ovulatory disorders, infertility, premature labor, and cervical incompetence in women who were exposed to DES in utero. These women are also subject to increased risk of adenocarcinoma of the vagina later in life.

J. Ethisterone, norethisterone, and megestrol (Megace) are synthetic **progesterone derivatives.** These drugs can cause masculinization of genitalia in female embryos, hypospadias in males, and cardiovascular anomalies.

K. Norethindrone (Ovcon; Norinyl) and levonorgestrol (Levlen) are **oral conceptives** that contain a combination of estrogen (e.g., ethinyl estradiol or mestranol) and progesterone (e.g., norethindrone or levonorgestrel) derivatives. These drugs can cause an increase of fetal abnormalities, particularly the **VACTERL syndrome**, consisting of vertebral, anal, cardiac, tracheoesophageal, renal, and limb malformations.

L. Nicotine is a **poisonous, additive alkaloid** delivered to the fetus through **cigarette smoking** by pregnant women (cigarette smoke also contains **hydrogen cyanide** and **carbon monoxide**). This drug can cause intrauterine growth retardation, premature delivery, low birth weight, and fetal hypoxia due to reduced uterine blood flow and diminished capacity of the blood to transport oxygen to fetal tissue.

M. Alcohol is an **organic compound** delivered to the fetus through **recreational or addictive** (i.e., **alcoholism**) **drinking** by pregnant women. This drug can cause: **fetal alcohol syndrome**, which results in mental retardation, microcephaly, holoprosencephaly, limb deformities, craniofacial abnormalities (i.e., hypertelorism, smooth philtrum, short palpebral fissures, flat nasal bridge, maxillary (midface) hypoplasia, and a thin upper lip), and cardiovascular defects (i.e., ventricular septal defects). Fetal alcohol syndrome is the leading cause of preventable mental retardation. The threshold dose of alcohol has not been established, so "no alcohol is good alcohol" during pregnancy.

VI. Category D Drugs

Definite evidence of risk to fetus.

A. Tetracycline (Achromycin) and doxycycline (Vibramycin) are **antibiotics** in the tetracycline family. These drugs can cause permanently stained teeth and hypoplasia of enamel.

B. Streptomycin, amikacin, and tobramycin (Nebcin) are **antibiotics** in the aminoglycoside family. These drugs can cause **CN VIII toxicity** with permanent bilateral deafness and loss of vestibular function.

C. Phenobarbital (Donnatal) and pentobarbital (Nembutal) are **barbiturates** used as **sedatives.** Studies have suggested a higher incidence of fetal abnormalities with maternal barbiturate use.

D. Valproic acid (Depakene) is an **antiepileptic** drug. This drug can cause neural tube defects, cleft lip, and renal defects.

E. Diazepam (Valium), chlordiazepoxide (Librium), alprazolam (Xanax), and lorazepam (Ativan) are **anticonvulsant** or **antianxiety** drugs. These drugs can cause cleft lip and cleft palate especially if used in the first trimester of pregnancy.

F. Lithium is used in treatment of **manic-depressive disorder.** This drug can cause fetal cardiac defects (i.e., Ebstein anomaly and malformations of the great vessels).

G. Hydrochlorothiazide (Diuril) is a **diuretic** and **antihypertensive** drug. This drug can cause fetal jaundice and thrombocytopenia.

VII. Chemical Agents

A. Organic mercury Consumption of organic mercury during pregnancy results in fetal neurologic damage including seizures, psychomotor retardation, cerebral palsy, blindness, and deafness.

B. Lead Consumption of lead during pregnancy results in abortion due to embryotoxicity, growth retardation, increased perinatal mortality, and developmental delay.

C. Polychlorinated biphenyls (PCBs) Consumption of PCBs during pregnancy results in intrauterine growth retardation, dark brown skin pigmentation, exophthalmos, gingival hyperplasia, skull calcification, mental retardation, and neurobehavioral abnormalities.

D. Potassium iodide (PI) PI is found in over-the-counter cough medicines and radiograph cocktails for organ visualization. PI is involved in thyroid enlargement (goiter) and mental retardation (cretinism).

E. Bisphenol A (BPA) is a common ingredient in plastics (e.g., reusable water bottles, computer housings, dental sealants). It has been reported *in mice* that exposure to bisphenol A during fetal development results in higher rates of breast cancer later in life.

F. Phthalates are a common ingredient in many household products (e.g., vinyl floor covering, detergents, shampoo, deodorants, nail polish, food storage bags, inflatable toys). It has been reported in humans that high levels of phthalates in pregnant women are associated with incomplete testicular descent in infant sons, suggesting anti-androgenic activity.

G. Methoxychlor (an insecticide) and **vinclozolin** (a fungicide) are both endocrine disruptors. It has been reported *in mice* that exposure to these endocrine disruptors during fetal development caused changes in mice that affected not only the mice exposed in utero but also all male mice for at least four subsequent generations (i.e., a transgenerational effect).

VIII. Recreational Drugs

A. Lysergic acid (LSD) has not been shown to be teratogenic.

B. Marijuana has not been shown to be teratogenic.

C. Caffeine has not been shown to be teratogenic.

D. Cocaine results in an increased risk of various congenital abnormalities, stillbirths, low-birth weight, and placental abruption.

E. Heroin has not been shown to be teratogenic. It is the drugs that are often taken with heroin that produce congenital anomalies. The principal adverse effect is **severe neonatal withdrawal**, causing death in 3%–5% of neonates. **Methadone** (used to replace heroin) is not teratogenic but is also associated with severe neonatal withdrawal.

IX. Ionizing Radiation

A. Acute high dose (over 250 rads) of radiation results in microcephaly, mental retardation, growth retardation, and leukemia. After exposure to **greater than 25 rads**, classic fetal defects will be observed so that termination of pregnancy should be offered as an option. Much information concerning acute high-dose radiation has come from studies of the atomic explosions over Hiroshima and Nagasaki.

B. Diagnostic radiation   Even if several radiographic studies are performed, rarely does the dose add up to significant exposure to produce fetal defects. **Radioactive iodine cocktails** for organ visualization should be avoided after week 10 of gestation because fetal thyroid development can be impaired.

X.   Selected Photographs

A. The photographs in Figure 27-1 illustrate the **TORCH** infections.

B. The photographs in Figure 27-2 illustrate sequelae of **neonatal syphilis**.

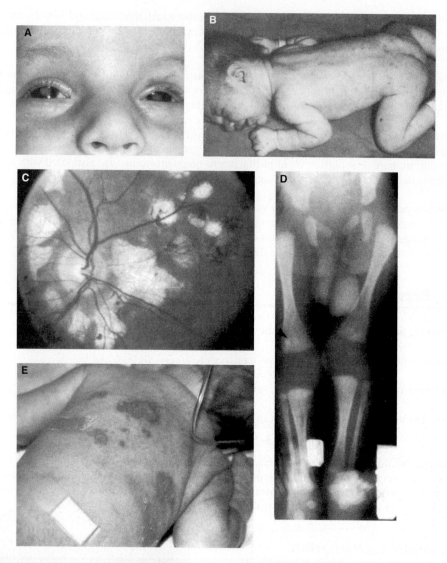

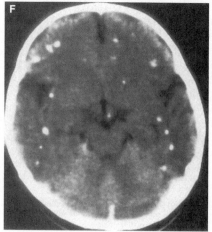

Figure 27-1. TORCH infections. **(A)** Example of cataracts seen with congenital rubella and herpes simplex virus infections. **(B)** Blueberry muffin spots seen with congenital rubella and cytomegalovirus infections due to extramedullary hematopoiesis. **(C)** Patchy, yellow-white lesions of chorioretinitis seen with congenital cytomegalovirus, herpes simplex virus, and *Toxoplasma gondii* infections. **(D)** Celery-stalk appearance of the femur (*arrowhead*) and tibia seen with congenital rubella, cytomegalovirus, and syphilis infections. The alternating bands of longitudinal translucency and density indicate a disturbance in normal bone metabolism. **(E)** Cutaneous vesicular lesions surrounded by an erythematous border on the back and right arm seen with congenital herpes simplex virus infection. **(F)** Diffuse cerebral calcifications seen with congenital cytomegalovirus and *Toxoplasma gondii* infections.

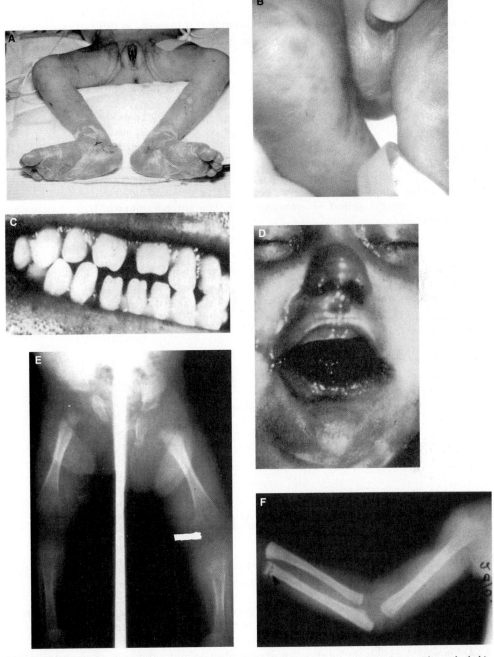

Figure 27-2. Congenital syphilis. **(A)** Vesiculobullous blisters on the legs and feet along with marked skin peeling are shown. **(B)** A copper-brown rash on the extremities is shown. **(C)** Hutchinson teeth that are small and widely spaced with notched upper central incisors are shown. **(D)** Nasal discharge with rhinitis is shown. **(E)** Wimberger sign shows focal erosions of the proximal medial tibia. **(F)** Saw-toothed appearance of the distal radius is shown. The radiolucent area represents syphilitic granulation tissue.

STUDY QUESTIONS FOR CHAPTER 27

Directions: Each of the numbered items or incomplete statements in this section is followed by answers or by completions of the statement. Select the **one** lettered answer or completion that is **best** in each case.

1. Which of the following time intervals best describes the maximum susceptibility period of embryonic development?

(A) Week 1
(B) Weeks 3–8
(C) Weeks 9–38

2. Which of the following time intervals best describes the resistant period of embryonic development?

(A) Week 1
(B) Weeks 3–8
(C) Weeks 9–38

3. The most common viral infection is

(A) cytomegalovirus
(B) rubella virus
(C) herpesvirus type 2
(D) varicella-zoster virus
(E) HIV

4. Which of the following is a parasite found in cats?

(A) *Treponema pallidum*
(B) *Toxoplasma gondii*
(C) Rubella virus
(D) Cytomegalovirus
(E) Varicella-zoster virus

5. Warfarin falls into which category of drugs?

(A) Category X drugs
(B) Category D drugs

6. Valium falls into which category of drugs?

(A) Category X drugs
(B) Category D drugs

 ANSWERS AND EXPLANATIONS

1. B. The embryonic period (weeks 3–8) is the time when the embryo is most susceptible to teratogens because all organ morphogenesis occurs at this time.

2. A. Week 1 is the resistant period when the conceptus demonstrates the "all-or-none" phenomenon (i.e., the conceptus either dies as a result of the teratogen or survives unaffected).

3. A. Cytomegalovirus is the most common fetal infection and is the cause of cytomegalic inclusion disease.

4. B. *Toxoplasma gondii* is a protozoan parasite found in cats and may be transmitted to the fetus transplacentally.

5. A. Warfarin is a Category X drug.

6. B. Valium is a Category D drug.

A Partial List of Inherited Diseases by Type

Autosomal Dominant	Autosomal Recessive	X-Linked	Mitochondrial	Multifactorial
Achondroplasia	α_1-Antitrypsin deficiency	**Recessive**	Cardiac rhythm disturbances?	Cancer
Acrocephalosyndactyly	Adrenogenital syndromes	Duchenne muscular	Cardiomyopathies?	Cleft lip
Adult polycystic kidney	Albinism	dystrophy	Infantile bilateral striated	Cleft palate
disease	Alpha thalassemia	Ectodermal dysplasia	necrosis	Clubfoot
Alport syndrome	Alkaptonuria	Ehlers-Danlos (Type IX)	Kearns-Sayre syndrome	Congenital heart defects
Apert syndrome	Argininosuccinic aciduria	Fabry disease	Leber hereditary optic	Coronary artery disease
Bor syndrome	Ataxia telangiectasia	Fragile X syndrome	neuropathy	Epilepsy
Brachydactyly	Beta thalassemia	G6PD deficiency		Hemochromatosis
Charcot-Marie-Tooth disease	Bloom syndrome	Hemophilia A and B		Hirschsprung disease
Cleidocranial dysplasia	Branched chain ketonuria	Hunter syndrome		Hyperlipoproteinemia
Crouzon craniofacial	Childhood polycystic kidney	Ichthyosis		(Types I, IIb, III, IV, V)
dysplasia	disease	Kennedy disease		Hypertension
Craniostenosis	Cystic fibrosis	Kinky hair syndrome		Legg-Calvé-Perthes disease
Diabetes associated with	Cystinuria	Lesch-Nyhan syndrome		Pyloric stenosis
defects in genes for	Dwarfism	Testicular feminization		Rheumatic fever
glucokinase, HNF-1α,	Ehlers-Danlos syndrome	Wiskott-Aldrich syndrome		Type 1 diabetes (associated
and HNF-4α	(Type VI)			with islet cell antibodies)
Ehlers-Danlos syndrome	Erythropoietic porphyria	**Dominant**		Type 2 diabetes (associated
(Type IV)	Fanconi anemia	Goltz syndrome		with insulin resistance
Epidermolysis bullosa simplex	Friedreich ataxia	Hypophosphatemic rickets		and obesity)
Familial adenomatous	Fructosuria	Incontinentia pigmenti		
polyposis	Galactosemia	Orofaciodigital syndrome		
Familial hypercholesterolemia	Glycogen storage disease			
(Type IIa)	Von Gierke (Type Ia)			
Goldenhar syndrome	Pompe (Type II)			
Heart-hand syndrome	Cori (Type IIIa)			
Hereditary nonpolyposis	Andersen (Type IV)			
colorectal cancer (HNPCC)	McArdle (Type V)			
Hereditary spherocytosis	Hers (Type VI)			
Huntington disease	Tarui (Type VIII)			
Marfan syndrome	Hemoglobin C disease			

APPENDIX | *A Partial List of Inherited Diseases by Type (continued)*

Autosomal Dominant	Autosomal Recessive	X-Linked	Mitochondrial	Multifactorial
Monilethrix	Hepatolenticular degeneration			
Myotonic dystrophy	Histidinemia			
Neurofibromatosis	Homocystinuria			
Noonan syndrome	Hypophosphatasia			
Osteogenesis imperfecta	Hypothyroidism			
(Types I and IV)	Junctional epidermolysis			
Pfeiffer syndrome	bullosa			
Piebaldism	Laurence-Moon syndrome			
Retinoblastoma	Lysosomal storage diseases			
Treacher Collins syndrome	Tay Sachs			
Uncombable hair syndrome	Gaucher			
Von Willebrand disease	Niemann-Pick			
Waardenburg syndrome	Krabbe			
Williams-Beuren syndrome	Sandhoff			
	Schindler			
	GM1 gangliosidosis			
	Metachromatic			
	Leukodystrophy			
	Mucopolysaccharidoses			
	Hurler			
	Sanfilippo A–D			
	Morquio A and B			
	Maroteaux-Lamy			
	Sly			
	Osteogenesis imperfecta			
	(Types II and III)			
	Oculocutaneous albinism			
	(Types I and II)			
	Peroxisomal disorders			
	Phenylketonuria			
	Premature senility			
	Pyruvate kinase deficiency			
	Retinitis pigmentosa			
	Sickle cell anemia			
	Trichothiodystrophy			
	Tyrosinemia			
	Xeroderma pigmentosa			

1. A 25-year-old woman comes into you office complaining of "spotting" and having "stomach pains" as she points to her lower abdominal area. She noted that she and her husband were trying to have a baby and that she had her last period about 5 weeks ago. She said that after talking with her girlfriends about her symptoms she was a little afraid of what it could be so she decided to see a physician. Her chart shows that she has had a history of pelvic inflammatory disease. Relevant physical exam findings include: a tender palpable pelvic mass, amenorrhea, light vaginal bleeding, and lower abdominal pain. Relevant laboratory findings include: elevated β-hCG levels but lower than expected for pregnancy, lower than normal progesterone levels, and a mass in the ampulla of the left uterine tube (shown by ultrasound). Which of the following is the most likely diagnosis?

A.   Choriocarcinoma
B.   A bleeding corpus luteum
C.   A spontaneous abortion
D.   Ectopic tubal pregnancy
E.   Appendicitis

2. A 31-year-old woman comes into the office complaining of "running a fever," being nauseated, and losing weight ("about 15 pounds or so") over the last month. She tells you that she had a miscarriage about 2 months ago and "all of a sudden these other problems come up." She adds that the doctors said she had "preeclampsia" during her first trimester of that pregnancy. She says she was supposed to come back in but didn't because she "felt depressed about losing the baby." She remarks that she hasn't had any changes in her diet and remarked she "thought she would have gained weight with all the food she was eating." Relevant physical exam findings include: normal thyroid gland upon palpation, no coughing of blood, and no diarrhea. Relevant laboratory findings include: elevated hCG levels, and normal T_4 and TSH (thyroid stimulating hormone) levels. Which of the following is the most likely diagnosis?

A.   Achalasia
B.   Hyperthyroidism
C.   Pelvic inflammatory disease
D.   Hydatidiform mole

E.   Gestational trophoblastic neoplasia (or choriocarcinoma)

3. A 37-year-old woman who is in her third trimester comes into your clinic complaining of bleeding that lasted for about "an hour or two." She remarks that she noticed the bleeding was "very bright red" in color, but felt no noticeable pain. She says she did nothing to cause the bleeding and "is concerned for the safety of her baby." Relevant physical exam findings include: no abdominal or pelvic pain could be found upon palpation. Relevant laboratory findings include: transvaginal ultrasound shows an intact, normally implanted placenta; however, the placenta is located in close proximity of the internal os. Which of the following is the most likely diagnosis?

A.   Placenta previa
B.   Placental abruption
C.   Placenta accreta
D.   Velamentous placenta
E.   Membranous placenta

4. A 34-year-old woman who is in her third trimester complains of her hands and face "swelling up a few days ago." She remarks that she has also felt like "her heart was racing a mile a minute." Relevant physical exam findings include: hypertension (>160/110 mm Hg) and edema of the hands and face. Relevant laboratory findings include: proteinuria (> 5 g/24 hours) and ultrasound are unremarkable. Which of the following is the most likely diagnosis?

A.   Molar pregnancy
B.   Severe preeclampsia
C.   Choriocarcinoma
D.   Ectopic tubal pregnancy
E.   Placental abruption

5. A distraught mother brings her 2-month-old daughter into your office, saying that she noticed a "lump growing from her child's bottom." She states she "noticed it about 2 weeks ago while changing her daughter's diaper." The lump was small and she so didn't think much of it, but over time it has "grown to the size of a baseball." Relevant physical exam findings include: a large spheroid mass that appeared to be very firm upon palpation. Relevant labora-

tory findings include: biopsy of the mass shows tissue containing hair, teeth, muscle fibers, and thyroid follicular cells. Which of the following is the most likely diagnosis?

A. Spina bifida with meningocele
B. Sacrococcygeal teratoma
C. Spina bifida with meningomyelocele
D. Chordoma
E. Caudal dysplasia (Sirenomelia)

6. After the delivery of a healthy baby girl, a physician noticed a tuft of hair on the lower back of the child. The physician asked the mother about her prenatal health care and she said she did not take folic acid until the second month of pregnancy because she didn't know she was pregnant until then. Relevant physical exam findings include: a tuft of hair on the lower back with no noticeable sac formation. Relevant laboratory findings include: radiograph shows a defect in the vertebral arches but no sac filled with fluid or spinal cord. Which of the following is the most likely diagnosis?

A. Spina bifida with meningocele
B. Spina bifida with meningomyelocele
C. Spina bifida occulta
D. Spina bifida with rachischisis
E. Caudal dysplasia (Sirenomelia)

7. A distraught father comes in with his 10-year-old son, saying that his son began "turning blue" when he was out playing catch with him. His son remarked that he "just felt really tired" when he was running after the ball. He is concerned that his son will not be able to play in the big game this weekend. Relevant physical exam findings include: loud holosystolic ejection murmur on auscultation, cyanosis, and clubbing of fingernails. Relevant laboratory findings include: ECG shows right ventricular hypertrophy. Which of the following is the most likely diagnosis?

A. Membranous ventricular septal defect
B. Eisenmenger's complex
C. Atrial septal defect
D. Patent ductus arteriosus
E. Coarctation of the aorta

8. A 39-year-old man comes to your office complaining of "heartburn after trying to eat" and not being able to swallow anything. He states, "I have tried everything from water to steaks; it doesn't matter what I eat I always have trouble swallowing it down." Relevant physical exam findings include: dysphagia and normal thyroid upon palpation. Relevant laboratory findings include: barium swallow radiograph shows a dilated esophagus with an area of distal stenosis (almost looks like a "bird's beak") and normal T_4 levels. Which of the following is the most likely diagnosis?

A. Esophageal atresia
B. Thyroid tumor
C. Esophageal stenosis
D. Reflux esophagitis
E. Achalasia

9. A mother brings her 1-month-old son into the clinic complaining of her son "vomiting all over the place when he tries to eat something." She says her son's vomiting looks like it was "shot out of a cannon." Relevant physical findings include: a small non-tender palpable mass on right costal margin. Relevant laboratory findings include: barium swallow radiograph shows a narrow pyloric channel and abdominal ultrasound shows a hypertrophic pylorus. Which of the following is the most likely diagnosis?

A. Esophageal hiatal hernia
B. Hypertrophic pyloric stenosis
C. Malrotation of the midgut with volvulus
D. Esophageal stenosis
E. Biliary atresia

10. A man brings his 3-year-old son into the office complaining that his son is having "bad stomach pains" and talks about him "running a fever" and "being thirsty all the time." He remarks that his son has not had a bowel movement lately. Relevant physical exam findings include: painless rectal bleeding, dark red stools, and abdominal distention. Relevant laboratory findings include: radiograph shows a remnant of the vitelline duct that was estimated to be about 2 feet from the ileocecal valve and a biopsy shows ectopic gastric and pancreatic mucosal tissue. Which of the following is the most likely diagnosis?

A. Volvulus
B. Intussusception
C. Foreign body obstruction
D. Meckel's diverticulum
E. Biliary atresia

11. A nurse comes into your office informing you that the child you delivered yesterday failed to pass meconium. The nurse remarks that the child also cries upon palpation of the

abdominal area. Relevant physical exam finding include: abdominal distention, megacolon upon palpation, and gushing of fecal material upon a rectal digital exam. Relevant laboratory findings include: barium enema shows dilated proximal segment and a narrow distal segment of the sigmoid colon. Which of the following is the most likely diagnosis?

A. Rectal atresia
B. Rectovesical fistula
C. Hirschsprung's disease
D. Anorectal agenesis
E. Intussusception

12. A 33-year-old man comes in complaining of "fever and chills" and that he "has to constantly go to the bathroom." He also indicates that he has pain just below the abdominal area on the right side. He states he has not had sexual intercourse in over 6 months. He suspects that it may be a urinary tract infection because he "has had a lot of them over the years." Relevant physical exam findings include: flank pain and costovertebral angle tenderness. Relevant laboratory findings include: normal calcium levels and CT scan shows an unusual kidney appearance. Which of the following is the most likely diagnosis?

A. Urachal fistula
B. Horseshoe kidney
C. Pyelonephritis
D. Kidney stones
E. Polycystic kidney disease

13. A 16-month-old boy has had recurrent bouts of cyanosis since birth. His parents tell you that "he cannot keep up with the other children his age." The parents indicate that their boy frequently turns blue, breathes heavily upon exertion, and sometimes experiences these difficulties for no reason. On many occasions, they have observed their son in a squatting position. Relevant physical exam findings include: systolic ejection murmur, cyanosis, clubbing of the fingernails, and a parasternal heave. Relevant laboratory findings include: radiographs show an enlarged right ventricle and "boot-shaped" heart, EKG shows right ventricular hypertrophy, echocardiogram shows pulmonary stenosis, right ventricular hypertrophy, overriding aorta, and a ventricular septal defect. Which of the following is the most likely diagnosis?

A. Tetralogy of Fallot
B. Tricuspid atresia

C. Total anomalous pulmonary venous return
D. Transposition of the great arteries
E. Persistent truncus arteriosus

14. A 40-year-old mother brings in her new 4-week-old baby boy and tells you that "my baby's face looks funny and he keeps sticking his tongue out." The mother recalls that during the pregnancy she had low α-fetoprotein (AFP) levels. Relevant physical exam findings include: a flat occiput; white spots in his iris (Brushfield spots); a large, protruding tongue; small, low-set ears; short feet and hands; a flexion crease across his palms (simian crease); curvature of the fifth digit; systolic ejection murmur; and hypotonia. Relevant laboratory findings include: echocardiogram shows an endocardial cushion defect (atrioventricular septal defect), karyotype analysis shows an extra chromosome 21. Which of the following is the most likely diagnosis?

A. Cri du chat syndrome
B. Edwards syndrome
C. Fragile X syndrome
D. Down syndrome
E. Patau syndrome

15. A 25-year-old woman who is a CEO of a new biotech company has been under considerable stress this past year trying to negotiate a contract with a major drug company. She has also been under a very rigorous exercise program because "she just can't stand any fat on her body" and ran in the Boston marathon 4 months ago. Because of her busy schedule, her eating habits have radically changed and sometimes "the sight of food just disgusts me." She is not on any drug medication. She tells you that recently she met "the guy" and has been sexually active with him for "about 2 months now." She comes to you because her menstrual cycle is 2 weeks late and sometimes she feels nauseous, especially in the morning. Relevant physical exam findings are unremarkable. Relevant laboratory findings include: a positive β-human chorionic gonadotropin (hCG) test. Which of the following is the most likely diagnosis?

A. Secondary amenorrhea resulting from stress
B. Secondary amenorrhea resulting from anorexia nervosa
C. Pregnancy
D. Turner syndrome
E. Secondary amenorrhea resulting from antipsychotic drug therapy

16. A father brings his 1-month-old daughter into the clinic complaining that his daughter frequently "throws up after she eats," and "it just shoots across the room." Relevant physical exam findings include: projectile vomiting when the infant is laid on its back after a feeding. Relevant laboratory findings include: radiograph shows a portion of the stomach located in the pleural cavity. Which of the following is the most likely diagnosis?

A. Hypertrophic pyloric stenosis
B. Gastroesophageal reflux disease
C. Esophageal hiatal hernia
D. Congenital diaphragmatic hernia
E. Tracheoesophageal fistula

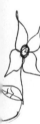

17. A father brings his 4-year-old daughter into the clinic. He says he noticed "a lump on her lower right side" and that "it has gotten bigger over time." Relevant physical exam findings include: a large, palpable mass on the right flank and no evidence of a urinary tract infection (UTI). Relevant laboratory findings include: normal catecholamine levels, normal androgen levels, and genetic testing reveals a deletion of a tumor suppression gene on chromosome 11. Which of the following is the most likely diagnosis?

A. Neuroblastoma
B. Pheochromocytoma
C. Congenital adrenal hyperplasia
D. Wilms' tumor
E. Childhood polycystic kidney disease

18. A 45-year-old man comes in complaining of chest and abdominal pain. He also says that his "blood pressure rises every so often" even when he is relaxing at home and that "it's been happening more and more." He says he exercises often and tries to stay in shape because he has a family history of obesity. Relevant physical exam findings include: profuse sweating, hypertension, abdominal discomfort, and lungs clear on auscultation. Relevant laboratory findings include: radiograph is negative for a pulmonary embolism, hyperglycemia, increased urinary vanillylmandelic acid (VMA) and metanephrine levels, and inability to suppress catecholamines with clonidine. Which of the following is the most likely diagnosis?

A. Angina
B. Pneumothorax
C. Myocardial infarction

D. Neuroblastoma
E. Pheochromocytoma

19. A woman comes in with her 16-year-old daughter and states that her daughter "has not had a menstrual period yet." The daughter says that she is not sexually active and that she is not on any form of birth control. Relevant physical exam findings include: ambiguous genitalia, amenorrhea, and early appearance of axillary and pubic hair. Relevant laboratory findings include: elevated urinary 17-ketosteroids, elevated serum DHEA sulfate, normal or decreased 17-hydroxycorticosteroids, genetic testing reveals 46, XX genotype, and CT head scan reveals no sign of tumor. Which of the following is the most likely diagnosis?

A. Female pseudointersexuality
B. Turner syndrome
C. Complete androgen insensitivity
D. Pituitary tumor
E. Male pseudointersexuality

20. A concerned couple brings their 3-week-old son into your office stating that they think something is wrong with his genital area. They noticed that his testicles appeared to be swollen when they were changing his diaper a week ago. They said that his scrotum felt like a "water-filled balloon." Neither parent could recall any traumatic episode with their son, saying that they have been very protective of him. Relevant physical exam findings include: an enlarged, nontender scrotum, testicles are not immediately palpable, no herniated bulge found, and flashlight test through the enlarged area showed illumination. Relevant laboratory findings include: absence of blood upon fluid collection. Which of the following is the most likely diagnosis?

A. Hypospadias
B. Hematocele
C. Congenital inguinal hernia
D. Cryptorchidism
E. Hydrocele of the testes

21. A mother brings her 5-year-old son into your office for a follow-up visit. The child previously had a bout with pneumonia and the mother remarked that the child has been coughing up "yellow and green stuff." The mother mentions that he has had a number of coughs and colds that were just like this in the past. Relevant physical exam findings include: foul-smelling greenish sputum with speckles of blood, orthopnea, and fever; and his chart is remarkable for cystic fibrosis. Relevant laboratory findings include: spirometry shows a reduced FEV_1/FVC ratio; radiograph shows multiple cysts that have a "honeycomb" appearance; and CT scan shows a dilation of bronchi. Which of the following is the most likely diagnosis?

A. Asthma
B. Bronchitis
C. Bronchiectasis
D. Pneumonia
E. Influenza

22. While delivering a newborn baby girl, you notice that she has abnormal facies but otherwise the delivery was uncomplicated. About 48 hours after birth, the baby girl developed seizures and muscle spasms. The baby girl is lethargic, mildly tachypneic, and jittery. Relevant physical findings include: peculiar facies, low-set ears, widely spaced eyes, small mandible, no detectable thymus upon palpation, muscle rigidity, harsh holosystolic murmur along the lower left sternal border, and a slight cyanotic tinge to the skin. Relevant laboratory findings include: hypocalcemia, a low T lymphocyte count, radiograph shows absent thymic shadow, and cardiac ultrasound shows a congenital heart defect in the conotruncal region, and genetic testing reveals a deletion on chromosome 22q. Which of the following is the most likely diagnosis?

A. Patau syndrome
B. DiGeorge syndrome
C. Miller-Diecker syndrome
D. Prader-Willi syndrome
E. Treacher Collins syndrome

23. After delivery of a baby boy, you notice that the infant has microcephaly, polydactyly, hypotelorism, cleft lip and palate, and an omphalocele. Unfortunately, the baby boy dies soon after birth. The mother of the baby boy is 43 years old and tells you, "I can't believe God did this to me, I took such good care of myself while I was pregnant." Relevant physical findings include: small head (microcephaly), polydactyly, close set eyes (hypotelorism), cleft lip and palate, and omphalocele. Relevant laboratory findings include: ultrasound shows congenital heart defects, CT scan shows holoprosencephaly, and karyotype analysis shows an extra chromosome 13. Which of the following is the most likely diagnosis?

A. Down syndrome
B. Fragile X syndrome
C. Patau syndrome
D. Cri du chat
E. Angelman syndrome

24. A mother brings in her 2-year-old son to the clinic stating that she "thinks her son can't hear her when she calls to him." She also indicates that he seems "slower mentally than the other kids" and he isn't "saying any words like 'Mommy.'" Her son has been in and out of the hospital a lot because of congenital heart defects and recently had his cataracts removed. She remarks that while she was pregnant toward the beginning she was a little sick and "broke out in a rash," but she thinks that "was caused by a new lotion she was using." Relevant physical exam findings include: microcephaly, deafness, hepatosplenomegaly, blueberry muffin spots, and a hint of jaundice. Which of the following is the most likely diagnosis?

A. HIV infection
B. Herpes simplex virus infection
C. Rubella virus infection
D. Patau syndrome
E. Down syndrome

25. A young mother brings in her 3-year-old son because of "a white spot in his right eye" that she first noticed in a photograph taken 2 weeks ago. She also tells you that "he seems to be always squinting with his right eye." She remembers hearing about a distant family member with the same sort of spot who eventually went blind. Relevant physical exam findings include: leukocoria (whitish spots in the pupillary area behind the lens), strabismus (squinting; deviation of the eye that the patient cannot overcome), poor vision in the right eye, and curious family history. Relevant laboratory findings include: CT scan shows a solid intraocular tumor with intratumoral calcifications and genetic testing reveals a deletion on chromosome 13q. Which of the following is the most likely diagnosis?

A. Congenital cataract
B. Congenital glaucoma
C. Retinitis pigmentosa
D. Papilledema
E. Retinoblastoma

26. A father brings his 8-year-old son to the clinic and tells you that "he is bleeding a lot" and that "the kid comes in from playing with a lot of bruises." When talking to the son, he tells you that he is "one of the coolest kids in school" because "he can pull his skin out all over the place." Then, he proceeds to demonstrate this fact by pulling his ears out several inches away from his body. His father tells you that last year his son was rushed to the hospital and had emergency surgery because "he had a hole in his intestines." Relevant physical findings include: highly elastic, velvety skin; fragile skin that bruises easily; loose, unstable, hypermobile joints. Relevant laboratory findings include: Genetic testing reveals a mutation in the gene for peptidyl lysine hydroxylase. Which of the following is the most likely diagnosis?

A. Ehlers-Danlos syndrome
B. Marfan syndrome
C. Junctional epidermolysis bullosa
D. Osteogenesis imperfecta
E. Achondroplasia

27. A frantic father rushes his 1-year-old daughter to your clinic saying that he "thinks his daughter's leg is broken." He says, "this is the third time my daughter has broken a bone in the last 2 months;" and he thinks his wife may be abusing the child while he is at work. Relevant physical exam findings include: short, deformed limbs, blue sclera of the eye, kyphoscoliosis, and medical history indicates that there may have been bone fractures at birth. Relevant laboratory findings include: radiographs show multiple, healed fractures of the limbs; and genetic testing reveals a mutation in the gene for Type 1 collagen on chromosome 7q22. Which of the following is the most likely diagnosis?

A. Marfan syndrome
B. Child abuse
C. Osteogenesis imperfecta
D. Ehlers-Danlos syndrome
E. Achondroplasia

28. A 22-year-old man comes into the office complaining of blurred vision. He states that he "has not had problems seeing before." He remarks that "his dad and sister had the same problem around his age." Relevant physical exam findings include: long, spidery fingers (arachnodactyly), hypermobile joints, arm span much greater than body height, and dislocation of lens (ectopia lentis). Relevant laboratory findings include: CT scan shows a dilated aorta; and genetic testing reveals a mutation for the fibrillin-1 gene on chromosome 15q21.1. Which of the following is the most likely diagnosis?

A. Marfan syndrome
B. Klippel-Feil syndrome
C. Osteogenesis imperfecta
D. Ehlers-Danlos syndrome
E. Achondroplasia

29. A father brings his 12-year-old son in and tells you that "his son is feeling weakness in his legs and is beginning to fall a lot." The father says "he can't run as good as he used to." He also says it's gotten so bad that when "he is sitting down he has to put his hands on his thighs just to stand up." Relevant physical exam findings include: rapidly progressive muscle weakness with frequent falls; muscle wasting in the legs and pelvis and progressing to shoulders and neck; and, pseudohypertrophy of calf muscles. Relevant laboratory findings include: no sign of myoglobulinuria, highly elevated creatine phosphokinase (CPK), EMG (electromyography) shows weakness resulting from muscle tissue destruction and not nerve damage, and genetic testing reveals a mutation on chromosome Xp21. Which of the following is the most likely diagnosis?

A. Achondroplasia
B. Myasthenia gravis
C. McArdle disease
D. Polymyositis
E. Duchenne muscular dystrophy

30. A mother comes in with her 16-year-old daughter. Her daughter tells you that "she has not had a menstrual period yet." The daughter indicates to you that she is not sexually active and that she is not on any form of birth control. The mother informs you that her daughter had surgery to repair a coarctation of the aorta when she was 6 months old but that "is probably not related to this menstrual problem." Relevant physical findings include: short stature, webbed neck, indications of a fetal cystic hygroma, absent menstruation (primary amenorrhea), shield-shaped chest with widely spaced pinpoint nipples, a low posterior hairline, and a small uterus. Relevant laboratory findings include: ultrasound shows small,

fibrous "streak" ovaries bilaterally; CT scan shows no signs of a tumor; karyotype analysis reveals a 45, XO genotype; buccal smear shows no Barr body; and high follicle-stimulating hormone (FSH) levels. Which of the following is the most likely diagnosis?

A. Congenital adrenal hyperplasia
B. Turner syndrome
C. Klinefelter syndrome
D. Female pseudointersexuality
E. Pituitary tumor

31. A mother brings in her 5-year-old son at the request of his summer camp counselor, who claims, "the boy is hyperactive and doesn't seem to be as smart as the other kids." The mother agrees, but has not done anything about until now. The mother indicates that her son was "pretty small at birth" and had a ventricular septal defect that was repaired soon after birth. The mother further tells you that "except for being small and the heart problem everything else in the pregnancy was just fine; but you know I did have a drink every now and then." Relevant physical exam findings include: hypertelorism, smooth philtrum, short palpebral fissures, flat nasal bridge, maxillary (midface) hypoplasia, and a thin upper lip. Relevant laboratory findings include: MRI shows holoprosencephaly. Which of the following is the most likely diagnosis?

A. Alcohol consumption during pregnancy
B. Thalidomide consumption during pregnancy
C. Phenytoin consumption during pregnancy
D. Prader-Willi syndrome
E. Wolf-Hirschhorn syndrome

32. A 25-year-old woman who is 32 weeks pregnant comes into the emergency room while in labor. The infant is stillborn. The mother is obviously upset and says "I want to know what happened." Although the mother had no prenatal care, she says "I am shocked that something went wrong because I had no problems with my first pregnancy; that baby is fine." The mother is sincere when she states that she did not smoke or drink alcohol during the pregnancy. The mother says, "Everything was going along just fine with this pregnancy until just a few hours ago." The mother requests an autopsy on the infant. Relevant physical findings of the autopsy include: the

body is swollen and jaundiced; yellow deposits in several areas of the brain, especially the basal ganglia; and ascites. Relevant laboratory findings of the autopsy include: severe anemia, high serum bilirubin levels, infant's blood type O positive. Further lab tests were done on the blood of the mother and father. The mother's blood was O negative. The father's blood was O positive. Which of the following is the most likely diagnosis?

A. Oligohydramnios
B. Polyhydramnios
C. Severe preeclampsia
D. Erythroblastosis fetalis
E. Placental abruption

33. A mother brings in her 6-week-old infant son because "I just want him to get checked out." She further tells you that "You know, he was born prematurely and thank God he didn't have any serious breathing problems; but I'm still worried." Relevant physical exam findings include: the infant is small but active, appears to be mildly short of breath, and a harsh, machine-like, continuous murmur in the upper left parasternal area. Which of the following is the most likely diagnosis?

A. Coarctation of the aorta
B. Membranous ventricular septal defect
C. Patent ductus arteriosus
D. Double aortic arch
E. Tetralogy of Fallot

34. A mother brings in her newborn baby girl and says, "my baby coughs and gags every time I try to feed her; one time she even turned blue and it scared me." The mother also indicates that her baby always has a "mouthful of saliva." Relevant physical exam findings include: a distended stomach, excessive saliva accumulation, a hint of pneumonitis, and inability to pass a catheter into the infant's stomach. Relevant laboratory findings include: radiograph shows a large amount of air in the stomach. Which of the following is the most likely diagnosis?

A. Esophageal hiatal hernia
B. Hypertrophic pyloric stenosis
C. Tracheoesophageal fistula
D. Respiratory distress syndrome
E. Congenital diaphragmatic hernia

35. A 30-year-old man comes to your office for a routine checkup. He has not real specific complaints but tells you, "my wife and I have been trying to have a baby for 3 years now; but no luck." Relevant physical exam findings include: the man is quite tall, thin, long legs, with a youthful appearance; little facial or axillary hair; gynecomastia is quite noticeable; testicles are small and firm; and penis is normal. Relevant laboratory findings include: low testosterone levels; high follicle-stimulating hormone (FSH) levels; no sperm in semen sample; and buccal smear reveals occasional cells with Barr bodies. Which of the following is the most likely diagnosis?

A. Turner syndrome
B. Klinefelter syndrome
C. Complete androgen insensitivity syndrome
D. Female pseudointersexuality
E. Congenital adrenal hyperplasia

ANSWERS AND EXPLANATIONS

1. D. Ectopic tubal pregnancy (ETP). ETP occurs when the blastocyst implants within the uterine tube because of delayed transport. The ampulla of the uterine tube is the most common site of an ectopic pregnancy. The rectouterine pouch (pouch of Douglas) is a common site for an ectopic abdominal pregnancy. ETP is most commonly seen in women with endometriosis or pelvic inflammatory disease. ETP leads to uterine tube rupture and hemorrhage if surgical intervention (i.e., salpingectomy) is not performed. ETP presents with abnormal uterine bleeding and unilateral pelvic pain, which must be differentially diagnosed from appendicitis, an aborting intrauterine pregnancy, or a bleeding corpus luteum of a normal intrauterine pregnancy.

2. E. Gestational trophoblastic neoplasia (GTN; or choriocarcinoma). GTN is a malignant tumor of the trophoblast that may occur following a normal or ectopic pregnancy, abortion, or hydatidiform mole. With a high degree of suspicion, elevated hCG levels are diagnostic. Nonmetastatic GTN (i.e., confined to the uterus) is the most common form of the neoplasia and treatment is highly successful. However, the prognosis of metastatic GTN is poor if it spreads to the liver or brain.

3. A. Placenta previa. Placenta previa occurs when the placenta attaches in the lower part of the uterus, covering the internal os. The placenta normally implants in the posterior superior wall of the uterus. Uterine (maternal) blood vessels rupture during the later part of pregnancy as the uterus begins to gradually dilate. The mother may bleed to death, and the fetus will also be placed in jeopardy because of the compromised blood supply. Because the placenta blocks the cervical opening, delivery is usually accomplished by cesarean section. This condition is clinically associated with repeated episodes of bright, red vaginal bleeding. Placental abruption would have shown a separation of the placenta and showed dark red bleeding accompanied by abdominal pain. Placenta accreta would have shown the placenta implanted much deeper in the myometrium.

4. B. Severe preeclampsia. Preeclampsia is a complication of pregnancy characterized by hypertension, edema, and/or proteinuria. Severe preeclampsia refers to the sudden development of maternal hypertension (>160/110 mm Hg), edema (hands and/or face), and proteinuria (>5 g/24 hr) usually after week 32 of gestation (third trimester). Eclampsia includes the additional symptom of convulsions. The pathophysiology of preeclampsia involves a generalized arteriolar constriction that impacts the brain (seizures and stroke), kidneys (oliguria and renal failure), liver (edema), and small blood vessels (thrombocytopenia and disseminated intravascular coagulation). Treatment of severe preeclampsia involves magnesium sulfate (for seizure prophylaxis) and hydralazine (blood pressure control). Once the patient is stabilized, delivery of the fetus should ensue immediately. Risk factors include: nulliparity, diabetes, hypertension, renal disease, twin gestation, or hydatidiform mole (produces first trimester preeclampsia). Her symptoms of hypertension, proteinuria, and edema are all telltale signs of preeclampsia. Also her advancing age makes her susceptible to this condition. A molar pregnancy is normally seen in the first trimester. Renal disease is unlikely because there were no other findings other than proteinuria.

5. B. Sacrococcygeal teratoma (ST). ST is a tumor that arises from remnants of the primitive streak, which normally degenerates and disappears. ST is derived from pluripotent cells of the primitive streak and often contains various types of tissue (e.g., bone, nerve, hair). ST occurs more commonly in female infants and usually becomes malignant during infancy (must be removed by age 6 months). Caudal dysplasia (sirenomelia) refers to a constellation of syndromes ranging from minor lesions of lower vertebrae to complete fusion of the lower limbs. Caudal dysplasia is caused by abnormal gastrulation, in which the migration of mesoderm is disturbed. Spina bifida occurs when the bony vertebral arches fail to form properly, thereby creating a vertebral defect usually in the lumbosacral region.

6. C. Spina bifida occulta. Spina bifida occurs when the bony vertebral arches fail to form properly, thereby creating a vertebral defect usually in the lumbosacral region. Spina bifida occulta is evidenced by a tuft of hair in the lumbosacral region. Spina bifida occulta is the least severe variation and occurs in 10% of the population. Spina bifida with meningocele occurs when the meninges protrude through a vertebral defect and form a sac filled with CSF. The spinal cord remains in its normal position. Spina bifida with meningomyelocele occurs when the meninges and spinal cord protrude through a vertebral defect and form a sac filled with CSF. Spina bifida with rachischisis occurs when the posterior neuropore of the neural tube fails to close during week 4 of development. This condition is the most severe type of spina bifida causing paralysis from the level of the defect caudally.

7. A. Membranous ventricular septal defect (VSD). Membranous VSD is caused by faulty fusion of the right bulbar ridge, left bulbar ridge, and AV cushions. It results in a condition in which an opening between the right and left ventricles allows free flow of blood. A large VSD is initially associated with an L → R shunting of blood, increased pulmonary blood flow, and pulmonary hypertension. One of the secondary effects of a large VSD and its associated pulmonary hypertension is proliferation of the tunica intima and tunica media of pulmonary muscular arteries and arterioles resulting in a narrowing of their lumen. Ultimately, pulmonary resistance may become higher than systemic resistance and cause R → L shunting of blood and cyanosis. At this stage, the characteristic of the patient has been termed the Eisenmenger complex. This is the most common type of VSD. An atrial septal defect (ASD) would have a fixed, split S2, systolic ejection murmur. A patent ductus arteriosus (PDA), which is normally detected in infants, would have a continuous machine-like murmur. Coarctation of the aorta would show a holosystolic murmur; however, there was no finding of a lack of a femoral pulse or rib notching.

8. E. Achalasia. Achalasia occurs because of the loss of ganglion cells in the myenteric (Auerbach) plexus and is characterized by the failure to relax the lower esophageal sphincter, which causes progressive dysphagia and difficulty in swallowing. The "bird's beak" appearance on the radiograph is a telltale sign of achalasia. Another telltale sign is that patients have a dysphagia involving both solids and liquids. The physical and lab findings exclude both thyroid disease and masses. Although reflux esophagitis would present with heartburn, it is limited to dysphagia of solids only; not solids and liquid.

9. B. Hypertrophic pyloric stenosis. Hypertrophic pyloric stenosis occurs when the muscularis externa in the pyloric region hypertrophies, causing a narrow pyloric lumen that obstructs food passage. It is associated clinically with projectile, non-bilious vomiting after feeding and a small, palpable mass at the right costal margin. An increased incidence of hypertrophic pyloric stenosis has been found in infants treated with the antibiotic erythromycin.

10. D. Meckel's diverticulum. Meckel's diverticulum (ileal diverticulum) occurs when a remnant of the vitelline duct persists, thereby forming an outpouching located on the antimesenteric border of the ileum. The outpouching may connect to the umbilicus via a fibrous cord or fistula. A Meckel's diverticulum is usually located about 30 cm proximal to the ileocecal valve in infants and varies in length from 2 to 15 cm. Heterotopic gastric or pancreatic mucosa may be present, which leads to ulceration, perforation, or gastrointestinal bleeding, especially if a large number of parietal cells are present. It is associated clinically with symptoms resembling appendicitis and bright-red or dark-red stools (i.e., bloody).

11. C. Hirschsprung disease (colonic aganglionosis). Hirschsprung disease is caused by the arrest of the caudal migration of neural crest cells. The hallmark is the absence of ganglionic cells in the myenteric and submucosal plexuses, most commonly in the sigmoid colon and rectum, resulting in a narrow segment of colon (i.e., the colon fails to relax). Although the ganglionic cells are absent, there is a proliferation of hypertrophied nerve fiber bundles. The most characteristic functional finding is the failure of internal anal sphincter to relax after rectal distention (i.e., abnormal rectoanal reflex). Mutations of the RET protooncogene (chromosome 10q.11.2) have been associated with Hirschsprung disease. It is associated clinically with a distended abdomen, inability to pass meconium, gushing of fecal material upon a rectal digital exam, and loss of peristalsis in the colon segment distal to the normal innervated colon.

12. B. Horseshoe kidney. The man's symptoms (fevers, chills, flank pain, and costovertebral angle tenderness) are classic signs of pyelonephritis resulting from a urinary tract infection (UTI). In this case, the UTI results from a urinary tract obstruction caused by a horseshoe kidney. The most common type of renal fusion is the horseshoe kidney. A horseshoe kidney occurs when the inferior poles of the kidneys fuse across the midline. Normal ascent of the kidneys is arrested because the fused portion gets trapped behind the inferior mesenteric artery. Kidney rotation is also arrested so that the hilum faces ventrally.

13. A. Tetralogy of Fallot (TF). TF is caused by an abnormal neural crest cell migration such that there is *skewed* development of the AP septum. TF results in a condition in which the pulmonary trunk obtains a small diameter while the aorta obtains a large diameter. TF is characterized by four classic malformations: **p**ulmonary stenosis, **r**ight ventricular hypertrophy, **o**verriding aorta, and a **ve**ntricular septal defect (VSD). Note the mnemonic PROVE. TF is associated clinically with marked cyanosis, whereby the clinical consequences depend primarily on the severity of the pulmonary stenosis.

14. D. Down syndrome (Trisomy 21). This is characterized by moderate mental retardation (the leading cause of inherited mental retardation), microcephaly, microphthalmia, colobomata, cataracts and glaucoma, flat nasal bridge, epicanthic folds, protruding tongue, simian crease in hand, increased nuchal skin folds, appearance of an "X" across the face when the baby cries as the upward slanted palpebral fissures run in a line with the nasolabial folds, and congenital heart defects. Alzheimer neurofibrillary tangles and plaques are found in Down syndrome patients after 30 years of age. Acute megakaryocytic leukemia (AMKL) is frequently present. Trisomy 21 is the most common type of trisomy whose frequency increases with advanced maternal age. Trisomy 21 is associated with low α-fetoprotein levels in amniotic fluid or maternal serum. A specific region on chromosome 21 seems to be markedly associated with numerous features of Trisomy 21. This region is called DSCR (Down syndrome critical region). The following genes have been mapped to the DSCR (although their role is far from clear): carbonyl reductase, SIM2 (a transcription factor), p60 subunit of chromatin assembly factor, holocarboxylase synthetase, ERG (a protooncogene), GIRK2 (a K^+ ion channel), and PEP19 (a Ca^{2+} dependent signal transducer). Trisomy 21 may also be caused by a chromosomal translocation between chromosomes 14 and 21 [i.e., t(14;21)].

15. C. Pregnancy. Amenorrhea can be primary or secondary. Primary amenorrhea is the complete absence of menstruation in a woman from puberty. The most common cause of primary amenorrhea is Turner syndrome. Secondary amenorrhea is the absence of menstruation for at least 3 months in a woman who previously had normal menstruation. Many factors can cause secondary amenorrhea, including stress, anorexia nervosa, elevated prolactin levels (e.g., prolactinoma or antipsychotic drug therapy), and pregnancy. Of these factors, only pregnancy is associated with a positive hCG test.

16. C. Esophageal hiatal hernia. Esophageal hiatal hernia is a herniation of the stomach through the esophageal hiatus into the pleural cavity caused by an abnormally large esophageal hiatus. An esophageal hiatal hernia renders the esophagogastric sphincter incompetent so that stomach contents reflux into the esophagus. Clinical signs in the newborn include vomiting (frequently projectile) when the infant is laid on its back after feeding.

17. D. Wilms' tumor (WT). WT is the most common renal malignancy of childhood. WT presents as a large, solitary, well-circumscribed mass that on cut section is soft, homogeneous, and tan-gray in color. WT is interesting histologically in that this tumor tends to recapitulate different stages of embryological formation of the kidney so that three classic histological areas are described: a stromal area; a blastemal area of tightly packed embryonic cells; and a tubular area. Neuroblastoma is ruled out because there was no mention of an increase in urine VMA and metanephrine levels.

18. E. Pheochromocytoma (PH). PH is a relatively rare neoplasm that contains both epinephrine and norepinephrine. PH occurs mainly in adults 40 to 60 years old and is generally found in the region of the adrenal gland but may be found in extra suprarenal sites. PH is associated with persistent or paroxysmal hypertension, anxiety, tremor, profuse sweating, pallor, chest pain, and abdominal pain. Laboratory findings include: increased urine VMA and metanephrine levels, inability to suppress catecholamines with clonidine, and hyperglycemia. PH is treated by surgery or phenoxybenzamine (an α-adrenergic antagonist).

19. A. Female pseudointersexuality (FP). FP occurs when an individual has only ovarian tissue histologically and masculinization of the female external genitalia. These individuals have a 46,XX genotype. FP is most often observed clinically in association with a condition in which the fetus produces an excess of androgens [e.g., congenital adrenal hyperplasia (CAH)]. CAH is caused most commonly by mutations in genes for enzymes involved in adrenocortical steroid biosynthesis (e.g., 21-hydroxylase deficiency, 11β-hydroxylase deficiency). In 21-hydroxylase deficiency (90% of all cases), there is virtually no synthesis of the cortisol or aldosterone so that intermediates are funneled into androgen biosynthesis, thereby elevating androgen levels. The elevated levels of androgens lead to masculinization of a female fetus. FP produces the following clinical findings: mild clitoral enlargement, complete labioscrotal fusion with a phalloid organ, or macrogenitosomia (in the male fetus). Since cortisol cannot be synthesized, negative feedback to the adenohypophysis does not occur, so ACTH continues to stimulate the adrenal cortex resulting in adrenal hyperplasia. Since aldosterone cannot be synthesized, the patient presents with hyponatremia ("salt-wasting") with adjoining dehydration and hyperkalemia. Treatment includes: immediate infusion of intravenous saline and long-term steroid hormone replacement, both cortisol and mineralocorticoids (9α-fludrocortisone). Although Turner syndrome is also a cause of primary amenorrhea, individuals with Turner syndrome have a 45,XO genotype. A pituitary tumor can be excluded because of negative CT scan findings.

20. E. Hydrocele of the testes. Hydrocele of the testes occurs when a small patency of the processus vaginalis remains so that peritoneal fluid can flow into the processus vaginalis, which results in a fluid-filled cyst near the testes. Peritoneal fluid drains from the abdomen through the tunica vaginalis. The fluid accumulates in the scrotum, becomes trapped, and causes the scrotum to enlarge. A hydrocele is usually harmless and in most cases resolves within a few months after birth. A hydrocele is normally treated only when there is discomfort or the testicular blood supply is threatened. A hematocele could have been considered also, but a hematocele is typically caused by trauma and blood would have been seen upon fluid collection. Inguinal hernias usually accompany hydroceles but there was no bulge detected upon physical examination.

21. C. Bronchiectasis. Bronchiectasis is the abnormal, permanent dilatation of bronchi resulting from chronic necrotizing infection (e.g., *Staphylococcus, Streptococcus, Haemophilus influenzae*), bronchial obstruction (e.g., foreign body, mucous plugs, or tumors), or congenital conditions (e.g., Kartagener syndrome, cystic fibrosis, immunodeficiency disorders). The lower lobes of the lung are predominantly affected and the affected bronchi have a saccular appearance. Clinical signs include: cough, fever, and expectoration of large amounts of foul-smelling purulent sputum. Bronchiectasis may also be classified to a group of disorders known as chronic obstructive pulmonary disease (COPD), which are characterized by increased resistance to airflow during both inspiration and expiration because of airway obstruction. Other members of COPD include: emphysema, chronic bronchitis, and asthma.

22. B. DiGeorge syndrome (DS). DS is caused by a microdeletion in the long arm of chromosome 22 (22q11), which is also called the DiGeorge chromosomal region (DGCR). DS occurs when pharyngeal pouches 3 and 4 fail to differentiate into the thymus and parathyroid glands. DS is usually accompanied by facial anomalies resembling first arch syndrome (micrognathia, low-set ears) resulting from abnormal neural crest cell migration, cardiovascular anomalies resulting from abnormal neural crest cell migration during formation of the aorticopulmonary septum, immunodeficiency resulting from absence of thymus gland, and hypocalcemia resulting from absence of parathyroid glands. DS has a phenotypic and genotypic similarity to velocardiofacial syndrome (VCFS); that is, both DS and VCFS are manifestations of a microdeletion at 22q11. The following genes have been mapped to 22q11 or the DGCR (although their role is far from clear): catechol-O-methyltransferase (COMT; an enzyme used in catecholamine metabolism); GPIIb (the receptor for von Willebrand factor); DGCR3 (a leucine zipper transcription factor); and citrate transport protein (CTP).

23. C. Patau syndrome. Aneuploidy is the addition of one chromosome (trisomy) or loss of one chromosome (monosomy). Trisomy results in spontaneous abortion of the conceptus. However, trisomy 13 (Patau syndrome), trisomy 18 (Edwards syndrome), trisomy 21 (Down syndrome), and Klinefelter syndrome (47, XYY) are found in the liveborn population. Monosomy results in spontaneous abortion of the conceptus. However, monosomy X chromosome (45, X; Turner syndrome) is found in the liveborn population. Aneuploidy occurs as a result of nondisjunction during meiosis. Trisomy 13 (Patau syndrome) is characterized by profound mental retardation, polydactyly, congenital heart defects, cleft lip and palate, and omphalocele. Infants usually die soon after birth.

24. C. Rubella virus infection. Rubella virus (German measles; member of TORCH) belongs to the Togaviridae family, which are enveloped, icosahedral positive single-stranded RNA viruses. The rubella virus is transmitted to the fetus transplacentally. The risk of fetal Rubella infection is greatest during the first month of pregnancy and apparently declines thereafter. Fetal rubella infection results in the classic triad of cardiac defects [e.g., patent ductus arteriosus, pulmonary artery stenosis, and atrioventricular (AV) septal defects], cataracts, and low birth weight. With the pandemic of rubella in 1964, the complexity of this syndrome became apparent and the term expanded. Rubella syndrome became standard. The clinical manifestations include: intrauterine growth retardation (most common manifestation), hepatosplenomegaly, generalized adenopathy, hemolytic anemia, hepatitis, jaundice, meningoencephalitis, eye involvement (e.g., cataracts, glaucoma, retinopathy), bluish-purple lesions on a yellow jaundiced skin ("blueberry muffin spots"), osteitis (celery stalk appearance of long bones), and sensorineural deafness. Exposure of pregnant women requires immediate assessment of their immune status. If the exposed pregnant woman is known to be immune (i.e., antibodies present), the woman can be assured of no risk. Postexposure prophylaxis of pregnant women with immune globulin (IG) is not recommended and should be considered only if abortion is not an option. Control measures for rubella prevention should be placed on immunization of children. Other members of TORCH include: *Toxoplasma gondii* (a protozoan parasite), cytomegalovirus (CMV), herpes simplex virus, varicella-zoster virus, treponema pallidum (a spirochete), and hepatitis B virus. TORCH infections are caused by toxoplasma (T), rubella (R), cytomegalovirus (C), Herpes virus (H), and other (O) bacterial and viral infections that are grouped together because they cause similar clinical and pathologic manifestations. See above discussion for specifics.

25. E. Retinoblastoma (RB). RB is a tumor of the retina that occurs in childhood and develops from precursor cells in the immature retina. The RB gene is located on chromosome 13q and encodes for RB protein that binds to a gene regulatory protein and causes suppression of the cell cycle, i.e., the RB gene is a tumor-suppressor gene (also called an anti-oncogene). A mutation in the RB gene will encode an abnormal RB protein such that there is no suppression of the cell cycle. This leads to the formation of RB. Hereditary RB causes multiple tumors in both eyes. Non-hereditary RB causes one tumor in one eye.

26. A. Ehlers-Danlos syndrome. Ehlers-Danlos syndrome is an autosomal-dominant genetic disorder involving the gene for peptidyl lysine hydroxylase, which is an enzyme necessary for the hydroxylation of lysine residues of collagen. It affects mainly Types I and III collagen. It is characterized by extremely stretchable and fragile skin, hypermobile joints, aneurysms of blood vessels, and rupture of the bowel.

27. C. Osteogenesis imperfecta (OI). OI is an autosomal-dominant (Types I–IV) or -recessive (Types II–III) genetic disorder caused by a mutation in the gene for Type I collagen on chromosome 7q22 or 17q22. OI is characterized by extreme bone fragility with spontaneous fractures occurring when the fetus is still in the womb and blue sclera of the eye. Severe forms of OI are fatal *in utero* or during the early neonatal period. Milder forms of OI may be confused with child abuse.

28. A. Marfan syndrome (MS). MS is an autosomal-dominant genetic disorder caused by a mutation in the gene for the protein fibrillin-1 on chromosome 15q21.1, which is an essential component of elastic fibers. These individuals are unusually tall and have exceptionally long, thin limbs, ectopia lentis (dislocation of the lens), severe near-sightedness, and heart valve incompetence.

29. E. Duchenne muscular dystrophy (DMD). DMD is an X-linked recessive disorder caused by a mutation in the gene for dystrophin on the short arm of chromosome X (Xp21). X-linked recessive inheritance means that males who inherit only one defective copy of the DMD gene from the mother have the disease. Dystrophin anchors the cytoskeleton (actin) of skeletal muscle cells to the extracellular matrix through a transmembrane protein (α-dystroglycan and β-dystroglycan) and stabilizes the cell membrane. A mutation of the DMD gene destroys the ability of dystrophin to anchor actin to the extracellular matrix. The characteristic dysfunction in DMD is progressive muscle weakness and wasting. Death occurs as a result of cardiac or respiratory failure, usually in the late teens or twenties. The description of how the boy arose from a seated position is called the Gower maneuver, which is classically seen in Duchenne muscular dystrophy. Becker muscular dystrophy normally begins around the third decade of life, whereas Duchenne can begin much earlier. McArdle disease is excluded because there was no sign of myoglobinuria, which would be a result of muscle glycogen phosphorylase deficiency.

30. B. Turner syndrome. Turner syndrome (monosomy X; 45,X) is a monosomic condition found only in females and characterized by: short stature, low-set ears, ocular hypertelorism, ptosis, low posterior hairline, webbed neck caused by a remnant of a fetal cystic hygroma, congenital hypoplasia of lymphatics causing peripheral edema of hands and feet, shield chest, pinpoint nipples, congenital heart defects, aortic coarctation, female hypogonadism, and ovarian fibrous streaks (i.e., infertility). This syndrome is a common cause of primary amenorrhea.

31. A. Alcohol consumption during pregnancy. Alcohol is an organic compound delivered to the fetus through recreational or addictive (i.e., alcoholism) drinking by pregnant women. This drug can cause: fetal alcohol syndrome, which results in mental retardation, microcephaly, holoprosencephaly, limb deformities, craniofacial abnormalities [i.e., hypertelorism, smooth philtrum, short palpebral fissures, flat nasal bridge, maxillary (midface) hypoplasia, and a thin upper lip], and cardiovascular defects (i.e., ventricular septal defects). Fetal alcohol syndrome is the leading cause of preventable mental retardation. The threshold dose of alcohol has not been established, so "no alcohol is good alcohol" during pregnancy.

32. D. Erythroblastosis fetalis. The Rh factor is clinically important in pregnancy. If the mother is Rh−, she will produce Rh antibodies if the fetus is Rh+. This situation will not affect the first pregnancy, but will affect the second pregnancy with an Rh+ fetus. In the second pregnancy with an Rh+ fetus, a hemolytic condition of RBCs occurs known as Rh−hemolytic disease of newborn (erythroblastosis fetalis). This causes destruction of fetal RBCs, which leads to the release of large amounts of bilirubin (a breakdown product of hemoglobin). This causes fetal brain damage resulting from a condition called kernicterus, which is a pathologic deposition of bilirubin in the basal ganglia. Severe hemolytic disease whereby the fetus is severely anemic and demonstrates total body edema (i.e., hydrops fetalis) may lead to death. In these cases, an intrauterine transfusion is indicated. Rh_0 (D) immune globulin (RhoGAM, MICRhoGAM) is a human immunoglobulin (IgG) preparation that contains antibodies against Rh factor and prevents a maternal antibody response to Rh+ cells that may enter the maternal bloodstream of an Rh− mother. This drug is administered to Rh− mothers within 72 hours after the birth of an Rh+ baby to prevent erythroblastosis fetalis during subsequent pregnancies.

33. C. Patent ductus arteriosus. Patent ductus arteriosus occurs when the ductus arteriosus, a connection between the left pulmonary artery and aorta, fails to close. Normally the ductus arteriosus functionally closes within a few hours after birth via smooth muscle contraction to ultimately form the ligamentum arteriosum. A patent ductus arteriosus causes an L → R shunting of oxygen-rich blood from the aorta back into the pulmonary circulation. This can be treated with prostaglandin synthesis inhibitors (e.g., indomethacin), which promote closure. It is very common in premature infants and maternal rubella infection. Clinical signs include: a harsh, machine-like, continuous murmur in the upper left parasternal area.

34. C. Tracheoesophageal fistula. Tracheoesophageal fistula is an abnormal communication between the trachea and esophagus that results from improper division of foregut by the tracheoesophageal septum. It is generally associated with esophageal atresia and polyhydramnios. Clinical features include: excessive accumulation of saliva or mucus in the nose and mouth; episodes of gagging and cyanosis after swallowing milk; abdominal distention after crying; and reflux of gastric contents into lungs, causing pneumonitis. Diagnostic features include: inability to pass a catheter into the stomach and radiographs demonstrating air in the infant's stomach.

35. B. Klinefelter syndrome. Klinefelter syndrome (47, XXY) is a trisomic condition found only in males and characterized by: varicose veins, arterial and venous leg ulcer, scant body and pubic hair, male hypogonadism, sterility with fibrosus of seminiferous tubules, marked decrease in testosterone levels, elevated gonadotropin levels, gynecomastia, dull mentality, antisocial behavior, delayed speech as a child, and eunuchoid habitus.

Figure Credits

CHAPTER 1

Figure 1-1. Modified from Dudek R, Fix J. BRS Embryology, 2nd ed. Philadelphia: Lippincott Williams & Wilkins, 1998:1, Fig 1-1.

Figure 1-2. From Dudek R, Fix J. BRS Embryology, 2nd ed. Philadelphia: Lippincott Williams & Wilkins, 1998:4, Fig 1-2.

CHAPTER 2

Figure 2-1. From Dudek R, Fix J. High-Yield Embryology. Philadelphia: Lippincott Williams & Wilkins, 1996:5, Fig 2-1.

CHAPTER 3

Figure 3-1. **(A–D)** From Dudek R, Fix J. BRS Embryology, 2nd ed. Philadelphia: Lippincott Williams & Wilkins, 1998:22, Fig 3-1. **(E)** From Sauerbrei EE, et al. A Practical Guide to Ultrasound in Obstetrics and Gynecology, 2nd ed. Philadelphia: Lippincott Williams & Wilkins, 1997:115, Fig 7-4F.

Figure 3-2. **(A, B)** From Sternberg SS. Diagnostic Surgical Pathology, vol 2, 3rd ed. Philadelphia: Lippincott Williams & Wilkins, 1999:2070, Figs 2 and 3. **(C)** From Sternberg SS. Diagnostic Surgical Pathology, vol 2, 3rd ed. Philadelphia: Lippincott Williams & Wilkins, 1999:2078, Fig 12. **(D)** From Sternberg SS. Diagnostic Surgical Pathology, vol 2, 3rd ed. Philadelphia: Lippincott Williams & Wilkins, 1999:2077, Fig 10.

CHAPTER 4

Figure 4-1. From Dudek R, Fix J. BRS Embryology. Philadelphia: Lippincott Williams & Wilkins, 1995:30, Fig 4-1.

Figure 4-2. **(A, B)** From Johnson KE. NMS Human Developmental Anatomy. Baltimore: Williams & Wilkins, 1988:79, Fig 6-1. **(C)** From Sadler TW. Langman's Medical Embryology, 7th ed. Baltimore: Williams & Wilkins, 1995:77, Fig 5.11C.

Figure 4-3. From Dudek R, Fix J. BRS Embryology, 2nd ed. Philadelphia: Lippincott Williams & Wilkins, 1998:33, Fig 4-3.

Figure 4.4. **(A)** From Sadler TW. Langman's Medical Embryology, 7th ed. Baltimore: Williams & Wilkins, 1995:62, Fig 4-7. **(B)** From Sadler TW. Langman's Medical Embryology, 7th ed. Baltimore: Williams & Wilkins, 1995:61, Fig 4-6.

CHAPTER 5

Figure 5-1. **(A–D)** From Dudek R, Fix J. BRS Embryology, 2nd ed. Philadelphia: Lippincott Williams & Wilkins, 1998:42, Fig 5-1.

Figure 5-2. **(A)** From Dudek R, Fix J. BRS Embryology, 2nd ed. Philadelphia: Lippincott Williams & Wilkins, 1998:43, Fig 5-2. Table from Dudek R. High-Yield Embryology, 2nd ed. Philadelphia: Lippincott Williams & Wilkins, 2001:27, Fig 6-1. **(B, C)** From Johnson KE. NMS Human Developmental Anatomy. Baltimore: Williams & Wilkins, 1988:147, Fig 10-2D, E. **(D)** From Kirks DR. Practical Pediatric Imaging, 3rd ed. Philadelphia: Lippincott Williams Wilkins, 1997:591, Fig 6-77B.

Figure 5-3. **(A)** From Dudek R, Fix J. BRS Embryology, 2nd ed. Philadelphia: Lippincott Williams & Wilkins, 1998:46, Fig 5-4A–C. **(B)** From Dudek R, Fix J. BRS Embryology, 2nd ed. Philadelphia: Lippincott Williams & Wilkins, 1998:49, Fig 5-8. **B(1)** From Avery GB, et al. Neonatology Pathophysiology and Management of the Newborn, 5th ed. Philadelphia: Lippincott Williams & Wilkins, 1999:602, Fig 33-17. **B(2)** From Donnelly LF, Higgin CB. MR imaging of conotruncal abnormalities. AJR 1996;166:925–928. **B(3)** From Avery GB, et al. Neonatology Pathophysiology and Management of the Newborn, 5th ed. Philadelphia: Lippincott Williams & Wilkins, 1999:605, Fig 33-20A. **B(4)** From Bisset GS III. Magnetic Resonance Imaging of the Pediatric Cardiovascular System. In: Cohen MD, Edwards MK, eds. Pediatrics Magnetic Resonance Imaging. Philadelphia: BC Decker, 1990:541–548.

Figure 5-4. **(A)** Modified from Johnson KE. NMS Human Developmental Anatomy. Baltimore: Williams & Wilkins, 1988:149, Fig 10-3. **(B)** From Dudek R, Fix J. BRS Embryology, 2nd ed. Philadelphia: Lippincott Williams & Wilkins, 1998:50, Fig 5-9. **B(1)** From McMillan JA, et al, eds. Oski's Pediatrics, 3rd ed. Philadelphia: Lippincott Williams & Wilkins, 1999:1349, Fig 273-2.

Figure 5-5. **(A)** From Dudek R, Fix J. BRS Embryology, 2nd ed. Philadelphia: Lippincott Williams & Wilkins, 1998:47, Fig 5-6. **(B)** From Dudek R, Fix J. BRS Embryology, 2nd ed. Philadelphia: Lippincott Williams & Wilkins, 1998:52, Fig 5-10. **B(1)** From Kirks DR. Practical Pediatric Imaging, 3rd ed. Philadelphia: Lippincott Williams & Wilkins, 1997:555, Fig 6-41. **B(2)** From Kirks DR. Practical Pediatric Imaging, 3rd ed. Philadelphia: Lippincott Williams & Wilkins, 1997:553, Fig 6-39.

Figure 5-6. **(A)** From Dudek R, Fix J. BRS Embryology, 2nd ed. Philadelphia: Lippincott Williams & Wilkins, 1998:47, Fig 5-7A, B. **(B)** From Dudek R, Fix J. BRS Embryology, 2nd ed. Philadelphia: Lippincott Williams & Wilkins, 1998:53, Fig 5-11. **B(1)** From Kirks DK. Practical Pediatric Imaging, 3rd ed. Philadelphia: Lippincott Williams & Wilkins, 1997:519, Fig 6-8A. **B(2)** From McMillan JA, et al, eds. Oski's Pediatrics, 3rd ed. Philadelphia: Lippincott Williams & Wilkins, 1999:1356, Fig 274-2.

Figure 5-7. **(A, B)** From Johnson KE. NMS Human Developmental Anatomy. Baltimore: Williams & Wilkins, 1988:154, Fig 10-6. **(D, E)** From Dudek R, Fix J. BRS Embryology, 2nd ed. Philadelphia: Lippincott Williams & Wilkins, 1998:55, Fig 5-12A, B. **D(1)** From McMillan JA, et al, eds. Oski's Pediatrics, 3rd ed. Philadelphia: Lippincott Williams & Wilkins, 1999:1369, Fig 278-1.

Figure 5-8. **(A–C)** Modified from Johnson KE. NMS Human Developmental Anatomy. Baltimore: Williams & Wilkins, 1988:159, Fig 10-7.

CHAPTER 6

Figure 6-1. **(A, E)** From Dudek R, Fix J. BRS Embryology, 2nd ed. Philadelphia: Lippincott Williams & Wilkins, 1998:66, Figs A, D. **(B–D left part only)** From Johnson KE. NMS Human Developmental Anatomy. Baltimore: Williams & Wilkins, 1988:96, Fig 7-3.

Figure 6-2. **(A–C)** Modified from Dudek R, Fix J. BRS Embryology, 2nd ed. Philadelphia: Lippincott Williams & Wilkins, 1998:67, Fig 6-2A. **(D, E)** From Sadler TW. Langman's Medical Embryology, 7th ed. Baltimore: Williams & Wilkins, 1995:108, Fig 7-8A, B. **Sonogram in A** from Sauerbrei EE: A Practical Guide to Ultrasound in Obstetrics and Gynecology, 2nd ed. Philadelphia: Lippincott Williams & Wilkins, 1997:116, Fig 7-5C.

Figure 6-3. **(A, B)** Drawn from Dudek R, Fix J. BRS Embryology, 2nd ed. Philadelphia: Lippincott Williams & Wilkins, 1998:68, Fig 6-3. **(C)** From Ross, et al. Histology: A Textbook and Atlas, 4th ed. Philadelphia: Lippincott Williams & Wilkins, 2003:781, plate 96. **(D)** From Thornberg KL, Faber JJ. Placental Physiology. New York: Raven Press, 1983:19. **(E)** From Dudek R. High-Yield Embryology, 2nd ed. Philadelphia: Lippincott Williams & Wilkins, 2000:21, Table 5-1.

Figure 6-4. From Dudek R. High-Yield Embryology, 2nd ed. Philadelphia: Lippincott Williams & Wilkins, 2000:24, Fig 5-4 and Table 5-2.

Figure 6-5. **(A–C)** From Dudek R. High-Yield Embryology, 2nd ed. Philadelphia: Lippincott Williams & Wilkins, 2000:8, Fig 2-2. **A(1)** From Dudek R. High-Yield Embryology, 2nd ed. Philadelphia: Lippincott Williams & Wilkins, 2000:20, Fig 5-2. **A(2)** Courtesy of Dr. R. W. Dudek. **B(1)** From Dudek R. High-Yield Embryology, 2nd ed. Philadelphia: Lippincott Williams & Wilkins, 2000:20, Fig 5-2. **B(2)** Courtesy of Dr. R. W. Dudek. **C(1)** Sadler TW. Langman's Medical Embryology, 6th ed. Baltimore: Williams & Wilkins, 1990:156, Fig 7.16B.

Figure 6-6. **(A)** From Sternberg SS. Diagnostic Surgical Pathology, vol 2, 3rd ed. Philadelphia: Lippincott Williams & Wilkins, 1999:2091, Fig 6. **(B)** From Sternberg SS. Diagnostic Surgical

Pathology, vol 2, 3rd ed. Philadelphia: Lippincott Williams & Wilkins, 1999:2089, Fig 1. **(C)** From Fletcher MA. Physical Diagnosis in Neonatology. Philadelphia: Lippincott Williams & Wilkins, 1997:85, Fig 16. **(D)** From Sternberg SS. Histology for Pathologists, 2nd ed. Philadelphia: Lippincott Williams & Wilkins, 1997:967, Fig 7. **(E)** From Benirschke K, Kaufmann P. The Pathology of the Human Placenta, 3rd ed. New York: Springer-Verlag, 1995. **(F)** Courtesy of M. C. Edwards.

CHAPTER 7

Figure 7-1. **(A–E)** Modified from Truex RC, Carpenter MB. Human Neuroanatomy. Baltimore, MD: Williams & Wilkins, 1969:91.

Figure 7-2. **(A, B)** Modified from Johnson KE. NMS Human Developmental Anatomy. Baltimore: Williams & Wilkins, 1988:177, Fig 11-7.

Figure 7-3. **(A–C)** From Dudek R, Fix J. BRS Embryology, 2nd ed. Philadelphia: Lippincott Williams & Wilkins, 1998:85, Fig 7-3.

Figure 7-4. **(A–C)** From Dudek R, Fix J. BRS Embryology, 2nd ed. Philadelphia: Lippincott Williams & Wilkins, 1998:87, Fig 7-5. **(D)** Modified from Patten BM. Human Embryology, 3rd ed. New York: McGraw-Hill, 1969, p 298.

Figure 7-5. **(A)** From Dudek R, Fix J. BRS Embryology, 2nd ed. Philadelphia: Lippincott Williams & Wilkins, 1998:88, Fig 7-6. **(B)** From Dudek R, Fix J. BRS Embryology, 2nd ed. Philadelphia: Lippincott Williams & Wilkins, 1998:89, Fig 7-7. **(C)** From Dudek R, Fix J. BRS Embryology, 2nd ed. Philadelphia: Lippincott Williams & Wilkins, 1998:90, Fig 7-8. **(D)** Modified from Sadler TW. Langman's Medical Embryology, 6th ed. Baltimore: Williams & Wilkins, 1990:373.

Figure 7-6. **(A–E)** From Johnson KE. NMS Human Developmental Anatomy. Baltimore: Williams & Wilkins, 1988:181, Fig 11-10.

Figure 7-7. **(A)** Modified from Haines DE. Fundamental Neuroscience. New York: Churchill Livingstone, 1997:69, Fig 5-5B, C, D. **(B)** From Siegel MJ. Pediatric Sonography, 3rd ed. Philadelphia: Lippincott Williams & Wilkins, 2002:677, Fig 15.6A. **(C)** From Haines DE. Fundamental Neuroscience. New York: Churchill Livingstone, 1997:69, Fig 5-5A. **(D)** Courtesy of Dr. T. Naidich, Miami, FL. **(E)** From Papp Z. Atlas of Fetal Diagnosis. Amsterdam, Netherlands: Elsevier, 1992:128.

Figure 7-8. **(A)** From Haines DE. Fundamental Neuroscience. New York: Churchill Livingston, 1997:68, Fig 5-3. **(B)** From Carlson BM. Human Embryology and Developmental Biology, 2nd ed. St. Louis: Mosby, 1999:244, Fig 10-43A. **(C)** From Haines DE. Fundamental Neuroscience. New York: Churchill Livingston, 1997:69, Fig 5-3G. **(D)** From Dudek R. High-Yield Embryology, 2nd ed. Philadelphia: Lippincott Williams & Wilkins, 2001:76, Fig 12-6F. **(E)** From Swischuk LE. Imaging of the Newborn, Infant, and Young Child, 5th ed. Philadelphia: Lippincott Williams & Wilkins, 2004:1016, Fig 7.52.

Figure 7-9. **(A)** From Swischuk LE. Imaging of the Newborn, Infant, and Young Child, 5th ed. Philadelphia: Lippincott Williams & Wilkins, 2004:1017, Fig 7.53A. **(B)** From Swischuk LE. Imaging of the Newborn, Infant, and Young Child, 5th ed. Philadelphia: Lippincott Williams & Wilkins, 2004:1017, Fig 7.53B. **(C)** From Swischuk LE. Imaging of the Newborn, Infant, and Young Child, 5th ed. Philadelphia: Lippincott Williams & Wilkins, 2004, p. 1017, Fig 7.53D. **(D)** From Swischuk LE. Imaging of the Newborn, Infant, and Young Child, 5th ed. Philadelphia: Lippincott Williams & Wilkins, 2004:1011, Fig 7.45B. **(E)** From Siegel MJ. Pediatric Sonography, 3rd ed. Philadelphia: Lippincott Williams & Wilkins, 2001:111, Fig 3.95B. **(F)** From Siegel MJ. Pediatric Sonography, 3rd ed. Philadelphia: Lippincott Williams & Wilkins, 2001:92, Fig 3.72D. **(G)** From Siegel MJ. Pediatric Sonography, 3rd ed. Philadelphia: Lippincott Williams & Wilkins, 2001:90, Fig 3.70A.

Figure 7-10. **(A)** From Siegel MJ. Pediatric Sonography, 3rd ed. Philadelphia: Lippincott Williams & Wilkins, 2001, p. 103, Fig 3.86. **(B)** From Swischuk LE. Imaging of the Newborn, Infant, and Young Child, 5th ed. Philadelphia: Lippincott Williams & Wilkins, 2004:1018, Fig 7.54A. **(C)** From Siegel MJ. Pediatric Sonography, 3rd ed. Philadelphia: Lippincott Williams & Wilkins, 2001:103, Fig 3.85A. **(D)** From Siegel MJ. Pediatric Sonography, 3rd ed. Philadelphia: Lippincott

Williams & Wilkins, 2001:102, Fig 3.84B. **(E)** From Papp Z. Atlas of Fetal Diagnosis. Amsterdam: Elsevier, 1992:101. **(F)** From Siegel MJ. Pediatric Sonography, 3rd ed. Philadelphia: Lippincott Williams & Wilkins, 2001:97, Fig 3.78A. **(G)** Courtesy of Dr. James E. Rytting.

CHAPTER 8

Figure 8-1. **(A, B, D)** From Dudek R. High-Yield Embryology. Philadelphia: Lippincott Williams & Wilkins, 1996:80, Fig 13-1. **(C)** Redrawn from Moore and Persaud. The Developing Human, 6th ed. Philadelphia: WB Saunders, 1998:505, Fig 19-18A. **(E)** From Rohen JW, et al. Color Atlas of Anatomy, 4th ed. Philadelphia: Lippincott Williams & Wilkins, 1998:124.

Figure 8-2. **(A)** From Fletcher MA. Physical Diagnosis in Neonatology. Philadelphia: Lippincott Williams & Wilkins, 1998:285, Fig 2. **(B)** From Fletcher MA. Physical Diagnosis in Neonatology. Philadelphia: Lippincott Williams & Wilkins, 1998:288, Fig 7-A. **(C)** From Fletcher MA. Physical Diagnosis in Neonatology. Philadelphia: Lippincott Williams & Wilkins, 1998:288, Fig 7-B. **(D)** From Fletcher MA. Physical Diagnosis in Neonatology. Philadelphia: Lippincott Williams & Wilkins, 1998:289, Fig 8-A. **(E)** From Fletcher MA. Physical Diagnosis in Neonatology. Philadelphia: Lippincott Williams & Wilkins, 1998:289, Fig 5. **(F)** From Fletcher MA. Physical Diagnosis in Neonatology. Philadelphia: Lippincott Williams & Wilkins, 1998:294, Fig 11-A. **(G)** From Fletcher MA. Physical Diagnosis in Neonatology. Philadelphia: Lippincott Williams & Wilkins, 1998:295, Fig 12. **(H)** From Fletcher MA. Physical Diagnosis in Neonatology. Philadelphia: Lippincott Williams & Wilkins, 1998:292, Fig 10. **H(2)** From Kirks DR. Pediatric Imaging, 3rd ed. Philadelphia: Lippincott Williams & Wilkins, 1998:231, Fig 3-41A. **(I)** From Kirks DR. Pediatric Imaging, 3rd ed. Philadelphia: Lippincott Williams & Wilkins, 1998:236, Fig 3-46. **I(2)** From Sternberg SS. Diagnostic Surgical Pathology, vol 1, 3rd ed. Philadelphia: Lippincott Williams & Wilkins, 1999:963, Fig 32. **(J)** From Fletcher MA. Physical Diagnosis in Neonatology. Philadelphia: Lippincott Williams & Wilkins, 1998:296, Fig 13B.

CHAPTER 9

Figure 9-1. From Dudek R. High-Yield Embryology. Philadelphia: Lippincott Williams & Wilkins, 1996:47, Fig 15-1 A-C.

Figure 9-2. **(A, B)** From Dudek R, Fix J. BRS Embryology, 2nd ed. Philadelphia: Lippincott Williams & Wilkins, 1998:116, Fig 9-2. **(C)** From Rohen JW, et al. Color Atlas of Anatomy, 4th ed. Philadelphia: Lippincott Williams & Wilkins, 1998:130.

Figure 9-3. **(A)** From Bergsma D. Birth Defects: Atlas and Compendium. Philadelphia: Lippincott Williams & Wilkins, 1973, Fig 6-47. **(B–D)** From Gilbert-Barness E: Potter's Atlas of Fetal and Infant Pathology. St. Louis, Mosby, 1998:366, 370. **(E)** From Avery GB. Neonatology: Pathophysiology and Management of the Newborn, 5th ed. Philadelphia: Lippincott Williams & Wilkins, 1999:1286, Fig 52-1. **(F)** From Kirks DR. Practical Pediatric Imaging, 3rd ed. Philadelphia: Lippincott Williams & Wilkins, 1997:205, Fig 3-3. **G(1)** From Kirks DR. Practical Pediatric Imaging, 3rd ed. Philadelphia: Lippincott Williams & Wilkins, 1997:211, Fig 3-14. **G(2)** From Sternberg SS. Diagnostic Surgical Pathology, vol 1, 3rd ed. Philadelphia: Lippincott Williams & Wilkins, 1999:993, Fig 26.

CHAPTER 10

Figure 10-1. **(A, B, C, E)** From Dudek R, Fix J. BRS Embryology, 2nd ed. Philadelphia: Lippincott Williams & Wilkins, 1998:124, Fig 10-1, and 1998:125, Fig 10-2. **(D)** From Dudek R. High-Yield Embryology, 2nd ed. Philadelphia: Lippincott Williams & Wilkins, 2000:35, Fig 7-1.

Figure 10-2. **(A)** From Fenoglio-Preiser CM. Gastrointestinal Pathology: An Atlas and Text, 2nd ed. Philadelphia: Lippincott Williams & Wilkins, 1998:33, Fig 3.5A. **(B)** From Fenoglio-Preiser CM. Gastrointestinal Pathology: An Atlas and Text, 2nd ed. Philadelphia: Lippincott Williams & Wilkins, 1998:37, Fig 3.10B. Courtesy of Dr. Cooley Butler, Scripps Memorial Hospital, La Jolla, CA. **(C, D)** From Fenoglio-Preiser CM. Gastrointestinal Pathology: An Atlas and Text, 2nd ed. Philadelphia: Lippincott Williams & Wilkins, 1998:36, Fig 3.8A, B. **(E, F)** From Yamada T, et al. Textbook of Gastroenterology, vol 1. Philadelphia: Lippincott Williams & Wilkins, 1999:1189, Fig 56-8A, B.

Figure 10-3. **(A)** From Johnson KE. NMS Human Developmental Anatomy. Baltimore: Williams & Wilkins, 1988:211, Fig 13-4. **(B)** From Fenoglio-Preiser CM. Gastrointestinal Pathology: An Atlas and Text, 2nd ed. Philadelphia: Lippincott Williams & Wilkins, 1998:155, Fig 6.3A. Courtesy of Dr. K. Bove, Children's Hospital Medical Center, Cincinnati, OH. **(C)** From Yamada T, et al. Textbook of Gastroenterology, vol 1. Philadelphia: Lippincott Williams & Wilkins, 1999:1337, Fig 62-13.

Figure 10-4. **(A)** Modified from Johnson KE. NMS Human Developmental Anatomy. Baltimore: Williams & Wilkins, 1988:215, Fig 13-9. **(B)** From Yamada T, et al. Textbook of Gastroenterology, vol 2, 3rd ed. Philadelphia: Lippincott Williams & Wilkins, 1999:2250, Fig 98-7. **(C, D)** From Lindner H. Embryology and anatomy of the biliary tree. In Way LW. Surgery of the Gallbladder and Bile Ducts. Philadelphia: WB Saunders, 1987.

Figure 10-5. **(A)** Modified from Johnson KE. NMS Human Developmental Anatomy. Baltimore: Williams & Wilkins, 1988:215, Fig 13-9. **A(1)** From Henrikson RC. NMS Histology. Philadelphia: Lippincott Williams & Wilkins, 1997:368, Fig 33-2. **A(2)** Redrawn from Pictet R, Rutter W. Handbook of Physiology. Section 7: Endocrinology, vol 1. Washington, DC: American Physiological Society, 1972:25–66. **(B–D)** Redrawn and modified from Cubilla AL, Fitzgerald PJ. Tumors of the exocrine pancreas. In: Hartman WH, Sobin LH, eds. Atlas of Tumor Pathology, 2nd ed. Washington, DC: Armed Forces Institute of Pathology, 1984. **(E)** From Yamada T, et al. Textbook of Gastroenterology, vol 2, 3rd ed. Philadelphia: Lippincott Williams & Wilkins, 1999:2118, Fig 92-9. Courtesy of Peter B. Cotton, MD, Durham, NC. **(F)** From Yamada T, et al. Atlas of Gastroenterology, 2nd ed. Philadelphia: Lippincott Williams & Wilkins, 1999:458, Fig 50-2. Courtesy of Dr. J. Rode. **(G)** From Misiewicz JJ, Bartram CI. Atlas of Clinical Gastroenterology. London, Gower Medical Publishing, 1987.

Figure 10-6. **(A)** From Johnson KE. NMS Human Developmental Anatomy. Baltimore: Williams & Wilkins, 1988:218, Fig 13-12. **(B)** From Sadler TW. Langman's Medical Embryology, 8th ed. Baltimore: Lippincott Williams & Wilkins, 2000:294, Fig 13.29B, C. Courtesy of Dr. S. Shaw, Department of Surgery, University of Virginia. **(C)** From Sadler TW. Langman's Medical Embryology, 8th ed. Baltimore: Lippincott Williams & Wilkins, 2000, p 294, Fig 13.29C. Courtesy of Dr. S. Lacey, Department of Surgery, University of North Carolina. **(D, E)** From Fenoglio-Preiser CM. Gastrointestinal Pathology: An Atlas and Text, 2nd ed. Philadelphia: Lippincott Williams & Wilkins, 1989:321, Fig 9.23A, and 1989:310, Fig 9.1B. **(F)** From Yamada T, et al. Atlas of Gastroenterology, 2nd ed. Philadelphia: Lippincott Williams & Wilkins, 1999:259, Fig 26-7. **(G)** From Fenoglio-Preiser CM. Gastrointestinal Pathology: An Atlas and Text, 2nd ed. Philadelphia: Lippincott Williams & Wilkins, 1989:315, Fig 9.10C. **(H)** From Yamada T, et al. Atlas of Gastroenterology, 2nd ed. Philadelphia: Lippincott Williams & Wilkins, 1999:258, Fig 26-4. **(G and H *insets*)** From Smith GH, Glasson M. Intestinal atresia: factors affecting survival. Aust N Z J Surg 1989;59:151. **(I)** From Fenoglio-Preiser CM. Gastrointestinal Pathology: An Atlas and Text, 2nd ed. Philadelphia: Lippincott Williams & Wilkins, 1989:318, Fig 9.15B. **(I *inset*)** From Fenoglio-Preiser CM. Gastrointestinal Pathology: An Atlas and Text, 2nd ed. Philadelphia: Lippincott Williams & Wilkins, 1989:318, Fig 9.15B.

Figure 10-7. **(A)** Line drawings from Sadler TW. Langman's Medical Embryology, 8th ed. Baltimore: Lippincott Williams & Wilkins, 2000:299, Fig 13.34A, B, C. **(A)** Photo from Sternberg SS. Histology for Pathologists, 2nd ed. Philadelphia: Lippincott Williams & Wilkins, 1997:554, Fig 6. **(B)** From Yamada T, et al. Atlas of Gastroenterology, 2nd ed. Philadelphia: Lippincott Williams & Wilkins, 1999:362, Fig 38.11 (histology), and 1999:363, Fig 38.13 (radiograph and chromosome). **(C)** From Larsen WJ. Human Embryology, 2nd ed. New York, Churchill Livingstone, 1997:268.

CHAPTER 11

Figure 11-1. **(A–C [tops])** From Dudek R. BRS Embryology, 2nd ed. Philadelphia: Lippincott Williams & Wilkins, 1998:139, Fig 11-1. **(A–C [bottoms])** From Dudek R. High-Yield Embryology, 2nd ed. Philadelphia: Lippincott Williams & Wilkins, 2000:56, Fig 10.1. **(D–H)** Diagrams from Yamada T, et al. Textbook of Gastroenterology, vol 1, 3rd ed. Philadelphia: Lippincott Williams & Wilkins, 1999:1186, Fig 56-6. **(D)** Radiograph from Kirks DR. Practical

Pediatric Imaging, 3rd ed. Philadelphia: Lippincott Williams & Wilkins, 1997:845, Fig 8-19A. **(F)** Radiograph from Avery GB. Neonatology Pathophysiology and Management of the Newborn, 5th ed. Philadelphia: Lippincott Williams & Wilkins, 1999:1018, Fig 44-6C.

Figure 11-2. **(A)** From Rohen JW, et al. Color Atlas of Anatomy, 4th ed. Philadelphia: Lippincott Williams & Wilkins, 1998:235. **(B)** From Kirks DR. Practical Pediatric Imaging, 3rd ed. Philadelphia: Lippincott Williams & Wilkins, 1997:671, Fig 7-58B. **(C)** From Kirks DR. Practical Pediatric Imaging, 3rd ed. Philadelphia: Lippincott Williams & Wilkins, 1997, p 674, Fig 7-61A.

Figure 11-3. **(A)** Left side is modified from Rohen JW, et al. Color Atlas of Anatomy, 4th ed. Philadelphia: Lippincott Williams & Wilkins, 1998:235. **A(1)** Redrawn from Sweeney LJ. Basic Concepts in Embryology. New York: McGraw Hill, 1998:321, Fig 13-5. **(B)** Left side is modified from Rohen JW, et al. Color Atlas of Anatomy, 4th ed. Philadelphia: Lippincott Williams & Wilkins, 1998:235. **B(2)** Redrawn from Sweeney LJ. Basic Concepts in Embryology. New York: McGraw Hill, 1998:321, Fig 13-5. **(C)** Left side is modified from Rohen JW, et al. Color Atlas of Anatomy, 4th ed. Philadelphia: Lippincott Williams & Wilkins, 1998:235. **C(2)** Redrawn from Sweeney LJ. Basic Concepts in Embryology. New York: McGraw Hill, 1998:321, Fig 13.5. **(D)** Left side is modified from Rohen JW, et al. Color Atlas of Anatomy, 4th ed. Philadelphia: Lippincott Williams & Wilkins, 1998:235. **D(2)** From Ross. Histology: A Text and Atlas, 4th ed. Baltimore: Lippincott Williams & Wilkins, 2003:599, plate 68, Fig 3.

Figure 11-4. **(A)** From Dudek R. High-Yield Embryology, 2nd ed. Philadelphia: Lippincott Williams & Wilkins, 2000:59, Fig 10-4. **(B)** From Kirks DR. Practical Pediatric Imaging, 3rd ed. Philadelphia: Lippincott Williams & Wilkins, 1997:695, Fig 7-78A.

CHAPTER 12

Figure 12-1. **(A, B)** From Dudek R. BRS Embryology, 2nd ed. Philadelphia: Lippincott Williams & Wilkins, 1998:149, Fig 12-1. **(C, D)** From Dudek R. BRS Embryology, 2nd ed. Philadelphia: Lippincott Williams & Wilkins, 1998:151, Fig 12-2.

Figure 12-2. **(A)** From Dudek R, Fix J. BRS Embryology, 2nd ed. Philadelphia: Lippincott Williams & Wilkins, 1998:153, Fig 12-3. **(B)** From Dudek R, Fix J. BRS Embryology, 2nd ed. Philadelphia: Lippincott Williams & Wilkins, 1998:154, Fig 12-4. **(C)** From Dudek R, Fix J. BRS Embryology, 2nd ed. Philadelphia: Lippincott Williams & Wilkins, 1998:155, Fig 12-5A. **C(1,4)** From Dudek R, Fix J. BRS Embryology, 2nd ed. Philadelphia: Lippincott Williams & Wilkins, 1998:153, Fig 12-5B, C. **C(2,3)** From Dudek R, Fix J. BRS Embryology, 2nd ed. Philadelphia: Lippincott Williams & Wilkins, 1998:156, Fig 12-6A, B. **(C[1–4]** *insets*) From Johnson KE. NMS Human Developmental Anatomy. Baltimore: Williams & Wilkins, 1988:307, Fig 18-4.

Figure 12-3. **(A)** From Smith DW. Recognizable Patterns of Human Malformation: Genetic Embryologic and Clinical Aspects, 3rd ed. Philadelphia: WB Saunders, 1982:185. **(B)** From Moore KL. The Developing Human: Clinically Oriented Embryology, 6th ed. Philadelphia: Lippincott Williams & Wilkins, 1998:228. **(C)** Courtesy of Dr. A. Shaw, Department of Surgery, University of Virginia. **(D, E)** From Laeung AKC. Ectopic thyroid gland simulating a thyroglossal duct cyst. Can J Surg 38:87, 1995. **(F)** From Fletcher A. Physical Diagnosis in Neonatology. Philadelphia: Lippincott Williams & Wilkins, 1997:225, Fig 62A. **(G)** From Kirks DW. Practical Pediatric Imaging, 3rd ed. Philadelphia: Lippincott Williams & Wilkins, 1997:246, Fig 3-54. **(H)** From Warkany J. Congenital Malformations: Notes and Comments. Chicago: Year Book Medical Publishers, 1971, Fig 44-4. **(I)** From Moore KL. The Developing Human: Clinically Oriented Embryology, 6th ed. Philadelphia: Lippincott Williams & Wilkins, 1998:248.

CHAPTER 13

Figure 13-1. **(A)** From Dudek R. High-Yield Embryology. Philadelphia: Lippincott Williams & Wilkins, 1996:33, Fig 10-1 (left side). **(B)** From Dudek R. BRS Embryology, 2nd ed. Philadelphia: Lippincott Williams & Wilkins, 1998:164, Fig 13.2. **C(1-3)** From Johnson KE. NMS Human Developmental Anatomy. Baltimore: Williams & Wilkins, 1988:269, Fig 16.6. **(D)** From Dudek R. High-Yield Embryology. Philadelphia: Lippincott Williams & Wilkins,

1996:42, Fig 8.2A. **D(1)** From Dudek R, Fix J. BRS Embryology, 2nd ed. Philadelphia: Lippincott Williams & Wilkins, 1998:165, Fig 13-3. **(E, F)** From Dudek R, Fix J. BRS Embryology, 2nd ed. Philadelphia: Lippincott Williams & Wilkins, 1998:165, Fig 13-3B, C.

Figure 13-2. **(A)** From Johnson KE. NMS Human Developmental Anatomy. Baltimore: Williams & Wilkins, 1988:269, Fig 16-6. **(C)** From Stevenson RE. Human Malformation and Related Anomalies. New York, Oxford University Press, 1993

Figure 13-3. **(A)** From Sternberg SS. Histology for Pathologists, SS Sternberg, 2nd ed. Philadelphia: Lippincott Williams & Wilkins, 1997:791, Fig 5. **(B)** From Kirks DR. Practical Pediatric Imaging, 3rd ed. Philadelphia: Lippincott Williams & Wilkins, 1997:1022, Fig 9-14. **(C)** From Stevenson RE. Human Malformations and Related Anomalies. New York: Oxford University Press, 1993. **(D)** From Kirks DR. Practical Pediatric Imaging, 3rd ed. Philadelphia: Lippincott Williams & Wilkins, 1997:1091, Fig 9-112. **(E)** From Kirks DR. Practical Pediatric Imaging, 3rd ed. Philadelphia: Lippincott Williams & Wilkins, 1997:1038, Fig 9-35. **(F)** From Kelalis PP, King LR. Clinical Pediatric Urology, vol 2. Philadelphia: WB Saunders, 1976:210. **(G)** From Kirks DR. Practical Pediatric Imaging, 3rd ed. Philadelphia: Lippincott Williams & Wilkins, 1997:1050, Fig 9-53A. **(H)** From Papp Z. Atlas of Fetal Diagnosis. New York, Elsevier, 1992:178. **(I, K)** Courtesy of Dr. R. W. Dudek. **(J)** From Sternberg SS. Diagnostic Surgical Pathology, vol 2, 3rd ed. Philadelphia: Lippincott Williams & Wilkins, 1999:1827, Fig 2. **(L)** From Belman AB. The Clinical Significance of Vesicoureteral Reflux. Pediatr Clin North Am 1976;23:707. **(M)** From Malek RS, Kelalis PP. Simple and ectopic ureterocele in infancy and childhood. Surg Gynecol Obstet 1972;134:611.

Figure 13-4. **B(1)** From Sternberg SS. Diagnostic Surgical Pathology, vol 1, 3rd ed. Philadelphia: Lippincott Williams & Wilkins, 1999:609, Fig 33. **B(2)** Courtesy of Dr. R. W. Dudek. **C(1)** From DeLellis RA. Diseases of the adrenal glands. In Murphy WM. Urological Pathology. Philadelphia: WB Saunders, 1997:539–584. **C(2)** From Sternberg SS. Diagnostic Surgical Pathology, vol 1, 3rd ed. Philadelphia: Lippincott Williams & Wilkins, 1999:616, Fig 47.

CHAPTER 14

Figure 14-1. **(A)** Modified from Dudek R, Fix J. BRS Embryology, 2nd ed. Philadelphia: Lippincott Williams & Wilkins, 1998:176, Fig 14-1A. **(B, C)** From Dudek R, Fix J. BRS Embryology, 2nd ed. Philadelphia: Lippincott Williams & Wilkins, 1998:176, Fig 14-1B, C. **(D)** From Ross MH, et al. Histology: A Text and Atlas, 4th ed. Baltimore: Lippincott Williams & Wilkins, 2003:765, plate 88, ovary 1, Fig 3.

Figure 14-2. **(A–C)** Modified from Shakzkes DR, Haller JO. Imaging of Uterovaginal Anomalies in the Pediatric Population. Urol Radiol 1991;13:58; and Markham SM, Waterhouse TB. Structural Anomalies of the Reproductive Tract. Curr Opin Obstet Gynecol 1992;4:867. **(D–F)** Modified from Dudek R, Fix J. BRS Embryology, 2nd ed. Philadelphia: Lippincott Williams & Wilkins, 1998:178, Fig 14-2. **(G)** From Janovski NA. Ovarian Tumors, vol 4. Major Problems in Obstetrics and Gynecology. Philadelphia: WB Saunders, 1973:191.

Figure 14-3. **(A, B)** From Dudek R, Fix J. BRS Embryology, 2nd ed. Philadelphia: Lippincott Williams & Wilkins, 1998:179, Fig 14-3A, B. **(C)** From Fletcher MA. Physical Diagnosis in Neonatology. Philadelphia: Lippincott Williams & Wilkins, 1997:369, Fig 29A. **(D)** From Sternberg SS. Histology for Pathologists, 2nd ed. Philadelphia: Lippincott Williams & Wilkins, 1997:852, Fig 1.

Figure 14-4. **(A–O)** Adapted from Goldstein DP, Laufer MR, Davis AJ. Gynecologic Surgery in Children and Adolescents: A Text Atlas. New York: Springer-Verlag; and American Fertility Society. The American Fertility Society classifications of adnexal adhesion, distal tubal occlusion, tubal occlusion secondary to tubal ligation, tubal pregnancies, müllerian anomalies, and intrauterine adhesions. Fertil Steril 1988;49:944. **(1–3, 5)** Courtesy of Dr. A. Gerbie. From Spitzer IB, Rebar RW. Counselling for women with medical problems: ovary and reproductive organs. In: Hollingsworth D, Resnik R, eds. Medical Counseling Before Pregnancy. New York: Churchill Livingstone, 1988:213–248. **(4)** From Gidwani G. Congenital Malformation of the Female Genital Tract. Philadelphia: Lippincott Williams & Wilkins, 1999:81, Fig 24. **(6)** Fleischer AC. Clinical Gynecologic Imaging. Philadelphia: Lippincott Williams & Wilkins, 1998:304, Fig 9-17E.

Figure 14-5. (**A, B**) From Pokorny SF. Configuration of the Prepubertal Hymen. Am J Obstet Gynecol 1987;157:950. **B(1)** From Emans SJ. Pediatric and Adolescent Gynecology, 4th ed. Philadelphia: Lippincott Williams & Wilkins, 1998:9, Fig 8A. (**C**) From Emans SJ. Pediatric and Adolescent Gynecology, 4th ed. Philadelphia: Lippincott Williams & Wilkins, 1998:9, Fig 8B. **C(1)** From Emans SJ. Pediatric and Adolescent Gynecology, 4th ed. Philadelphia: Lippincott Williams & Wilkins, 1998:9, Fig 8C. (**D, E**) From Goldstein DP, Iaufer MR, Davis AF. Gynecologic Surgery in Children and Adolescents: A Text Atlas. New York: Springer-Verlag (in press). (**F**) From Emans SJ. Pediatric and Adolescent Gynecology, 4th ed. Philadelphia: Lippincott Williams & Wilkins, 1998:11, Fig 11. **F(1)** From Emans SJ. Pediatric and Adolescent Gynecology, 4th ed. Philadelphia: Lippincott Williams & Wilkins, 1998:11, Fig 12. (**G**) From Emans SJ. Pediatric and Adolescent Gynecology, 4th ed. Philadelphia: Lippincott Williams & Wilkins, 1998:11, Fig 13. **G(1)** From Emans SJ. Pediatric and Adolescent Gynecology, 4th ed. Philadelphia: Lippincott Williams & Wilkins, 1998:11, Fig 14.

CHAPTER 15

Figure 15-1. (**A–C**) From Dudek R, Fix J. BRS Embryology, 2nd ed. Philadelphia: Lippincott Williams & Wilkins, 1998:184, Fig 15-1. (**D**) From Ross MH, et al. Histology: A Text and Atlas, MH Ross et al, 4th ed. Philadelphia: Lippincott Williams & Wilkins, 2003:717, Plate 83, Testes II, Fig 1, *inset.*

Figure 15-2. (**A–C**) Modified from Shakzkes DR, Haller JO. Imaging of Uterovaginal Anomalies in the Pediatric Population. Urol Radiol 1991;13:58 and Markham SM, Waterhouse TB. Structural Anomalies of the Reproductive Tract. Curr Opin Obstet Gynecol 1992;4:867. (**D, E**) From Dudek R, Fix J. BRS Embryology, 2nd ed. Philadelphia: Lippincott Williams & Wilkins, 1998:186, Fig 15-2A, B.

Figure 15-3. (**A, B**) From Dudek R, Fix J. BRS Embryology, 2nd ed. Philadelphia: Lippincott Williams & Wilkins, 1998:187, Fig 15-3.

Figure 15-4. (**A, C, D**) From Gilbert-Barness. Potter's Atlas of Fetal and Infant Pathology. St. Louis: Mosby, 1998:294. (**B, E**) Courtesy of Dr. T. Ernesto Figueroa.

Figure 15-5. (**A**) Courtesy of Dr. J. Kitchin, Department of Obstetrics and Gynecology, University of Virginia. (**B**) Wilkins L. The Diagnosis and Treatment of Endocrine Disorders in Childhood and Adolescence, 3rd ed. Springfield IL: Charles C Thomas, 1965:439. (**C**) From Warkany J. Congenital Malformations: Notes and Comments. Chicago, Year Book Medical Publishers, 1971:337. (**D**) From Jones. Hermaphroditism, Genital Anomalies and Related Endocrine Disorders. Philadelphia: Lippincott Williams & Wilkins, 1958.

CHAPTER 16

Figure 16-1. (**A**) From Pehamberger H, Honigsmann H. Dysplastic nevus syndrome with multiple primary amelanotic melanomas in oculocutaneous albinism. J Am Acad Dermatol 1984;11:731–735, Fig 1. (**B**) Courtesy of the Department of Dermatology, Columbia University, New York, NY. (**C**) Courtesy of Ingrid Winship, MBChB, MD, Cape Town, South Africa. (**D**) From Fletcher MA. Physical Diagnosis in Neonatology. . Philadelphia: Lippincott Williams & Wilkins, 1997:130, Fig 34B. (**E**) From Bernice R, Karachi ND, Toronto, Canada, from Mallory SB. What syndrome is this? Ehlers-Danlos syndrome. Pediatr Dermatol 1991;8:348–351, Fig 1. (**F**) From Bernice R, Krafchik ND, Toronto, Canada, from Mallory SB. What syndrome is this? Ehlers-Danlos syndrome. Pediatr Dermatol 1991;8:348–351, Fig 2. (**G**) From Avery GB. Neonatology, Pathophysiology, and Management of Newborn, 5th ed. Philadelphia: Lippincott Williams & Wilkins, 1999:1340, Fig 54-22. (**H**) From Reese V, Frieden IJ. Association of Facial Hemangiomas with Dandy-Walker and Other Posterior Fossa Malformations. J Pediatr 1993;122:379–384. (**I**) From Salmon MA, Lindenbaum RH. Developmental Defects and Syndromes. Aylesbury, England: HM & M Publishers, 1978:95. (**J**) Courtesy of Gilles G. Lestringant, MD, Abu Dhabi, United Arab Emirates. (**K**) From Sternberg SS. Diagnostic Surgical Pathology, vol 1, 3rd ed. Philadelphia: Lippincott Williams & Wilkins, 1999:24, Fig 32.

Figure 16-2. (**A**) From Junqueira LC, Carneiro J. Basic Histology, 9th ed. Stamford, CT: Appleton & Lange, 1998:335. (**B**) Courtesy of Dr. Antoine Petit, Argenteuil, France. (**C**) Courtesy of

Peter H. Itin, MD, Basel, Switzerland. **(D)** Courtesy of Marc E. Grossman, New York, NY. **(E)** From Spitz JL. Genodermatoses. Philadelphia: Lippincott Williams & Wilkins, 1996:241, Fig 10.13. **(F)** Courtesy of Paulus T. V. M. de Jong, MD, Rotterdam, the Netherlands.

Figure 16-3. **(A)** Adapted from Grumback MM, Styne DM. Puberty: Ontogeny, neuroendocrinology, physiology, and disorders. In: Wilson JD, Foster DW, eds. Williams Textbook of Endocrinology, 8th ed. Philadelphia: WB Saunders, 1992; and Marshall WA, Tanner JM. Variations in pattern of pubertal changes in girls. Arch Dis Child 1969;44:291. **(B)** From J Chronic Dis (July 1960); and Feinstein AR, ed. Medical Genetics, 1958–1960. St. Louis: Mosby, 1961. Reprinted with permission of the editors of the Journal of Chronic Diseases. **(C)** From Fletcher MA. Physical Diagnosis in Neonatology. Philadelphia: Lippincott Williams & Wilkins, 1997:330, Fig 10. **(D)** Courtesy of George E. Giffor, MD, Children's Hospital, Boston, MA. **(E)** From Fletcher MA. Physical Diagnosis in Neonatology. Philadelphia: Lippincott Williams & Wilkins, 1997:330, Fig 11A.

Figure 16-4. **(A–D)** From Dudek R, Fix J. BRS Embryology, 2nd ed. Philadelphia: Lippincott Williams & Wilkins, 1998:197, Fig 16-1. **(E, F)** Redrawn from Avery JK. Oral Development and Histology, 2nd ed. New York: Thieme Medical Publishers, 2002:131, Fig 8-3, and 2002:133, Fig 8-7. **(G)** Redrawn from McMillan JA, et al, eds. Oski's Pediatrics, 3rd ed. Philadelphia: Lippincott Williams & Wilkins, 1999:645, Fig 114-3.

CHAPTER 17

Figure 17-1. **(A)** From Dudek R, Fix J. BRS Embryology, 2nd ed. Philadelphia: Lippincott Williams & Wilkins, 1998:201, Fig 17-1. **(B)** Redrawn from Gray's Anatomy: The Anatomical Basis of Medicine and Surgery, 38th ed. Edinburgh, Scotland: Churchill Livingstone, 1995:372. **(C)** Modified from Sadler TW. Langman's Medical Embryology, 8th ed. Baltimore: Lippincott Williams & Wilkins, 2000:164, Fig 8.4A, B. **(D)** From Sadler TW. Langman's Medical Embryology, 8th ed. Baltimore: Lippincott Williams & Wilkins, 2000:169, Fig 8.8C. **(E)** From McMillan JA, et al, eds. Oski's Pediatrics, 3rd ed. Philadelphia: Lippincott Williams & Wilkins, 1999:396, Fig 66-8. **(F)** From Fletcher MA. Physical Diagnosis in Neonatology. Philadelphia: Lippincott Williams & Wilkins, 1997:188, Fig 16B. **(G)** From McMillan JA, et al, eds. Oski's Pediatrics, 3rd ed. Philadelphia: Lippincott Williams & Wilkins, 1999:398, Fig 66-16. **(H)** Courtesy of M. M. Cohen, Jr., Halifax, Nova Scotia, Canada. **(I)** Courtesy of M. M. Cohen, Jr., Halifax, Nova Scotia, Canada. **(J)** From McMillan JA, et al, eds. Oski's Pediatrics, 3rd ed. Philadelphia: Lippincott Williams & Wilkins, 1999, Fig 66-12.

Figure 17-2. **(A)** From Dudek R, Fix J. BRS Embryology, 2nd ed. Philadelphia: Lippincott Williams & Wilkins, 1998:204, Fig 17-3. **(B)** Redrawn from Larsen. Human Embryology, 2nd ed. New York: Churchill Livingston, 1997:77. **(C)** From Esses SI. Textbook of Spinal Disorders. Philadelphia: Lippincott Williams & Wilkins, 1994:44, Fig 2-14C. **(C inset)** from Dudek R, Fix J. BRS Embryology, 2nd ed. Philadelphia: Lippincott Williams & Wilkins, 1998:207, Fig 17-5. **(D)** From Kirks DR. Practical Pediatric Imaging, 3rd ed. Philadelphia: Lippincott Williams & Wilkins, 1997:314, Fig 4-66. **(E, F)** From Dudek R, Fix J. BRS Embryology, 2nd ed. Philadelphia: Lippincott Williams & Wilkins, 1998:207, Fig 17-5. **(G)** From Esses SI. Textbook of Spinal Disorders. Philadelphia: Lippincott Williams & Wilkins, 1994:259, Fig 14-2A. **(H)** From Jinkins JR. Neurodiagnostic Imaging. Philadelphia: Lippincott Williams & Wilkins, 1997:69, Fig 7-2A. **(I)** From Dudek R, Fix J. BRS Embryology, 2nd ed. Philadelphia: Lippincott Williams & Wilkins, 1998:207, Fig 17-5. **(J)** Courtesy of Derek C. Harwood-Nash, MD, Toronto, Ontario, Canada. **(J inset)** from Dudek R, Fix J. BRS Embryology, 2nd ed. Philadelphia: Lippincott Williams & Wilkins, 1998:207, Fig 17-5. **(K)** From McMillan JA, et al, eds. Oski's Pediatrics, 3rd ed. Philadelphia: Lippincott Williams & Wilkins, 1999:2118, Fig 432-26.

Figure 17-3. **(A)** Courtesy of Dr. A. E. Chudley, Professor of Pediatrics and Child Health, Children's Hospital, Winnipeg, Canada. **(B, C)** From McKusick VA. Heritable Disorders of Connective Tissue, 4th ed. St. Louis: CV Mosby, 1972:758. **(D)** From Salmon MA, Lindenbaum RH. Developmental Defects and Syndromes. Aylesbury, England: HM & M Publishers, 1978:172. **(E)** From McKusick VA. Heritable Disorders of Connective Tissue, 4th ed. St. Louis: CV Mosby, 1972:67. **(F, G)** From McMillan JA, et al, eds. Oski's Pediatrics, 3rd ed. Philadelphia: Lippincott Williams & Wilkins, 1999:2149, Fig 433-8A, B. **(H)** Courtesy of Daid A. Hanscom, MD, Seattle, Washington and Gillette Children's Hospital, St. Paul, Minnesota. **(I, J)** From Kaufman CE. Essentials of Pathophysiology. Philadelphia: Lippincott Williams & Wilkins, 1996:261, Fig 26-2. Used with permission of the patient.

CHAPTER 18

Figure 18-1. **(A)** From Dudek R, Fix J. BRS Embryology, 2nd ed. Philadelphia: Lippincott Williams & Wilkins, 1998:214, Fig 18-1. **(B, C)** From Fletcher MA. Physical Diagnosis in Neonatology. Philadelphia: Lippincott Williams & Wilkins, 1997:355, Fig 19, and 1997:309, Fig 1B. **(D)** From Avery GB. Neonatology: Pathophysiology and Management of the Newborn, 5th ed. Philadelphia: Lippincott Williams & Wilkins, 1999:1271, Fig 51-2. **(E)** From Nicholson LV, Davison K. Dystrophin in Skeletal Muscle. II. Immunoreactivity in Patients with Xp21 Muscular Dystrophy. J Neurol Sci 1989;94:137–146.

CHAPTER 19

Figure 19-1. **(A, B)** From Dudek R, Fix J. BRS Embryology, 2nd ed. Philadelphia: Lippincott Williams & Wilkins, 1998:218, Fig 19-1 and p. 222, Fig 19-3. **C(1)** From Sadler. Langman's Medial Embryology, 7th ed. Philadelphia: Williams & Wilkins, 1995:170. **C(2, 4)** From Dudek R, Fix J. BRS Embryology, 2nd ed. Philadelphia: Lippincott Williams & Wilkins, 1998:224, Fig 19-4. **C(3)** From Larson W. Human Embryology, 2nd ed. New York: Churchill Livingstone, 1997:323.

Figure 19-2. **(A, B, E)** From Dudek R, Fix J. BRS Embryology, 2nd ed. Philadelphia: Lippincott Williams & Wilkins, 1998:220, Fig 19.2. **(C, D, F, G)** From Keats TE, Smith TH. Atlas of Normal Developmental Roentgen Anatomy, 2nd ed. Chicago: Year Book Medical Publisher, 1977:33, 292, and 295.

CHAPTER 20

Figure 20-1. **(A, B)** From Dudek R, Fix J. BRS Embryology, 2nd ed. Philadelphia: Lippincott Williams & Wilkins, 1998:228, Fig 20.1, and 1998:232, Fig 20.3. **C(1)** From Sadler. Langman's Medical Embryology, 7th ed. Philadelphia: Lippincott Williams & Wilkins, 1995:170. **C(2, 4)** From Dudek R, Fix J. BRS Embryology, 2nd ed. Philadelphia: Lippincott Williams & Wilkins, 1998:234, Fig 20.4. **C(3)** From Larson W. Human Embryology, 7th ed. New York: Churchill Livingstone, 1995:323.

Figure 20-2. **(A, B, E)** From Dudek R, Fix J. BRS Embryology, 2nd ed. Philadelphia: Lippincott Williams & Wilkins, 1998:230, Fig 20-2. **(C, D, F, G)** From Keates TE, Smith TH. An Atlas of Normal Developmental Roentgen Anatomy, 2nd ed. Chicago, Year Book Medical Publishers, 1977:31, 237 and 289.

CHAPTER 21

Figure 21-1. **(A–C)** From Dudek R, Fix J. BRS Embryology, 2nd ed. Philadelphia: Lippincott Williams & Wilkins, 1998:327, Fig 21-1A–C. **(D)** From Dudek R, Fix J. BRS Embryology, 2nd ed. Philadelphia: Lippincott Williams & Wilkins, 1998:328, Fig 21-2. **(E)** From Dudek R, Fix J. BRS Embryology, 2nd ed. Philadelphia: Lippincott Williams & Wilkins, 1998:329, Fig 21-3.

Figure 21-2. **(A)** From Gilbert-Barness E. Potter's Atlas of Fetal and Infant Pathology. St. Louis: Mosby, 1998:172. **(B)** From Avery GB. Neonatology, Pathophysiology, and Management of the Newborn, 5th ed. Philadelphia: Lippincott Williams & Wilkins, 1999:149, Fig 11-7. **(C, D)** From Aladjen S, Vidyasagar D. Atlas of Perinatology. Philadelphia: WB Saunders, 1982:295 and 375. **(E)** From Fenoglio-Preiser CM. Gastrointestinal Pathology: An Atlas and Text, 2nd ed. 1998:43, Fig 3.19.

CHAPTER 23

Figure 23-1. From Dudek R. High-Yield Embryology, 2nd ed. Philadelphia: Lippincott Williams & Wilkins, 2000:125, Fig 22-1A.

Figure 23-2. **(A)** From deGrochy J, Turleau C. Clinical Atlas of Human Chromosomes. New York: John Wiley, 1977:131. **(B)** From McMillan JA, et al, eds. Oski's Pediatrics, 3rd ed. Philadelphia: Lippincott Williams & Wilkins, 1999:2229. **(C)** From Sadler. Langman's Medical Embryology, 7th ed. Baltimore: Williams & Wilkins, 1995:136, Fig 8-6. **(D)** From deGrochy J, Turleau C. Clinical Atlas of Human Chromosomes. New York: John Wiley, 1977:163. **(E, F, G, I)** From Smith DW. Recognizable Patterns of Human Malformation, 3rd ed. Philadelphia: WB Saunders, 1982:13, 75. **(H)** From Salmon MA, Lindenbaum RH. Developmental Defects and Syndromes. Aylesbury, England: HM & M Publishers, 1978:372. **(J)** From McMillan JA, et al, eds. Oski's Pediatrics, 3rd ed. Philadelphia: Lippincott Williams & Wilkins, 1999:2231.

CHAPTER 24

Figure 24-1. **(A)** From Smith DW. Recognizable Patterns of Human Malformation, 3rd ed. Philadelphia: WB Saunders, 1982:37. **(B)** From Salmon MA, Lindenbaum RH. Developmental Defects and Syndromes. Aylesbury, England: HM & M Publishers, 1978:321.

Figure 24-2. **(A, B)** From Salmon MA, Lindenbaum RH. Developmental Defects and Syndromes. Aylesbury, England: HM & M Publishers, 1978:321. **(C, D)** From Gilbert-Barness E. Potter's Atlas of Fetal and Infant Pathology. St. Louis: Mosby, 1998:254, 277. **(D [top])** From Jinkins. Neurodiagnostic Imaging. Philadelphia: Lippincott Williams & Wilkins, 1997:55, Fig 5-9A.

Figure 24-3. **(A-D)** From Dudek R. High-Yield Embryology, 2nd ed. Philadelphia: Lippincott Williams & Wilkins, 2000:134, Fig 23-3. **(C, D)** Photographs from Mufti GJ, Flandrin G. An Atlas of Malignant Haematology. Philadelphia: Lippincott Williams & Wilkins, 1996:73, 179.

Figure 24-4. **(A)** From Jacobs PA, Glover TW. X-linked mental retardation: a study of 7 families. Am J Med Genet 1980;7:471. **(B)** Courtesy of David R. Biocers, MD, New York, NY. **(C)** Courtesy of Gilles G. Lestringant, MD, Abu Dhabi, United Arab Emirates. **(D)** Courtesy of Marc E. Grossman, MD, New York, NY. **(E)** Courtesy of Gregory Pastores, MD, New York, NY. **(F)** Redrawn from Spitz. Genodermatoses. Philadelphia: Lippincott Williams & Wilkins, 1996:101. **(G)** From McMillan JA, et al, eds. Oski's Pediatrics, 3rd ed. Philadelphia: Lippincott Williams & Wilkins, 1999:2239. **(H)** Courtesy of David R. Bickers, MD, New York, NY.

CHAPTER 25

Figure 25-1. **(A, F)** From Friedman JM. Genetics. Philadelphia: Lippincott Williams & Wilkins, 1992:151, 51. **(B-D)** From Gelehrter TD. Principles of Medical Genetics, 2nd ed. Philadelphia: Lippincott Williams & Wilkins, 1997:25, Figs 3.3:34, 3.13:41, 3.22, and 1997:38, Fig 3.18.

CHAPTER 27

Figure 27-1. **(A)** From Avery GB. Neonatology, Pathophysiology and Management of the Newborn, 5th ed. Philadelphia: Lippincott Williams & Wilkins, 1999:1293, Fig 52.11. **(B)** From McMillan JA, et al, eds. Oski's Pediatrics, 3rd ed. Philadelphia: Lippincott Williams & Wilkins, 1999:687, Fig 116-9. **(C)** Courtesy of Dr. George H. McCrachen, Jr., Dallas, Texas. **(D)** Courtesy of Dr. Guido Currarinao, Dallas, Texas. **(E)** From Avery GB. Neonatology, Pathophysiology and Management of the Newborn, 5th ed. Philadelphia: Lippincott Williams & Wilkins, 1999:1154, Fig 47-4. **(F)** From Avery GB. Neonatology, Pathophysiology and Management of the Newborn, 5th ed. Philadelphia: Lippincott Williams & Wilkins, 1999:1136, Fig 47-2.

Figure 27-2. **(A)** From Fletcher MA. Physical Diagnosis in Neonatology. Philadelphia: Lippincott Williams & Wilkins, 1997:133, Fig 37B. **(B)** From Fletcher MA. Physical Diagnosis in Neonatology. Philadelphia: Lippincott Williams & Wilkins, 1997:133, Fig 37D. **(C)** From McMillan JA, et al, eds. Oski's Pediatrics, 3rd ed. Philadelphia: Lippincott Williams & Wilkins, 1999:440, Fig 79-5. **(D)** Courtesy of Dr. George H. McCracken, Jr., Dallas, Texas. **(E)** From Avery GB. Neonatology, Pathophysiology and Management of the Newborn, 5th ed. Philadelphia: Lippincott Williams & Wilkins, 1999:1129, Fig 47-1. **(F)** Courtesy of Dr. Guido Currarinao, Dallas, Texas.

Appendix From Dudek R. High-Yield Cell and Molecular Biology. Philadelphia: Lippincott Williams & Wilkins, 1999:70, Table 12.1.

Index

Page numbers in *italics* designate figures; page numbers followed by "t" designate tables or boxes.